Images and understanding

Images and understanding

THOUGHTS ABOUT IMAGES

IDEAS ABOUT UNDERSTANDING

A COLLECTION OF ESSAYS BASED ON A
RANK PRIZE FUNDS' INTERNATIONAL SYMPOSIUM
ORGANIZED WITH THE HELP OF

Jonathan Miller

HELD AT THE ROYAL SOCIETY IN OCTOBER 1986 AND

EDITED BY

HORACE BARLOW

COLIN BLAKEMORE

MIRANDA WESTON-SMITH

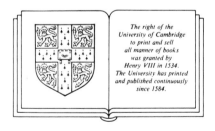

The right of the
University of Cambridge
to print and sell
all manner of books
was granted by
Henry VIII in 1534.
The University has printed
and published continuously
since 1584.

CAMBRIDGE UNIVERSITY PRESS

CAMBRIDGE

NEW YORK   PORT CHESTER

MELBOURNE   SYDNEY

Published by the Press Syndicate of the University of Cambridge
The Pitt Building, Trumpington Street, Cambridge CB2 1RP
40 West 20th Street, New York, NY 10011, USA
10 Stamford Road, Oakleigh, Melbourne 3166, Australia

First published 1990
Reprinted 1991

Printed in the United States of America

British Library cataloguing in publication data
Images and understanding.
1. Man. Visual perception. Cognition
I. Miller, Jonathan II. Barlow, H.B.
III. Blakemore, Colin IV. Weston-
Smith, Miranda V. Rank Prize Funds
152.1'4

Library of Congress cataloging in publication data
Rank Prize Funds' International Symposium (1986:
Royal Society)
Images and understanding.
"A collection of essays based on a Rank Prize Funds'
International Symposium, organized with the help of
Jonathan Miller, held at the Royal Society in
October 1986."
Bibliography: p.
Includes index.
1. Vision – Congresses. 2. Visual perception –
Congresses. 3. Imagery (Psychology) – Congresses.
I. Barlow, (Horace). II. Blakemore, Colin.
III. Weston-Smith, Miranda. IV. Rank Prize Funds.
V. Title.
QP474.R36 1986   152.1'4   88-11805

ISBN 0-521-34177-9 hardback
ISBN 0-521-36944-4 paperback

Contents

Preface

It is difficult to explain to a layman that there is a problem in how we see things. It seems so effortless. We look and, behold, we see. Yet the more we study the process, the more complex and unexpected we find it. Of one thing we can be sure: we do not see things in the way common sense says we should.

The initial steps in the process, and the bare outline of the subsequent steps, are fairly well understood. We see because light rays are focused onto our retina, because a million nerve cells in each eye send their own signal to the brain where the information is processed by the thousand million nerve cells of the visual system, analysing its features, putting them together and relating them to what we have seen before. As this volume shows, we already know a lot of details about these intricate devices, but many key aspects are still a mystery. We do not yet know enough to answer the layman's simple question: 'How do I see a dog?'

There are two other broad approaches to these problems. One is used by visual psychologists (called psychophysicists) who explore the limitations of our visual system – how we respond to colour, shape, movement, etc. – by studying it from the outside. They try to infer from our responses what is going on inside the head when we are shown some simple visual pattern or other. They find that the brain uses shortcuts, multiple parallel systems and other tricks so that it can do the job well enough and quickly enough to help us to survive. Visual illusions give us some insight into the devices the brain employs to help us make sense of the visual world.

But there is another approach to vision, that of people who employ it in various ways: to paint pictures, to draw caricatures, to make movies, to record body movements, etc. Their observations often draw our attention to the higher levels of visual processing.

ix

This book is unique in outlining all three approaches to the problem. Here, then, is a feast for everyone. The scientist will have new aspects of vision thrust upon him, as in Jonathan Miller's chapter on Moving Pictures. The layman can learn how, in principle, we see not only colour, but the permanent colour of an object. The problem of what it is like for an animal to see intrigues everyone. Another theme concerns computers and how they can be used to construct images of one sort or another.

It is fascinating to see the quirks and complexities of the visual system revealed from so many different angles. It will be no less fascinating when, finally, we understand just how it all works. This book shows vividly how far we have progressed and how far we still have to go. I commend it to everyone who has ever wondered about our wonderful gift of sight.

Francis Crick

Editors' introduction

Artists, designers and engineers share an age-old problem, how to move facts and ideas from one mind to another: how are these mental transfusions achieved? Through the use of *images* – not just in the form of pictures and diagrams but with words, demonstrations, even music and dance. Some of this idea-swapping is simple enough, such as telling someone else how to tie a knot or wire up an electric plug. But much of image-making is profound, even enigmatic. How do you paint a picture of God, or dance about death, or draw a diagram explaining infinity?

It is time for a new look at images through the eyes of both science and art, because modern technology is expanding the means of developing, communicating and interpreting images, while physiology and psychology are giving new insights into the internal mechanisms of coding, perceiving and interpreting messages from the senses. This book is the product of an international conference on this subject held at the Royal Society, London, during October 1986; how it happened deserves explanation.

The symposium was financed by The Rank Prize Funds, one of the many charities founded by the late Lord Rank. He was the youngest of three brothers who built up their father's flour milling business into a large and successful concern, and he was also a keen Methodist. As he was sitting through a rather lengthy sermon in about 1935 the thought occurred to him, 'This would be much better with pictures'. History does not record whether the sermon left any other impression in his mind, but the thought persisted, and being a man who acted on his thoughts he arranged for a film to be made. It was called *The Turn of the Tide*, and indeed it was the turn of the tide for the British movie industry. The film itself may have been rather a good one, for it won an award at Cannes, but what mattered was what happened when J. Arthur Rank subsequently tried to get it shown publicly. He expected to have no difficulty with a prize-winning film, but none of the distributors would even look at it. His experience with flour told him at once what to do: if you have a good product which no-one will buy, you must buy up those who are doing the buying; it's called 'vertical integration'. That was how he got into the movie-showing business, and it was not long before he had a very large part of the whole British film industry under his control.

That was Lord Rank's first contact with images, but very much later he again brought a new kind of image into everyday life, for he played an important part in helping the Xerox Corporation get off the ground. The xerographic process had been developed and the first copier was almost ready to be produced when Xerox ran out of money; Lord Rank provided the new injection of capital that was needed, and both sides have benefited greatly.

He founded very large charitable trusts, and towards the end of his life he gave enough money to start The Prize Funds. These were for awarding prizes to individuals who had made notable contributions to the two branches of science most closely related to his business successes – nutrition and opto-electronics. He had always had a keen interest in the technical and scientific aspects of both milling and image-production, so this was a natural gesture, and it was the section of the Funds dealing with opto-electronics that supported this symposium.

These Prize Funds have Scientific Advisory Committees to assist them in deciding how to use their resources, and the late Dr Frank Jones was approached to chair the Opto-Electronics Advisory Committee. Before accepting, he insisted that the eye be considered an opto-electronic device, and so it comes about that the whole business of seeing images and understanding them, as well as producing them, falls within the scope of opto-electronics. It was the generosity of Lord Rank that made possible the symposium, and hence this book, and it was the Opto-Electronics Advisory Committee that delegated one of its members, Horace Barlow, to set about organizing it; he sought help from three others.

As professors often do, he turned to those whom he had once tried to teach, and found two who have usurped the role of teacher and grabbed much bigger audiences, namely Colin Blakemore and Jonathan Miller. Then Miranda Weston-Smith joined us to help with the editing, and she has contributed much to shape the book that is in your hands.

It was a challenging task to assemble a collection of contributors from the arts and the sciences who could speak and write with authority and clarity about the vast subject of *Images and Understanding*. But as, one after another, our invitations were accepted, we felt again that we had hit on an idea that was both timely and exciting.

Of course, there are gaps in what has been covered. We wish that we could have included a master painter to tell us how Great Pictures are created, and likewise a director to tell us about the Great Movies. Maybe the growing field of cognitive psychology could have had more of a say. But despite these omissions, the conference was an exciting meeting of minds; one of those rare occasions when artists and scientists had a chance to present their ideas to each other. Now this book, the image of the meeting, presents those ideas to you.

H.B.B.

C.B.

M.W-S.

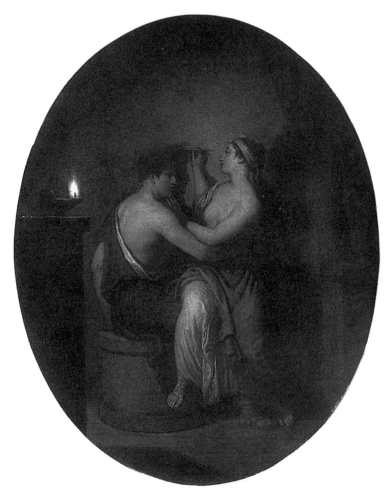

'The origin of drawing' by David Allen (1775). Reproduced by kind permission of the National Gallery of Scotland.

PART 1

The essence of images

JONATHAN MILLER

Horace Barlow divides our topic into images *before* the eye and images *behind* it [p. 5]. The problem is that the word 'image' is conventionally applied to configurations presented *to* the eye – photos, paintings, engravings, TV displays, shadows, reflections and projections – and although there are good reasons for applying the same term to patterns of nervous activity in the visual system, the logical connotations are recognisably different. When it comes to so-called *mental* images, the relevance of the word image is distinctly controversial and although it would be perverse to deny the existence of visual 'imaginings' there are those who insist that it is misleading to describe what is 'seen' as a visual image. But since photos etc. are widely regarded as 'typical' cases of imagery, that is to say as images in the *un*controversial sense, it might be useful to analyse their logical character to see in what respect the other examples differ from or fall short of the standard requirements.

For something to be identifiable as an image in the standard sense it must fulfil the following conditions. It must have a visible appearance since it is only by virtue of looking like something or other that it can look *like* whatever it happens to be an image of.

And yet mere resemblance is not enough since one thing can look like something else without either of them being the image of the other. Besides, resemblance is a reciprocal relationship and if visible similarity were a sufficient condition for being an image one would be tempted to say that the Duke of Wellington was the image of his portrait or that a tree was the image of its own shadow. There must therefore be an additional factor which *assigns* the role of being an image to one rather than the other member of a mutually resembling pair. The factor in question is the mode of production, or, to be more accurate, the spectator's recognition of the process responsible for the

1

likeness. When we identify a painting as an *image* of someone, it's not only because it looks like him or her, but more significantly because we have reason to believe that it has been fashioned for the express purpose of representing the sitter's likeness, of *being* his or her image. In other words, it's our understanding of the *convention* of portraiture that allows us to assign the role of image to a given configuration of pigment. And by exclusion the same convention allows us to *withold* the title of image when it comes to things like damp patches which merely *happen* to look like so and so.

The convention of representation is so robust that as long as we have reason to believe that something exemplifies it we can identify something as an image in the face of considerable *unlikeness*. Picasso's portrait of Kahnweiler is not immediately recognisable as a *person*, let alone as a particular person, but because it's immediately recognisable as a *painting*, and because such objects have a long-standing reputation for bearing images, we conclude, correctly as it happens, that this particular configuration of pigment is, after all, an image of *someone* and since the label says so we take it on trust that it's an image of Kahnweiler. In fact once we have identified something as an image, having recognised the intention that makes it one, a previously undetectable resemblance can become startlingly convincing – which is what Picasso must have meant when he assured Gertrude Stein that her portrait would come to look just like her. But this doesn't explain why shadows, silhouettes and reflections have acquired the reputation of being images: when it comes to *natural* configurations there's no question of anyone having fashioned the resemblance. Nevertheless the fact that we have an understanding, albeit an informal one, of the way in which shadows and reflections are produced guarantees that as long as we recognise something *as* a shadow or *as* a reflection we will automatically identify it as the image of whatever casts it. It's only in exceptional circumstances where we don't know that something is a reflection that we fail to see it as an *image* and *mis*identify it as something real. When Narcissus saw his reflection in the water he failed to recognise it as a reflection and in failing to identify it as a mere image, he fell in love with what he thought to be someone *else*. Whereas when a Narcissist looks into a mirror he knows perfectly well that he is seeing a reflection and knowingly falls in love with *himself*.

Now that we've summarised the requirements for something to be an image in the standard sense we are in a better position to enumerate the peculiarities of images occurring *within* the visual system. One peculiarity springs to mind immediately. The patterns of nervous activity which are detectable at various stations throughout the visual system are not like external images for they do not have to be presented to the eye to be seen by the spectator. Unlike a photograph or a painting whose appearance can always be compared with whatever it's supposed to be an image of, the pattern of nervous activity in the lateral geniculate nucleus is *within* the spectator and although its occurrence is responsible for his seeing so and so, he is not in a position to compare its appearance with the appearance of so and so. And for that reason alone its status as an image is epistemologically different from that of the standard cases.

The other respect in which post-retinal images differ from images presented to the eye is emphasised by Horace Barlow and Colin Blakemore when they distinguish non-topographic and non-isomorphic maps from topographic and isomorphic ones (see pp.21 and 271). In those parts of the visual tract where the distribution of fibres preserves the spatial arrangement of the sensory array, the pattern of nervous activity is legibly related to the pattern of light and shade falling on the retina, and for that reason its status as an image is not unrelated to that of a photograph, because although the format is *within* the spectator and not actually visible *to* him, the fact that it preserves some, though not all, of the spatial properties of the pre-retinal scene makes it an image in the standard sense of the term. But when it comes to those parts of the visual system in which elaborate decomposition occurs, such that all *legible* resemblance vanishes, then the sense in which the pattern of activity can be called an *image* of the visual scene is altogether different. In this context the word image has a much more sophisticated connotation, one which would not, I suspect, be readily understandable by anyone for whom paintings, photographs, shadows and reflections were canonical examples of imagery.

Nevertheless the mathematical connotation of the word image is just as legitimate as the traditional iconic one and anyone who can appreciate the concept of 'functions' will readily identify high level patterns of nervous activity as credible instances of imagery, in spite of the fact that the format in question bears no *visible* similarity to the pre-retinal scene of which it is said to *be* an image. The only reason why we feel reluctant to apply the term image to such a format of nervous activity, is that it's difficult to eliminate the homuncular theory of perception in which a phantom spectator scrutinises the nervous input as if it were a photograph. If perception were to be the result of an homunculus looking at the output of the transducers, we would expect him to behave as *we* do when confronted by something claiming to be an image of something else, i.e. he would require it to *look* like whatever it was an image of. But perception does *not* presuppose the existence of anything or anyone which *looks*, and as long as the format of nervous activity is *functionally* mappable on to the optical property of the distal array, veridical perception results.

But what happens about non-veridical perception, by which I do not mean hallucination, but simply the experience of visualising something – 'seeing' it as we say, with the mind's eye. The problem is, that in the absence of an actual object, scene or person, it's tempting to stipulate the existence of a substitute which supplies the transitive requirements of the verb to see. So that someone who imagines or 'sees' Helvellyn is said to be looking not at Helvellyn but at a mental image of it. Now although it's generally understood that visualising Helvellyn or whatever is not a case of looking at a diaphenous version of the real mountain, it's not all that easy to say what *is* going on. Although Roger Shepherd's experiments with mental rotation (see Postscript) prove that the concept of imagery is operationally inescapable, it cannot be denied that such images are conspicuously different from the standard examples. The most obvious difference is the impossibility of distinguishing between the intentional object and the medium which affords or hosts it. When I look at a photograph or a painting I recognise or 'see' Helvellyn *in* it, meaning that I can *also* identify visual properties which make it recognisable as a photo or as a painting. *A* more significant difference however is the peculiar indeterminacy of mental images. When *physical* images are indeterminate with regard to some visible feature of the object, person or scene which they represent, there is always a determinable reason for the deficit – bad focus, poor resolution, an inappropriate viewpoint or else the relevant part of the picture is missing – but when a *mental* image fails in this respect the deficit cannot be traced to a visible shortcoming in its appearance. The item in question is simply omitted and, as in a verbal description, the omission does not leave a visible gap. This, according to some authors (see Dennett, Chapter 19), violates the most basic rule of images in general and for that reason they are reluctant to apply the word image to whatever it is one 'sees' with the mind's eye. The so-called imagery 'debate' continues to occupy the psychological community and although the Postscript by Shepherd and Chapter 22 by Goodman are the only ones which address this topic explicitly it is to be hoped that some of the other contributions will throw a light on this controversial subject.

1

What does the brain see? How does it understand?

HORACE BARLOW

People interested in images, for whom this book is written, can be divided into two groups: those who are mainly concerned with images in the outside world before they are presented to the eye, and those, like myself, who investigate what happens to them after they have entered the eye. The first group includes artists who create all sorts of images, critics who examine them, historians who trace their origins, and a large group of people who use images for entertainment and utilitarian purposes – even commercial or political ones. The second group consists of those who try to find out how the images swallowed by the eye are digested to provide new insight and understanding in the hungry mind.

One reason for making this division is that the two groups use different languages, and it is sometimes hard for them to understand each other. The authors of this book are supposed to have presented their material in a non-technical way that is suitable for general readers, but we sometimes fail because it is so difficult to explain universally accepted preconceptions and to avoid buzzwords that one's colleagues understand perfectly well. What happens behind the eye is especially hard for in-front-of-the-eye experts to understand, and the first aim of this chapter is to give a brief account of the neural hardware that lies behind the eye and the way we think images are represented in it. Those who know all this should skip to Part 2 (p.20), where I attempt the more difficult task of defining what is meant by understanding an image, and indicate how I think the brain may start to do this.

Part 1 How the brain sees

There are philosophical difficulties in saying that the brain 'sees', and these are discussed further by Colin Blakemore (Chapter 17), Nelson Goodman (Chapter 22), and Roger Shepard (in his Postscript). Jonathan Miller (p.1)

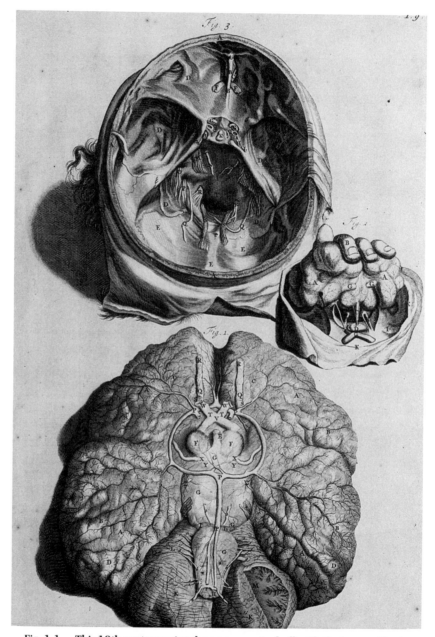

Fig. 1.1.   This 18th century print shows an empty skull with the inverted brain
beneath it. The optic nerves are marked W and T; the optic chiasma where some
of the fibres cross is V. Laterally one sees the lower surfaces of the two crinkled and
convoluted cerebral hemispheres with their rich vascular supply.

has already pointed out some of the ways images behind the eye differ from those in front of it, but anatomists and physiologists cheerfully ignore all these problems and talk about images in the brain in much the same way as they talk about a tasty meal that has just been consumed: this rapidly becomes something very different from the appetizing creation that tempted you to eat it, but we still refer to it as the *meal* because the chemical changes the food undergoes are the important matter, not the words used to describe them. It is these changes in the *image*, brought about by the mechanisms of the visual pathway and analysed by opening the skull, that I shall outline here. This knowledge should alter the way we think about 'seeing' in much the same way that astronomical observations changed our concepts of the universe, even though profound questions remain unanswered. Progress in understanding the brain has, however, been frustrating because one so rarely answers the question that prompted the search; but the answers that are obtained are the only ones available and we must be guided by them.

The cerebral cortex

The first figure shows what you see if you open the skull. The brain has been removed and its under-side is shown in the lower half of the figure. The prominent white X is the *optic chiasma* (marked V) where more than half of the fibres in the *optic nerves* cross over from one side of the brain to the other. The optic nerves have been severed at the top of the X and they plunge into the brain at the bottom of the X; in the brain they ultimately find their way, through a relay station called the *lateral geniculate nucleus*, to special regions of *cerebral cortex* at the back of the brain. These, it is generally agreed, are the structures that enable us to understand images.

The corrugated surfaces covered with blood vessels on either side of the optic chiasma are the under-sides of the cerebral hemispheres, and the *cortex* is the surface layer about one-tenth of an inch thick containing most of the cells. Since the total area on each side in humans is about one square foot it has to be crinkled to fit into the available space. Like everything else in this picture, what you can see is only a tiny fraction of what is there; in fact after the first moment of awe at seeing a human brain one cannot help being disappointed, for there is very little in its appearance to suggest what it does or how it works.

The cerebral cortex is surprisingly uniform in general appearance and microscopic structure, so if this is what enables one to understand images you will ask what ideas are held about its general function. Table 1.1 lists three suggestions. The first is from Judson Herrick, the great American comparative anatomist of the 1920s and 1930s of this century; he said the cortex is

Table 1.1. **THREE IDEAS ABOUT THE CEREBRAL CORTEX**

STORES KNOWLEDGE ACQUIRED ABOUT THE ENVIRONMENT

C.J. HERRICK, 1928

CONSTRUCTS WORKING MODEL OF THE ENVIRONMENT

K.J.W. CRAIK, 1943

REVERSE OPTICS – RECONSTRUCTING OBJECTS FROM THEIR IMAGES

T. POGGIO *et al.*, 1985

like the bank of filing cabinets in a government office, where all the records are kept[1]. This was based on rather superficial observations of what animals with large cortices can do, and ones without them cannot, but it must be admitted that more detailed experimentation and observation has not added very much. On this view the main job of the cortex is to *store* knowledge of the environment.

Next consider the idea advanced by Kenneth Craik, a Cambridge psychologist who died tragically in 1944. He proposed that it makes a *working model* of the environment that an animal lives in[2]. This is different from Herrick's view because it requires a component often missing in a government office, namely intelligent interpretation of the files. Anybody can jam things into a filing cabinet, but it is another matter to write a minute on each file that gives an account of the situation with the predictive power of a working model.

Finally consider what Tommy Poggio and his colleagues in Artificial Intelligence at M.I.T. say about the visual parts of the cortex. This is the group that the late David Marr[3] founded and did his best work with; they say it performs inverse optics – it *reconstructs* the objects that cause visual images from the images themselves[3]. At first this sounds radically different, but stored knowledge and models of the environment are what you need in order to make reconstruction possible, as is clearly brought out in Andrew Witkin's paper in this book (see Chapter 14). *Storage, modelling, reconstruction* are good ideas to have in mind as we proceed, but in the second part of this chapter (p.20) I shall amplify the view that *understanding* is the most fundamental cortical function, and that this depends upon detecting the relationships[1, 3] between the parts of an image, and between the image and the environment.

Localisation of function

How can one give substance to these ideas? The methods for finding out what the brain does are very restricted, so progress has been slow and tedious. You can look at the anatomy in ever-greater detail, but very often this yields facts that cannot be interpreted, giving no clues about function. However by combining the anatomical study of diseased or damaged brains with careful observations of the behavioural and psychic defects of patients it has been shown over the last hundred years that different parts of the cortex handle different aspects of higher behaviour. In many cases this parcellation of function has been confirmed by experiments and observations on animals with carefully controlled lesions. Also one can stimulate electrically and observe reactions, or inquire about the subjective sensations experienced and introspections aroused. Finally one can record the activity of nerve cells through electrodes, as we shall see in a minute. But there is no magic microscope to show one what a piece of the brain does and how it does it; it is a matter of piecing together incomplete scraps of evidence from varied sources.

Figure 1.2 is a side view of the human left cerebral hemisphere with some prominent anatomical terms listed on the left, and a resumé of functional localisations derived from the effects of damage, stimulation and recording

ANATOMICAL   **FUNCTIONAL**

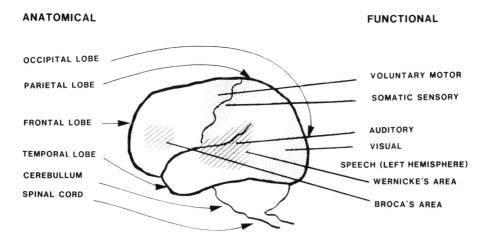

SIDE VIEW OF LEFT CEREBRAL HEMISPHERE

Fig. 1.2. Side view of the left cerebral hemisphere showing the anatomical terms and main functional areas. Evidence for the motor and sensory areas comes from knowledge of their anatomical connections and is amply confirmed by recording and by the effects of stimulation, damage, and disease. Knowledge of the speech areas comes mainly from clinical observation of patients with localised damage to the left hemisphere, often resulting from a stroke (cerebral thrombosis).

shown on the right. Stimulation of the three sensory areas in conscious humans causes sensations of sight, hearing, and touch, usually of a rather prosaic and uninteresting kind such as 'a luminous patch the size of a pea', or 'a faint buzzing sound', or 'light touch on the thumb'. Damage to one of these areas interferes with the corresponding sensation, and if one records electrically from these regions one detects signs of activity upon stimulation of the appropriate sense; I shall show some important results from the visual cortex in a moment.

More interesting, because more related to function, are the two cross-hatched areas. These are the approximate locations of two regions discovered more than 100 years ago, damage to which causes interference with speech – aphasia[4]. The surprising thing is that these areas are in the left hemisphere only; damage to corresponding areas in the right hemisphere leaves speech intact in the great majority of right-handed people. There are differences between the defects resulting from damage to the two regions, the anterior one – Broca's area – being more concerned with the production of speech, while the posterior region, named after Wernicke, has more to do with the conceptualisation of what is to be said. Marcus Raichle's chapter in this book (see p.284) tells us about some modern techniques that enable one to find which regions of the brain become active in normal humans performing various mental tasks, and this may open up a new subject – Psycho-Anatomy. But although this is a very exciting prospect, again one feels thwarted because it will only tell one *where* something is done, and will say little about *what* is done and *how*.

The visual pathways

In the hope of finding out more on the 'what' and 'how' the anatomy has been examined in greater detail, and Fig. 1.3 sketches some of these results in a diagram of the visual pathways seen from above. The eyes lie underneath the frontal lobes, and the optic nerves carry the image back from the eye to the brain.

Let me draw your attention to an interesting detail; light from objects in the right visual field is shown entering the eye as continuous lines, light from the left as dashed lines. These form images on the left and right halves of each retina respectively, because of inversion by the eyes' optics. As shown, at the chiasma only half the fibres cross: those from the right half of the visual field *of both eyes* go to the left half of the brain, while those from the left half-fields go to the right half of the brain. By this anatomical re-arrangement the images of the two half-fields seen through the two different eyes are brought together, and I think the brain's insistence that nervous activity which has the same

BRAIN FROM ABOVE

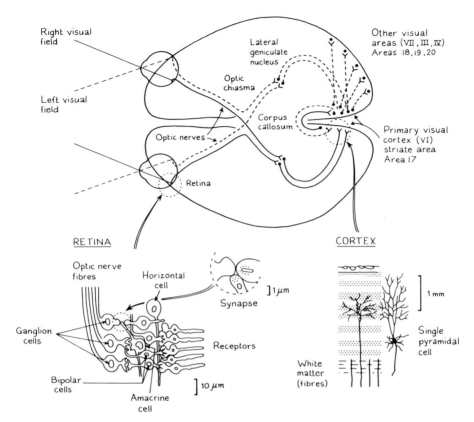

Fig. 1.3.   Diagrammatic view of the human visual pathways seen from above. Note how the light rays (dashed) from the left visual field entering each eye excite ganglion cells whose axons (also dashed) synapse in the right lateral geniculate nucleus, whence the information is carried to the primary visual cortex (also called VI, area 17, or the striate area) in the posterior pole of the right cerebral hemisphere. Similarly rays from the right visual field are reunited in the left hemisphere. This is achieved by the appropriate fibres crossing in the optic chiasma while the rest remain on the same side. A portion of the retina is magnified to show the retinal ganglion cells, of which there are 10^6 in each eye in the human. Their axons carry the image to the brain, and they pick up their messages from the receptors through other neurons in the retina. To the right a portion of visual cortex is magnified. There are at least 100 cells for each input fibre and more than 10^5 per sq.mm. The axons of the pyramidal cells carry information to other visual areas and more distant parts of the brain.

origin in the external world should be reunited at the same place in the brain
has an important message for us; I shall return to it.

Two regions of the pathway are shown in greater magnification in the
lower part of Fig. 1.3 The important components are the *nerve cells* and
synapses; thus it is the *ganglion cells* in the retina that pick up the messages
from the *receptors* which have been stimulated by light in the image. They do
this through junctions or synapses with intermediate cells called *bipolars*, and
the complex synaptic connections between the various cell types in the retina
do the computations that determine what property of the light, shade, and
colour in the image excites a ganglion cell. These cells then transmit their
messages to the brain as electrical impulses travelling along their long
processes called *axons*, which constitute the fibres of the optic nerve. Note that
what I told you about the optic chiasma proves that the long tails of these
retinal ganglion cells, their axons, have an uncanny capacity to find their
way to the right place in the brain: they seem to know exactly where to go.

After one more relay, or synapse, at the *Lateral Geniculate Nucleus* they
proceed to the *Primary visual cortex* (V 1), also called *area 17*, or *striate cortex*.
After further relays the information is disseminated to other visual cortical
areas and other regions of the brain which have a multiplicity of not very
illuminating names. On the right is shown an enlarged diagram of the cortex.
Again the nerve cell is the important component, and I've shown a single
example of one of the commonest types, the *pyramidal cell*. But there are in fact
a bewildering variety of different types, some of them shown in Fig. 1.9, and
also a bewildering number of actual cells. In the human retina there are
about a million ganglion cells, and consequently about a million axons reach
the brain on each side. But in the primary visual cortex alone there are at least
100 times as many cells as there are input fibres. Let us see how these cells are
arranged.

The map of the visual field

Figure 1.4 shows a postero-lateral view of the left cerebral hemisphere of a
monkey. In this species much of the primary visual cortex is visible from this
aspect, unlike the case in humans where the primary cortex is tucked round
the corner in the fissure between the two hemispheres, leaving only secondary areas visible from the side. The map of the central 8 degrees of the
contralateral hemifield is shown; it was constructed by noting whereabouts
in the visual field one must place a stimulus in order to excite the cells of that
region[5]. Note that it is very distorted in the sense that *equal* areas of the visual
field occupy very *unequal* areas of the cortical surface. The centre point of the
visual field maps to the point where the lines marked horizontal and vertical

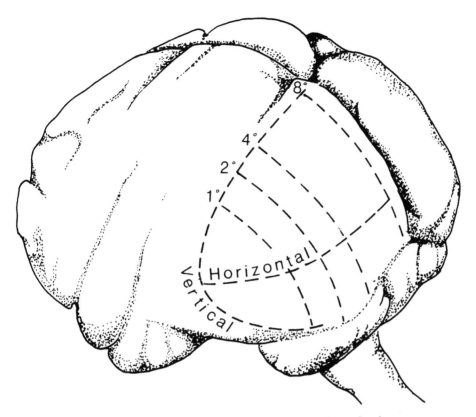

Fig. 1.4. Postero-lateral view of the left cerebral hemisphere of a *rhesus* monkey. In this animal (unlike *Homo sapiens*) the central 8° of the visual field is represented in a smooth, uncrinkled area visible from the side. The numbers give the degrees of eccentricity from the centre of the field, which corresponds to the left-most point on the map. The line marked horizontal shows where the horizontal meridian of the right visual field projects, and is itself roughly horizontal; the line marked vertical shows where the vertical meridian projects, and it is strongly curved as a result of the greatly expanded representation of the central parts of the visual field. The other half of the visual field is of course represented in the other hemisphere. Vertical positions (but not horizontal) are reversed, the upper part of the visual field projecting to the lower half of the map and vice versa. In spite of the distortions resulting from the expanded central representation the mapping is precise and accurate to about 1 mm.

intersect. Points along the vertical meridian in the visual field at various distances downwards plot along the upper part of the line marked vertical, while points along the horizontal meridian map along the line marked horizontal. Although distorted, the map is precise, so after a few points have been plotted one can predict where a new point will map on to the cortex with a precision of about a millimetre.

Maps within maps

That, however, is not the end of the story about the importance of position in the cortex. Hubel and Wiesel[6] showed in 1962 that different cortical neurons respond to different orientations of a visual stimulus (see Fig. 1.8). They also found from painstaking anatomical reconstructions of electrode positions that cells with different orientation preferences were not scattered at random over a square millimetre of cortex, but were grouped in an orderly manner[7]. This has recently been demonstrated in remarkable experiments using voltage-sensitive dyes.

Figure 1.5 is a photograph of a small region about 4 × 5 mm on the surface of the primary visual cortex of a monkey; note the two blood vessels and their branches, which is all the detail you can see. When Gary Blasdel and Guy Salama, who did these experiments[8], soaked the cortex with a voltage-sensitive dye and then stimulated it with gratings of differing orientations they generated the astonishing patterns shown in Fig. 1.6. Different parts of the cortex 'light up' when the eye is stimulated by stripes running in different directions, and the colour corresponding to each orientation is shown to the right of the figure. A good deal of wizardry is needed to do this, for the changes in luminance involved in generating this figure are of the order of a few hundredths of one per cent, but again we are seeing how modern techniques are opening a new vista on cortical function. Colin Blakemore (p.257) gives

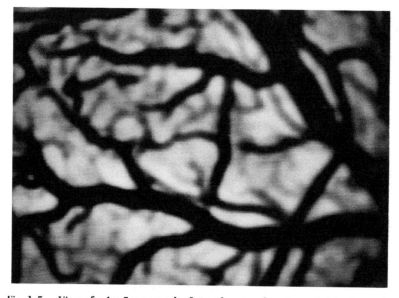

Fig. 1.5.   View of a 4 × 5 mm patch of visual cortex showing only blood vessels.

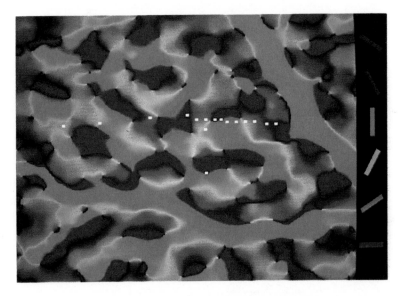

Fig. 1.6. The same region of cortex showing how orientation preference is mapped. Blasdel & Salama[8] obtained this by exposing the eye to stripes at six different orientations, measuring the very small changes of reflectance that occurred, and representing the differences between these changes according to the colour codes shown to the right. The two main blood vessels can still be seen, but the other details show there is structure in the mapping of orientation within the overall positional map.

more details of these cortical maps within maps, and of others elsewhere in the brain.

These are fascinating pictures, but is it churlish to feel disappointed again? I wanted to know *what* was going on, not *where* it was going on. But one must pay attention to the facts one finds, not those one wanted, and these facts seem to be saying loud and clear that the cortex attaches much importance to *position* in organising its function. To find out more about the *what* one must analyse in greater detail the responses of individual cells to different visual stimuli.

Responses from single neurons

Figure 1.7 shows the responses of two typical retinal ganglion cells – the type of nerve cell shown at bottom left of Fig. 1.3 that takes part in transmitting the retinal image up the optic nerve to the brain. One cell deals with one small part of the retina, so in order to excite it the light must be placed in exactly the right position in the visual field, which is called the *receptive field* of that cell. The responses consist of electrical impulses propagated along the nerve, and

H. Barlow

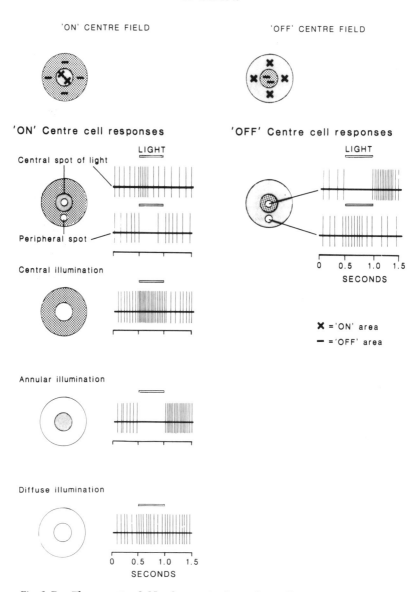

Fig. 1.7.   The receptive fields of two retinal ganglion cells, an 'on-centre' and an 'off-centre', are shown at the top. A cross indicates that light falling in this region increases the impulse rate from the cell, whereas light in the regions marked by minus signs slows the cell with a transient increase when it is extinguished. The next row shows the responses for centred spots and displaced spots for the two types. Below this the effects of illuminating the whole of the central region, and illuminating the surround without the centre are shown, while the lowest line shows that illumination of both parts together is relatively ineffective: the two zones inhibit each other. The two types can be thought of as signalling local 'whiteness' or 'blackness', and the ineffectiveness of uniform illumination shows that they respond to local contrast, not the absolute level of illumination. (After Kuffler & Nicholls[9])

it will be seen that only one of the cells increased its rate of impulse firing when the light came on; the rate of the other actually decreased during the stimulus, but increased when the light went off. The situation is actually more complicated than this, for if the stimulus spot had been displaced from the centre of the receptive field, or replaced by an annulus illuminating the region around the centre of the cell's receptive field, exactly the reverse pair of responses would have been recorded: the cell which increased in rate on illumination with a central spot would have slowed upon illumination in its annular surround, and speeded up on extinction of this light, while the other cell would have done the reverse. Further complications arise when colour is considered, as described by John Mollon (p.61), but I shall not attempt to describe these here.

On the whole records from this level in the visual pathway fit well both with our subjective impressions and with quantitative measurements of visual capacities. Thus it may seem intuitively right that we have separate cells that signal 'whiteness' and 'blackness' – the two types that respond as described above to increases and decreases in illumination. It also seems right that they respond to *contrast* rather than absolute illumination level, for we are all familiar with the fact that a level of luminance that looks white when surrounded by blackness can look black if the material surrounding it has its illumination greatly increased; in the former case 'on' cells would respond with increased firing, whereas in the latter it would be the 'off' cells. And in their sensitivity, spatial and temporal resolution, and capacity to adapt to different levels of ambient illumination, the properties of the retinal ganglion cells are what one might expect from scientific studies of visual performance. But it is always a surprise to remind oneself that this pattern of brief electrical impulses in two million optic nerve fibres is an obligatory stage in the representation of everything we see, intervening between the visual scene and our sensations of it.

Figure 1.8 shows the responses of a neuron in the visual cortex such as the pyramidal cell shown at bottom right of Fig. 1.3. These cells are usually responsive only if the stimulus is elongated and oriented correctly, as well as being positioned in the appropriate place in the visual field. They often respond to stimuli delivered to either eye, demonstrating the functional result of the arrangement whereby the information from the half-fields of each eye is brought together by the partial crossing over of fibres at the optic chiasma. In some cells there is strong interaction between the inputs from the two eyes, so that a stimulus object in the real world has to be placed in the appropriate depth plane as well as in the appropriate position[10]; selectivity for depth and orientation have been added to the requirements for activating a cell, with

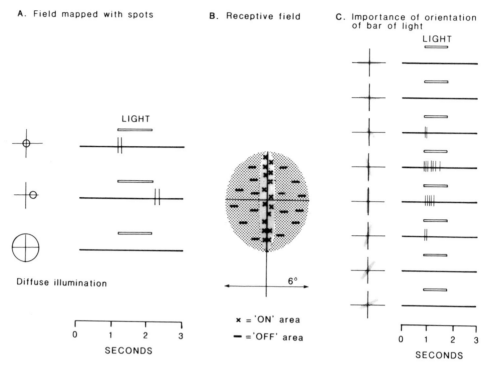

Fig. 1.8. The receptive field of a neuron in primary visual cortex and its responses to oriented stimuli. The convention for crosses and minus signs, indicating responses to a spot at on and off, are the same as in Fig. 1.7. The records of responses at the right show how many impulses were elicited by a bar at the orientations shown. This cell responded best to a nearly vertical stimulus, but there is a full range of cells at each position in the visual field, each responding best to a different orientation. Some of them respond best to stimulation through both eyes, provided that the stimulus is positioned exactly right for each of them; thus they require the stimulus to be at the correct *depth*, as well as the correct azimuth, elevation, and orientation in the visual field. (After Kuffler & Nicholls[9])

consequences for the frequency with which they are activated that will be considered shortly.

Is it possible to correlate structure and function at the level of the cell, or possibly even at the level of the individual synapse between one cell and another? Figure 1.9 shows drawings of some cells from the visual cortex made by Ramon Y Cajal almost 100 years ago and published in his monumental book on the histology of the nervous system in 1899[11]. Lack of the appropriate techniques made him completely blind to their function, but now one can combine the electrophysiological techniques whose results were shown in Figs. 1.7 and 1.8 with subsequent anatomical investigations of the same individual cells[12]. In this way it will be possible to work out much of the

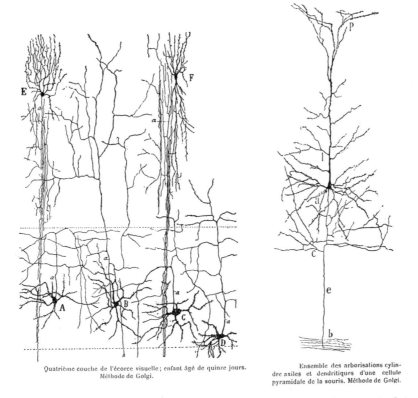

Quatrième couche de l'écorce visuelle; enfant âgé de quinze jours. Méthode de Golgi.

Ensemble des arborisations cylin-dre axiles et dendritiques d'une cellule pyramidale de la souris. Méthode de Golgi.

Fig. 1.9. Drawings by Ramon y Cajal[11] of cells from the cortex of a mouse (right) and from the central layers of the visual cortex of a 15-day human infant (left). The preparations from which they were drawn were stained by the Golgi method of silver impregnation, which picks out a single cell, apparently completely capriciously; if all the cells had been stained, they would have obscured each other hopelessly. One can now obtain even more complete pictures of single cells, and furthermore this can be done for cells whose properties have been determined by single unit recording[12].

circuitry of cerebral cortex, though it is a daunting task, for each square millimetre contains over 100,000 cells, and there are 100,000 square millimetres of cortex on each side of our brain!

In the optic nerve the image is carried as a pattern of electrical impulses in some million fibres from each eye, and at any given moment most of these fibres are carrying impulses at a rate between say 5 per second and their maximum of about 500 per second. In the cortex the image is still represented by a pattern of impulses, but at any one time only a small proportion of the vast array of cortical neurons is active, because cortical neurons are more selective about what each of them responds to. As a result, when a cell *does* respond it says something important and more specific about the image.

This is an interesting way to represent an image, and the fact that each individual nerve cell conveys an important piece of information makes us feel that we have made some progress in understanding how images are 'digested'. But there is also something profoundly unsatisfactory about it: what earthly use is an array of 100 million cells, each of which responds to some rather specific characteristic of a small part of the visual field? The images we are familiar with in our heads have a unity and usefulness that this representation, fragmented into a vast number of tiny pieces like a jig-saw puzzle, seems to lack. Why is it represented like this? How is the picture on the jig-saw puzzle detected, or rather what neural mechanisms carry the analysis of the image further, and what is the goal of these further steps? I want to suggest that the main obstacle here is that we have not grasped the true problem. The brain must do more than 'see' images, it must also 'understand' them, and perhaps it would help if we could clarify the meaning of understanding. Then we could take another look at this apparently fragmented representation of the image.

Part 2 Understanding understanding

Understanding is a matter of comprehending relationships. We understand a novel when we comprehend the interactions between the characters and their relationship with the events of the plot. Similarly with a picture, we understand it if we can relate its flat surface to a three-dimensional scene, and if we can then relate this scene to mythical or real people and events in the manner intended by the artist. In-front-of-the-eye experts know almost instinctively how to establish these relationships in the minds of others, and I believe these tricks of the trade may give valuable clues about the mental mechanisms of understanding. Jonathan Miller's discussion (p.191) of the factors that promote continuity between one shot and the next in a movie is particularly illuminating, for he shows how one particular detail, such as the direction of the actor's gaze, may be crucial. Establishing relationships depends entirely upon such links, and only when the recipient brain finds them can it collapse a whole sequence of otherwise disconnected scenes into a single plot or story. As viewers, we are completely unaware of the means used to draw our minds in the right direction – so it is hardly surprising that we are also unaware of the mechanisms of understanding at earlier stages in the whole process. But I believe the detection of linking features, and the way the brain uses them to assemble the information in images, is the key to understanding the anatomy and physiology of the visual pathways, and perhaps the key to much higher forms of understanding.

Vision is sometimes defined as the sense that tells one *what* is *where* in the space around us[3]; for that one needs to comprehend the relationship between something in the image and some property in the external world, like the position of an object, or its edibility. But there are many relationships to be understood *within* an image, and these must be taken into account before objects in the real world can be recognised effectively. On this view the first step must be to analyse the relationships of the pieces of an image to each other – to find the patterns and regularities it contains – and these are the steps that should be achieved by the bits of the brain I have been describing. Comprehending the relations between images and objects must come later, while the understanding required for a novel, picture, or movie is obviously at a higher level still.

The links that show relationships within images

The Gestalt school appreciated very clearly that it made no sense to consider images as a large number of separate fragments, and they were therefore much concerned with internal structure. They demonstrated that there are interactions between the parts of an image and described these in terms of principles such as 'grouping', 'good continuation', 'Pragnantz', or 'common fate'. Perhaps because these principles were given a somewhat mystical status by their proponents they were not very easily assimilated by many psychologists, but the attempts to perform visual tasks on computers now make it very clear what their role really is: they are the links within an image that the visual system uses, so they define the basis for image understanding.

If one considers how the Gestalt programme of perception might be achieved one sees that there are two stages: first, *local* properties of an image such as colour, direction of movement, texture, or binocular disparity, must be detected; second, the information so gained must be re-assembled. As I have argued elsewhere[15], the pattern selectivity of cells in primary visual cortex fits in well with the view that they are performing the first operation: neurons respond selectively to just the characteristics of the image that the Gestalt school drew attention to. How can the second step of re-assembly be achieved?

Selective addressing and non-topographical neural images

I suggest that reassembly is achieved by selective addressing: the cells in primary visual cortex, such as the pyramidal cell shown in Fig. 1.9, grow into other cortical areas where they create new patterns in which the information is brought together according to new principles that are not necessarily related to the topography of the original image. This is a speculation, but modern neuro-anatomy can trace the destination of these axons[14], so it should be testable in the near future.

Figure 1.10 shows how new *neural images* might be formed using this principle. Start with the formation of the optical image at the left, for it is an instructive analogy of the proposed neural process. Such an image is an array of light in which the intensity at a *point* in the image is proportional to the intensity of light that enters the eye at a particular *angle*, and therefore comes from a particular part of an object in the external world: direction of entry from the visual field is mapped to position in the image. The lens shown here is not the only way this can be done, as Michael Land describes in his contribu-

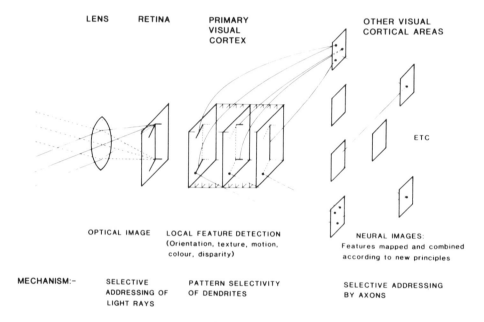

Fig. 1.10.   From optical to neural images. On the left is the familiar ray diagram showing the formation of an optical image on the retina. Note that the rays entering the edges of the lens must be brought to a focus by bending them to bring them to the right points in the image, this 'addressing' being selective according to the position of entry of the rays at the lens. The central block depicts the many types of feature detector, represented as successive layers each dealing in parallel with the same image. Here the three layers that respond selectively to the orientations of edges in the head, tail and shaft of the image of the arrow are shown. It is hypothesized that the next step is the formation of many different neural images, in which features of the original image are mapped and brought together according to the principles suggested by Gestalt psychology, and perhaps others yet unknown. It is thought that cortical neurons achieve this by addressing their axons to positions that depend upon their own pattern selectivity, as well as their position in the image. In this way parts of the image can become related by their properties, as well as by their positions in the visual field.

tion to this book (see p.197), but it seems a very simple and straightforward method as long as you confine your attention to the central ray. Because light normally travels in straight lines these central rays automatically find their ways to the appropriate point in the image, but the image-forming property of a lens results from its focussing action on light entering the edges of the lens: these rays would pass to the wrong points in the image if they travelled in straight lines and have to be bent downwards if they entered above the centre of the lens, upwards if below it.

Focussing by the lens ensures that light from a particular point on a distant object reaches a single position on the retina, and the necessary bending of the rays can be regarded as a form of *selective addressing*: rays are bent upwards under one condition, downwards under another. Can the selective addressing capability of nerve axons also focus information? Can it reunite information from external objects in the way that the lens reunites light rays that have become separated in their journey from a distant object?

An instructive step (not shown in Fig. 1.10) occurs in the optic nerve as the retinal image is being transmitted to the brain. As was shown in Fig. 1.1 and 1.3, the array of light on each retina is not simply copied as a pattern of nervous activity at the cerebral cortex. Instead the fibres from each retina rearrange themselves so that the left half of the visual field projects to the right cerebral hemisphere, the right half to the left hemisphere, this being brought about by some fibres crossing in the optic chiasma while the remainder continue to the hemisphere on their own side. So the rearrangement whereby nervous activity aroused by a single object reaches the same part of the cortex, whether it is seen by the left or the right eye, is achieved by selective addressing of the axons of retinal ganglion cells.

In the primary visual cortex the cells respond selectively to those particular features of the image that underlie Gestalt principles, as we have seen. There are many such features, and this is shown in Fig. 1.10 by depicting many planes of feature detectors, each plane specialising in a different feature; for instance vertical lines excite cells in the back plane, while the oblique lines on the head and tail of the arrow excite cells in two other planes. The information from each set of feature detectors is then projected on to another plane where similarity of *feature* determines position, not simply similarity of position in the original image. It is this re-assembly according to a different principle that is thought to be analogous to focussing by a lens, where different light rays were bent differently. There would also be planes of feature detectors for colour, depth, and motion, but these are not involved for this image and are not shown; the projections to other maps from these planes would also be organised according to similarity of feature, not only position. I think that it is the rôle of the axons of cells that respond to different features in the image to focus or assemble this information in new images.

The essence of such new images is that items of information that belong together, but have become separated, should be reunited – as the light rays were reunited by the lens and as the two images of each half visual field were reunited by the partial crossing at the optic chiasma. But in what ways do things 'belong together'? In many cases it is because the messages originate from the same place in the visual field and hence from the same object, but there are clues to the origin of a visual stimulus that do not depend upon position: they can for instance have the same colour, texture, or direction of motion, and this would often be the case if they arose from different parts of the same object. Though they might not express it this way I think the Gestalt psychologists spotted the links by which the visual system comprehends such probable relationships between separate pieces of the image, and this is the first step towards understanding it.

In new neural images formed according to these principles one must expect the topographical organisation of the image to be degraded, for the neighbours of a given axon terminal will tend to be the terminals of other axons responding to the same feature, not necessarily the axons of cells responding to nearby positions in the visual field. There is evidence for the degradation of the topographical mapping and for the segregation of different types of information in the pathways from the primary visual cortex[14], and some of this evidence is described by Colin Blakemore (Chapter 17) and Tony Movshon (Chapter 8). But at the moment all one can say for certain is that the combination of pattern selectivity and selective addressing has the potential for creating new neural images; in such non-topographical maps[15] information is assembled in new ways that make it relatively easy to understand how the Gestalt phenomena of segregation and figure/ground distinction might be performed. I believe it is these new neural images that enable us to analyse and understand what we see.

How about the more complex, higher levels, of image-understanding that naturally interest in-front-of-the-eye experts more than the primitive steps that we may be beginning to understand physiologically and anatomically? You will find more about the links that connect the shots of a movie from Jonathan Miller (Chapter 12), more hints about links in pictures in the chapters by Ernst Gombrich (Chapter 2) and John Willats (Chapter 16), and something about the links a novelist uses to draw the reader's mind in the right direction from David Lodge (Chapter 9). Those of us who deal with the world behind the eye would much appreciate explicit knowledge about these *links*, for more than anything else it is they that generate the knowledge of relationships that constitute understanding. I hope I have shown how they may enable us to understand the external world, and how the network of connections that our cunning neurons weave in our brains can embody them.

Conclusions

This book is being published in the belief that an account of what goes on inside the skull is relevant for those who are mainly concerned with the external world, and that the latter group have knowledge of the ways that images are linked, connected, and meaningfully manipulated that can aid scientific understanding of the mysteries of the mind. I hope the insights and questions of each group will be of mutual interest.

2

Pictorial instructions

ERNST GOMBRICH

I think it must be appropriate to start my study on images and understanding with one of the cases in which it may be a matter of life and death whether an image is correctly understood. I have in mind those leaflets or cards we all know from our air travels containing pictorial instructions on what to do in an emergency. Here are two examples (Figs. 2.1 and 2.2): one (removed by one of my accomplices) from a British Airways plane, another which I purloined from Lufthansa, illustrating the same contingency of what to do when the aircraft comes down on water. The British Airways sequence merely reminds you at first that you will find the vests for adults under the seat; the designer assumes that you know how to start putting them on, two stages illustrated in the Lufthansa leaflet. Both instructions then show the passenger from the back fastening a strap around their bodies, a movement explained by Lufthansa by means of two arrows. I confess that watching the air hostess demonstrating the next phase always worried me. Will I be able in the rush to tie the strap 'securely in a bow' on my side as I have often been told? I am not very good at this. Apparently there are no bows in the Lufthansa model, you are supposed to hook them in or up. In any case if British Airways lands you on the water you must apparently end up standing stock still and reflect on the meaning of the red cross symbol, unless you have understood the air hostess who told you that it points to the valve to be used for inflating the vest – but not yet, lest its bulk will impede your movement through the emergency door, graphically but not very reassuringly illustrated down below. The Lufthansa model is more detailed. It shows you extending the straps sideways – but not where to leave them – it also illustrates the movement of pulling with both hands for inflation and of topping up the air by blowing through a tube. Finally it reassures you by showing how a lamp will light up to facilitate your rescue as you float in the water.

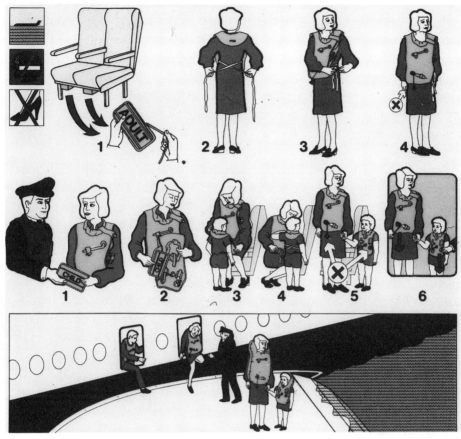

Fig. 2.1. Instruction leaflet, British Airways, Super one-eleven, Pine & Co. (P) Ltd., F407 (7th) – detail.

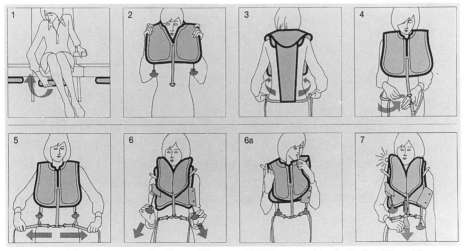

Fig. 2.2. Instruction leaflet, Lufthansa, A3120, printed in the Federal Republic of Germany, 7/83 – detail.

I have no wish to criticise these various instructions, only to point out that the task they are intended to teach is not all that easy to perform if you have never done it. The demonstrations by the hostesses surely help and I was happy on a recent flight across the Atlantic also to see a movie being shown which obviously relieved the cabin staff of a tedious task and seemed to me reassuringly clear, though the matter of the bow on my hip still eluded me. In any case it seems to me clear that the understanding of images, whether stills or movies, is vastly facilitated by the addition of verbal explanations.

You will have observed that the pictorial instructions issued on airlines which I have shown try to get on with the minimum of words or of other symbols which would not be intelligible to a passenger hailing from a foreign culture. One exception is the sequence of the panels which are to be read from left to right, and in most cases numbered in arabic numerals. Another exception is the use of the symbol of the arrow to indicate the direction of the required movement. Of course it takes the meaning of the symbol wholly for granted, but as an historian I have come to wonder when and where it assumed this universal significance as a pointer or vector. One need only ask such a question to find how poorly the world of the image is explored. I have not found such symbolic arrows before the 18th century, as in this illustration (Fig. 2.3) from a French treatise on *Hydraulic Architecture* of 1737 indicating the direction of rotation; in the same century topographical artists also sometimes used it to show the direction of the flow of the river by a discrete arrow[1].

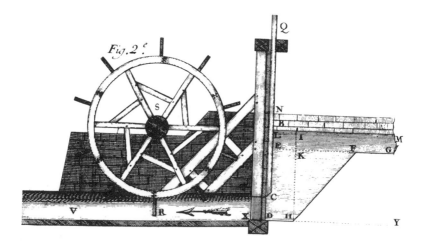

Fig. 2.3.   Diagram of waterwheel (with arrow) after Bernard Forest de Bélidor, *Architecture Hydraulic*, 1737.

Needless to say, the type of wordless pictorial instruction I have discussed is the exception rather than the rule in the genre. More frequently language is called in for the mutual elucidation of word and image in the interest of understanding. The method is employed to good effect in a Reader's Digest book of 400 pages called *What to do in an Emergency*, using more or less naturalistic illustrations supported by a text. I am afraid many of the emergencies illustrated are a little too unpleasant to contemplate but nobody will mind looking at Fig. 2.4 with an instruction on how to right an overturned caravan. True, the text tells us that the safest course in such a case is to get expert help from a garage or motoring organisation, but if you have at your disposal three fairly strong adults and at least 18 metres of stout rope you may try your luck in the way illustrated, which I have selected because the authors here take no chances over the tying of knots which are explained in comforting detail.

Even these few examples should suffice to remind you that in the genre of pictorial instruction the role of the designer, however important, still comes second after that of the inventor. In real life the performance of a particular task is usually learned by imitation and trial and error. You are shown how to ride a bicycle and then you try it till you get the hang of it. Whether you can then verbalise let alone illustrate the necessary movements is another matter.

There is a time-honoured story of the man who goes to the doctor who asks him what is wrong. "Doctor," he says "when I put my left hand behind my neck, and afterwards far down behind my back and stretch the arm swinging it round, my shoulder hurts terribly." "Why on earth are you performing such foolish antics?" "How else should I put on my overcoat?"

I have asked a young artist to illustrate the procedure for me in easy stages and here are our joint results (see Fig. 2.5), though I am sure Dr Jonathan Miller could improve on them.

The point, of course, is that the movement for seeking for the armhole behind your back is again one of trial and error. Kind bystanders sometimes try to help us senior citizens to perform the operation though this courtesy is more practised on the continent of Europe than in this country where it may be felt to be an unsolicited intrusion.

Engineers who are used to analysing motor skills have termed the components of such actions 'chunks'. The illustrator must learn to isolate the chunks and to show the performance from its most telling angle. As you see the genre of pictorial instruction is by no means as trivial as it may sound at first sight. It must break up the flow of the skilled movement into a fixed sequence of stationary positions.

Admittedly this need applies only to one special kind of pictorial instruc-

Righting an overturned caravan

If high winds topple a caravan onto its side, the safest course is to get expert help from a garage or motoring organisation. But it is possible to get the caravan back up on your own.

To use the technique, you need three fairly strong adults and at least 60ft (18m) of stout rope such as that used by climbers. You also need to practise the pulley knot shown here. It uses the rope to make a series of loops which act like pulleys, giving you extra leverage. Once you have mastered the knot, however, you can use it in any situation to move much heavier weights than you could otherwise handle: to help to free a car stuck in mud, for example.

• Remove as much equipment as possible from the caravan, and put it in the car. If the door is inaccessible, get into the caravan through an end window. Turn off any gas cylinders and disconnect the electricity as well.

• Raise the corner legs, or 'steadies', on the lower side. Put a block against the lower wheel, too, to stop it slipping. Lower the upper steadies slightly – not fully – so that they will make a three-point touchdown with the wheel.

• Tie the middle of the rope securely to the upper axle or a nearby part of the chassis. Then make the pulley knot shown here. Put the loop at the end of the knot round a sturdy stake driven into the ground at an angle.

• Throw the rope's other end over the caravan and wind it twice round a second stake to make a lowering line.

• Pull slowly and carefully on the free end of the rope. Ask at least two adults to pay out the lowering line gradually at the same time. Use as many adults as are available.

• Alternatively, you may be able to use the car either to help to pull the caravan up or in place of one of the stakes. Attach or loop the rope round the car's towing bracket.

• As the caravan comes upright, do not let it drop the last few feet; you could damage the axle and sub-frame. Let it down carefully.

HOW TO MAKE A PULLEY KNOT

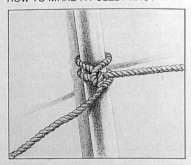

1 Attach the middle of the rope firmly to the caravan's axle or chassis. Throw one end over the caravan to make the lowering line.

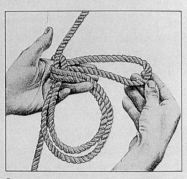

2 Make a fold in the other rope about 2ft (600mm) from the fixing point, and bring the doubled section across and behind the rope.

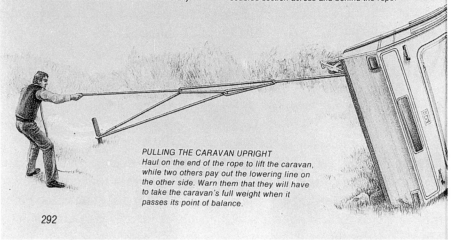

PULLING THE CARAVAN UPRIGHT
Haul on the end of the rope to lift the caravan, while two others pay out the lowering line on the other side. Warn them that they will have to take the caravan's full weight when it passes its point of balance.

292

Fig. 2.4. 'How to right a caravan', pp. 292/293, from *What to do in an Emergency*, Copyright 1986, The Reader's Digest Association Limited.

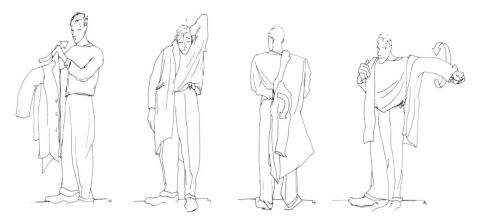

Fig. 2.5. How to put on an overcoat, drawn by Leonie Gombrich.

tion, the one I have chosen to deal with here. That there are other forms of pictorial instruction must be apparent in any case, for what else are a lecturer's 'visual aids' than a form of pictorial instruction? More relevant for historians is the fact that pictorial instruction was precisely the task assigned to the visual arts by the Christian Church to avoid the charge of idolatry. To quote the famous pronouncement by Pope Gregory the Great at the beginning of the Middle Ages: 'What writing is to the reader, pictures are to those who cannot read.'[2] I need hardly remind you of the application of this doctrine by the Church during a millenium of image-making in which the Last Judgement was displayed to the faithful in awe-inspiring compositions, and the lives of Christ and of the Saints told in many episodes in various media.

Not that all teaching was religious. The image had been used for instruction even before the development of sequential narrative. No system of the various possibilities can or need here be given; suffice it to remind you that there is a spectrum extending from the realistic portrayal of a specimen to a purely abstract diagram. The typical case of portrayal is to be found in herbals where the characteristics of a plant are represented as faithfully as possible[3]. On the opposite pole of the diagram we may think of cosmological images, notably calendar images like the Hellenistic Egyptian temple ceiling at Dendera representing the annual cycle with the images of the Zodiac and other symbolic figures such as the Decans representing units of ten days[4].

In the class of portrayal we may also place the marked or manipulated illustration of a specimen such as we find in the type of medical treatises demonstrating the point of the body suitable for cauterisation[5]. Closer still to a manual of instruction is that astounding treatise by the Hohenstaufen emperor, Frederick II, *De Arte Venandi cum Avibus*, on the art of hawking. The

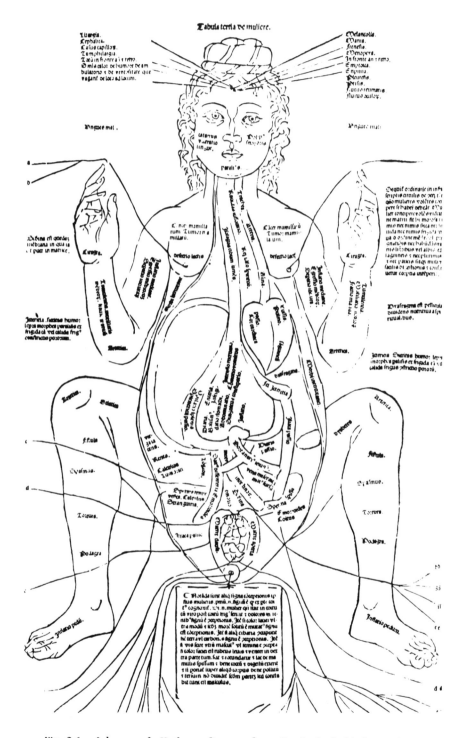

Fig. 2.6.   Johannes de Ketham, diagram from *Fasciculo de Medicina*, 1491.

magnificent illuminated manuscript of that treatise (in the Vatican) from the 13th century also illustrates the various forms of holding the hawk on the fist[6].

Somewhere in between the portrayal of a specimen and the abstract diagram of relationships we may place that vital instrument of visual instruction, the map, for the map is intended to represent the spatial relationship between locations on the globe in more or less schematic form[7]. Even so the abstract diagrammatic map merges almost imperceptibly with the bird's eye view of a territory as in certain drawings by Leonardo da Vinci of a part of central Italy[8]. These, of course, are imaginary bird's eye views for even Leonardo did not succeed in his dream of rivalling the birds. We may call such imaginary views visualisations.

Various forms of visualisation play a crucial role in images intended for pictorial instructions, though it is not always easy to establish where portrayal ends and visualisation begins. The history of anatomical illustration offers any number of examples. A well known woodcut from the *Fasciculo de Medicina* by Johannes de Ketham of 1491 purports to illustrate the main positions of the body organs (Fig 2.6). It has often and rightly been contrasted with the anatomical drawing by Leonardo da Vinci done only a few years later (Fig. 2.7), but even this exploration of the female body, though based on autopsy, is largely a visualisation and not even a wholly correct one. Even so it is clear that Leonardo's heroic visualisation excluded the insertion of labels and captions which characterise the earlier image. Here too Leonardo was a pioneer for in his scientific drawings he usually inserted a letter key to which he referred in his explanatory texts, a method surely derived from geometrical demonstrations in the tradition of Euclid[9]. This method which we too easily take for granted came to triumph in the many woodcuts of Georg Agricola's classic text book on mining, *De re Metallica*, from the middle of the 16th century. On the next plate (Fig. 2.8) we see under A a workman carrying broken rock in a barrow, under B the first chute, under C the first box with its handle marked D, and so all the way down to X, the third tub and Y the plugs.

With this example, however, I have moved out of the Middle Ages and strayed a little too far from my central problem of the teaching of manual skills. Even before the end of the 15th century we find an early example of a real pictorial instruction, demonstrating the sequence of a performance in easy stages. I am referring to a pattern book now kept in the Göttingen Library of how to paint the decorative scrolls that adorned manuscripts and even the early printed books of the period (Fig. 2.9). I owe the knowledge of this interesting manual, which has been published in facsimile, to Dr Michael Evans of the Warburg Institute[10]. The author demonstrates how to draw and

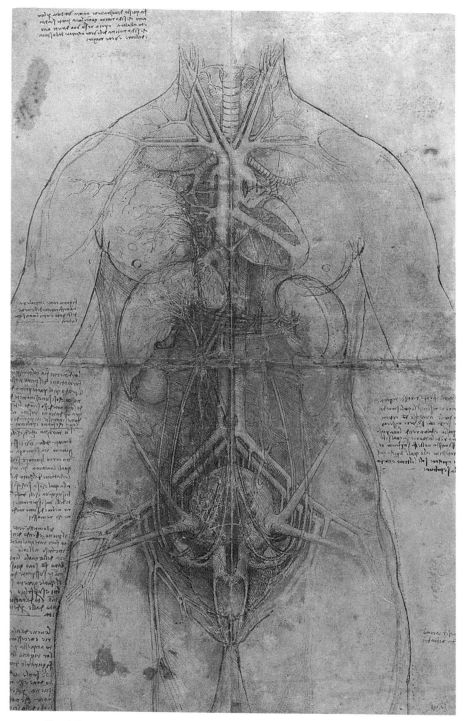

Fig. 2.7.   Leonardo, Anatomical Drawing of the Female Body, Windsor, Royal
Library, 12281, by gracious permission of Her Majesty the Queen, c. 1510.

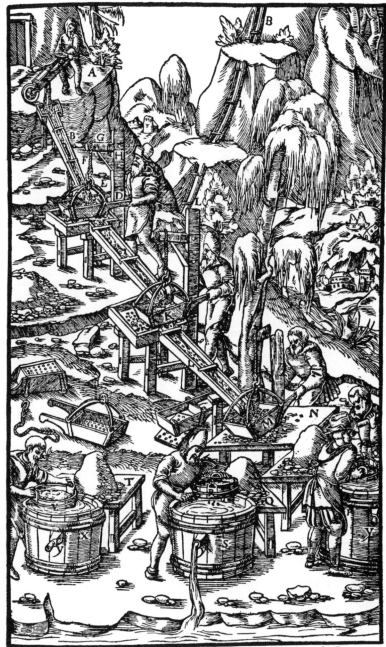

A—Workman carrying broken rock in a barrow. B—First chute. C—First box. D—Its handles. E—Its bales. F—Rope. G—Beam. H—Post. I—Second chute. K—Second box. L—Third chute. M—Third box. N—First table. O—First sieve. P—First tub. Q—Second table. R—Second sieve. S—Second tub. T—Third table. V—Third sieve. X—Third tub. Y—Plugs.

Fig. 2.8. G. Agricola. *De re Metallica.* Book VIII. 1556 (after the English translation. New York 1950).

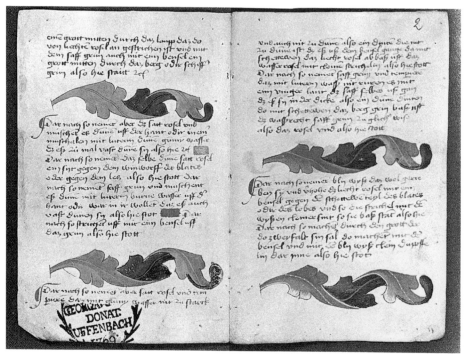

Fig. 2.9.   Page from the Göttingen Model Book, Niedersächsische Staats – und
Universitäts Bibliothek, Göttingen.

colour the scroll in successive stages until it gets the rounded and supple
appearance.

I did not know this early example when I wrote my book on *Art and Illusion*
in which I illustrated a number of somewhat later drawing manuals, like the
one by Odoardo Fialetti of 1608 which starts with this instruction of how to
draw eyes in profile (Fig. 2.10). Notice that this type of pictorial instruction
stands somewhat apart, because here every stage of the performance to be
taught leaves a permanent trace and can therefore be illustrated with ease.
Such books are still being produced in great numbers. Another method which
never died out is the demonstration by means of contrast of the right and
wrong way of setting about a task, for example on the correct and incorrect
way of holding the pen when drawing a map[11]. If you rest your hand on the
surface you will certainly smudge the drawing.

Maybe instructions in penmanship took second place to those in
swordmanship and similar skills in combat which formed part of the education of the gentleman. Quite a number of such manuals have been preserved from the 15th century onwards. Many of them are strictly utilitarian
lacking any artistic ambitions like the bulky fencing book drawn on paper by

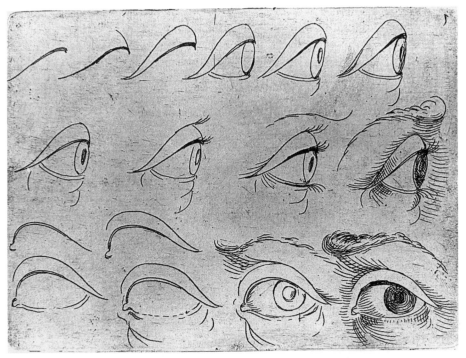

Fig. 2.10.   Odoardo Fialetti, *il vero Modo . . . per dissegnier*, Venice 1608.

one Thalhoffer, dated 1443, which also includes instructions in wrestling and unarmed combat (Fig. 2.11). Naturally there are also luxury editions for the use of princes[12].

I have greatly enjoyed the search for the *incunabula* of pictorial instructions much facilitated by the resources of the Warburg Institute, but I must restrict myself here to a few examples remarkable for individual devices.

The two illustrations you see in Fig. 2.12, come from the most sophisticated fencing book I know, appropriately called *A Treatise on the Science of Arms* of 1553 by Camillo Agrippa. One illustration shows within one frame four stages of the fencer's movement lettered successively A, B, C and D in almost cinematic sequence. The other gives a sample of the movements of the blade in a complex geometrical figure, though I must confess that I have so far failed to profit fully from this pictorial instruction in the complex science of thrust and parry.

What is relevant in these handbooks for my context is that the analysis of movements is part of the skill. They all have a name familiar to the fencing master. There is a natural transition therefore from the teaching of fencing to the teaching of the dance, the fencing master and the dancing master may have been one and the same person. This natural transition is evident in two

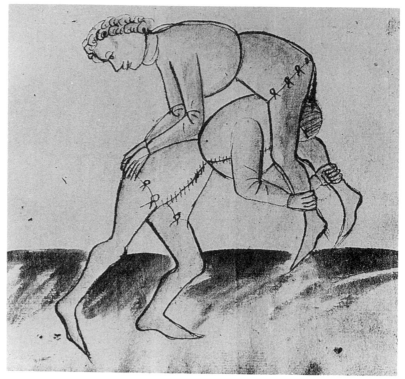

Fig. 2.11.   Hans Thalhofer, *Fechtbuch*, 1443, ed. G. Hergsell, Prague, 1901.

pages from the dialogue on dancing by Thoinot Arbeau of which an English translation came out in 1959 (Fig. 2.13). I quote:

> 'You see above four pictures of the gestures I have described to you, to wit;
> *Feinte, estocade, taille haute* and *revers haut*. There remain the pictures of
> the other two gestures which you see below. Besides these there are
> several other body movements but it seems to me it will suffice for you to
> have them in writing without necessitating pictures – Fencing has
> already acquainted me with all these gestures. Now tell me how to dance
> the buffens'[13]

Since we can look forward in this book to a contribution on dance notation (Chapter 5) I do not propose to pursue this type of literature any further but other forms of exercise also share with dancing and fencing the need for a technical vocabulary to describe relevant movements. We still use such a vocabulary when speaking of swimming for instance of the breast stroke or of crawling. The first illustrated swimming manual by one Everard Digby came out in England in Latin in 1587 and in English in 1595[14]. One of the most sophisticated and ambitious of such illustrated treatises on athletics is a work by one Giocondo Baluda of 1630 on various exercises to be performed on the

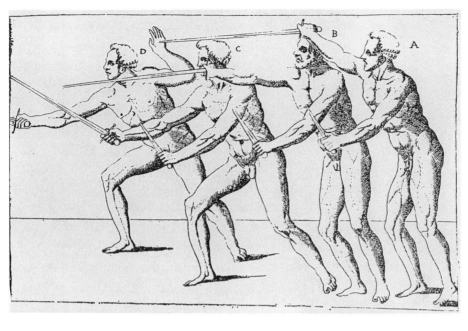

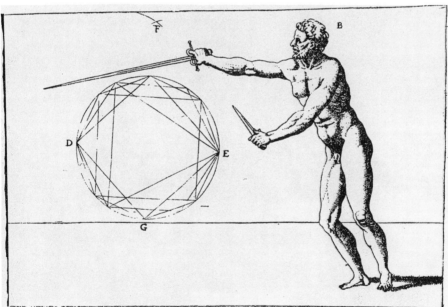

Fig. 2.12.   Camillo Agrippa, *Trattato di Scienzia d'Arme*, 1553 (after Bascetta, Vol. II).

You see above four pictures of the gestures I have described to you, to wit; *feinte, estocade, taille haute* and *revers haut.* There remain the pictures of the other two gestures which you see below. Besides these there are several other body movements but it seems to me it will suffice for you to have them in writing without necessitating pictures.

Feincte

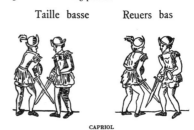

Eftocade

Taille basse

Reuers bas

CAPRIOL

Fencing has already acquainted me with all these gestures. Now tell me how to dance the buffens.

ARBEAU

Taille haulte

Reuers hault

Suppose that A, B, C and D represent four persons suitably attired, either as soldiers or Amazons, or two of each, and that they are about to enter the hall.

CAPRIOL

I visualize them as you depict. What would they do?

ARBEAU

First, A would enter alone and brandishing his sword in time to the music circle the hall, then returning to the entrance place the point of his sword on the ground as if he desired to challenge his companions to combat. This done, he would again circle the hall and B would follow him, and when they had completed the round B would summon his companions. Now

Fig. 2.13.   Thoinot Arbeau, *Orchésography,* English edn, pp. 184/5.

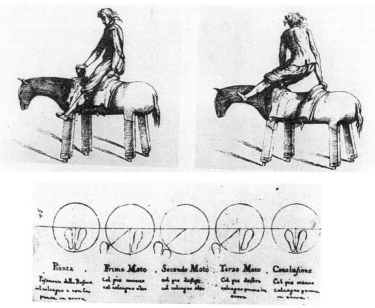

Fig. 2.14.   Giocondo Baluda, *Modo di Volteggiare il Cavallo di legno,* 1630 (after Bascetta, Vol. I).

wooden horse (Fig. 2.14). Like Agrippa before him he also illustrates the successive movements of the athletes, showing five phases of the action from various sides, but he adds another feature by indicating the position of the feet in schematic form.

A treatise on the art of catering of 1639 contains instructions on the folding of napkins (Fig. 2.15) which may be one of the first to illustrate the exact position of the hands in performing the task as well as the desired result that recalls the Japanese technique of Oregami[15].

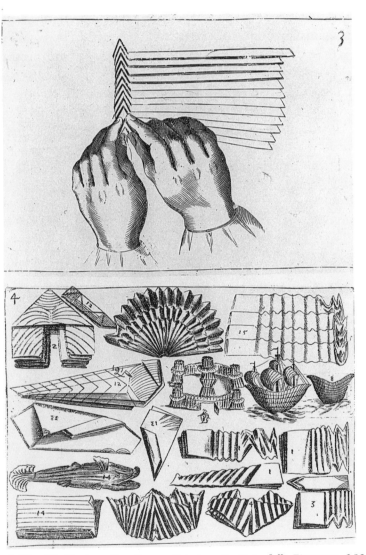

Fig. 2.15. M. Giegher, *Treatise on Catering, Trattato delle Piegature,* 1639 (after Facciolo II, 1966).

42 E. Gombrich

But all these individual examples are eclipsed by the greatest enterprise in pictorial instruction, the *Grande Encyclopédie* launched in 1751 by Diderot and D'Alembert in conscious imitation of *Chambers' Encyclopedia*; but as the preface of the French work proudly announces Chambers' had 30 pages of illustrations and they proposed to have 600. Indeed the large engraved folio plates of the ten volumes of the illustrated supplements of the *Encyclopédie* were an integral part of that great educational venture, for it was intended, among other things, to remove the secrecy from craft traditions and to demonstrate the importance of trade and industry to the public, invoking the spirit and example of Francis Bacon who had diagnosed so long ago the bias of education against manual skills. To turn the pages of these magnificent folio volumes is to be transported back to the 18th century at the threshold of the Industrial Revolution.

Here in Fig. 2.16 are the first two plates of the article on cotton from the section *Oeconomie Rustique* illustrating the interior of the workroom and the view of the machine which is then carefully analysed and measured for those who want to read the description. On the next plate you can follow the sequence of the manual operation from 1 to 6 with figure 1 having a subsidiary commentary.

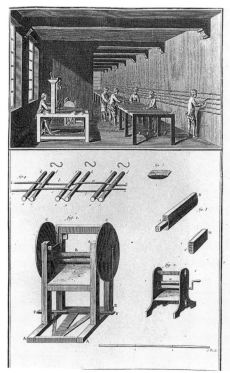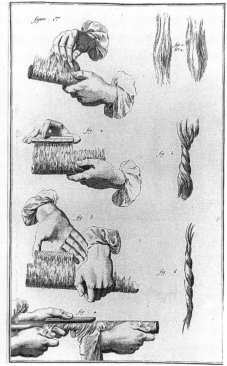

Fig. 2.16. *Grande Encyclopédie*, '*Cotton*', Pl.1 & 2, Vol. I.

Naturally the military arts are not neglected. The many plates devoted to the individual positions of parading soldiers would have gladdened the heart of any sergeant major. More theoretical are the plates devoted to the complex skill of manoeuvre in carrying out evolutions, that is turning movements in formation. Figure 2.17 illustrates the passing of a bridge and the reformation of the detachment.

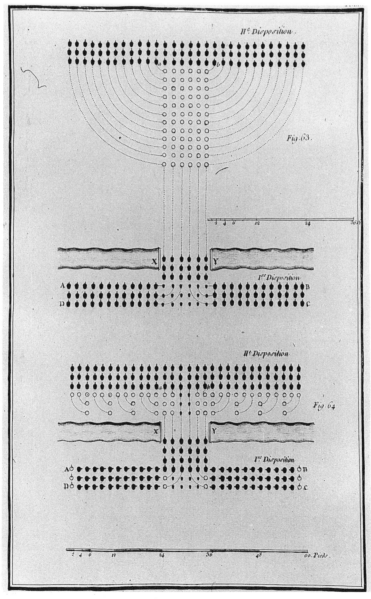

Fig. 2.17. *Grande Encyclopédie, 'Art Militaire'.*

The rest of my story would have to concern technology and sociology, in other words the means and the demands shaping the history of pictorial instruction up to the present day. The greatest contribution of technology is of course the use of the photographic camera for pictorial instruction. It has enabled teachers and writers of manuals to illustrate the hands of the great

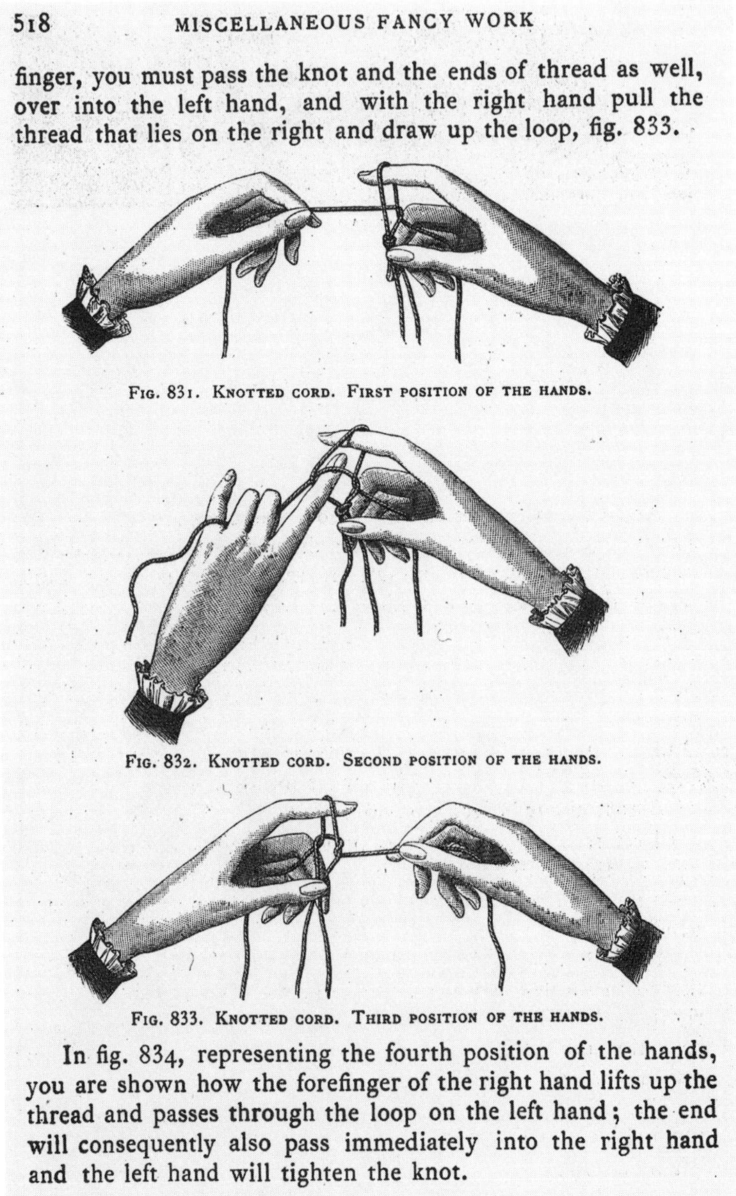

518   MISCELLANEOUS FANCY WORK

finger, you must pass the knot and the ends of thread as well, over into the left hand, and with the right hand pull the thread that lies on the right and draw up the loop, fig. 833.

FIG. 831. KNOTTED CORD. FIRST POSITION OF THE HANDS.

FIG. 832. KNOTTED CORD. SECOND POSITION OF THE HANDS.

FIG. 833. KNOTTED CORD. THIRD POSITION OF THE HANDS.

In fig. 834, representing the fourth position of the hands, you are shown how the forefinger of the right hand lifts up the thread and passes through the loop on the left hand; the end will consequently also pass immediately into the right hand and the left hand will tighten the knot.

Fig. 2.18.   Thérèse de Dillmont, *Encyclopedia of Needlework*, n.d.

masters, as Malvine Brée has illustrated the hands of the renowned peda-
gogue Leschetizky in her book demonstrating the position of the hands while
playing a scale. One wonders when we will get video-tapes showing the
hands of our master pianists, either taken from television performances or
made *ad hoc* for the purpose of 'master classes'.

The growing demand for visual instructions goes together with the popularity of handicrafts outside the workshop and in the home. Such a typical
manual as the *Encyclopedia of Needlework* brings to mind the busy hands of
Victorian ladies (Fig. 2.18). Of greater social significance are the manuals
issued with the first sewing machine for they remind us of the increase in
home industries which required such basic instructions in manual skills.

It must soon have been realised how much the marketing of tools and
instruments could benefit from the addition of instruction leaflets of various
kinds; indeed it is rare today to find an apparatus which is not also explained
in multilingual and pictorial instructions.

I should like to end by paying tribute to that great store in Chicago called
Marshall Field in which I bought a tie, for I have always treasured the leaflet
they sell with it (Fig. 2.19). Unlike other guides the designer shows himself
aware of the special problem presented by the mirror which fiendishly
changes right to left and left to right, forward to back and back to forward. I
know that motorists, dentists and engravers have overcome this difficulty
and can make the inverse movements of those they see in the mirror. I am not
one of them, and though I have studied the pictorial instruction about the
tying of the black tie for evening wear with special attention I shall here reveal
that I cowardly use a made-up tie.

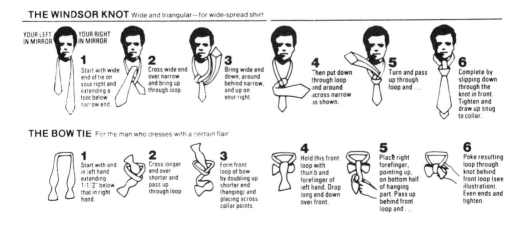

Fig. 2.19.   The Windsor Knot, and the Bow Tie, leaflet **Marshall Field, Chicago.**

3

Computer-generated cartoons

DON PEARSON, E. HANNA AND K. MARTINEZ

Introduction

The cartoon or line drawing is a very economical method of portraying a person or scene. Studies of the criteria used by humans in the recognition of faces have indicated that simple geometrical considerations (the distance between the eyes, the width of the mouth, and so on) predominate[1]; these can be adequately conveyed in a cartoon. Hand shapes can also be satisfactorily represented in this way; for example, the Royal National Institute for the Deaf publishes the standard manual alphabet used for finger-spelling in cartoon form[2].

We have become interested in generating cartoons electronically, as a way of transmitting moving images over the telephone network[3-7]. Since the telephone network has been designed to carry low-frequency speech signals, it can take up to several minutes to transmit a single frame of a conventional television picture. Experiments have shown, however, that enough small cartoon images can be transmitted every second to create the illusion of movement. As these images have only two levels of luminance, it is possible to use a very different code similar to that used in transmitting documents over telephone lines by facsimile. Such codes, termed 'run-length' or 'relative-address' codes, send the image information as a succession of numbers; each number represents the distance of a black/white transition from a neighbouring transition[8].

One of the aims of our work, which we share with others [9-11], is to enable the deaf to communicate over distances by signing or lip-reading. Since sign language relies on hand shape, orientation, position and movement, together with facial expression, it can be adequately conveyed in moving cartoons. Another of our aims is to use the cartoon as a foundation or primitive on which to build up shading and colour[12]. This may allow moving colour images for video-conferencing to be transmitted very economically over the new digital telephone and data networks which are now being introduced.

46

There is a double constraint which these engineering aims place on the cartoon: it should satisfactorily portray the face and hands of the person concerned, but it should do so with as few lines as possible. The more lines there are, the more the information which has to be transmitted per image or per second in the run-length code; a consequently greater 'channel capacity' is required to carry the signal. The channel capacity needed for a broadcast-standard studio television picture is about 20,000 times that available on a telephone line; extreme economy is therefore needed in the cartoon.

Electronic generation of cartoons

The subject of how to draw an economical cartoon was considered in the 1950s and 1960s in terms of information theory[13], the idea being that cartoon lines should be placed where the object is difficult to predict and the line therefore carries the most information. However, the validity of this approach has been questioned[14]. It also presupposes a more basic operation needed to convert an image into a line drawing (of whatever kind). The prescription for this basic operation is essential in any electronic implementation.

Our first approach to electronic generation was to try to detect edges in the image. An edge is a sudden change in the luminance of the image (Fig. 3.1a). It seemed reasonable to suppose that the locations of these changes would be useful to the eye. To detect the edges, a computer can be programmed to search for a particular pattern of lighter and darker image elements, indicated as + and − signs in Fig. 3.1b. This is accomplished by scanning the

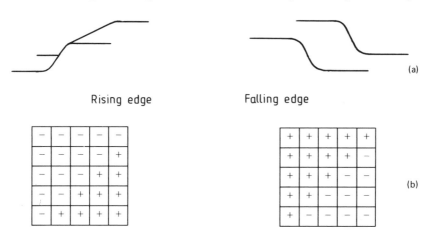

Fig. 3.1. (a) Luminance changes corresponding to an edge in the image.

(b) The pattern of lighter (+) and darker (−) image elements which a computer searches for in order to detect an edge at 45° to the vertical.

electronically sampled image using a 'window', shown in Fig. 3.1b as a 5×5 array of image elements. Since the edge can lie in any angular direction, this may have to be repeated with different patterns sensitive to different edge orientations.

After fairly lengthy experimental investigations which used many different published edge-detection procedures, we concluded that edge detection, when applied to the human form, does not succeed very well[4-6]. It tends to produce too many lines and at the same time to omit some key ones. Edge-detected images of humans look vaguely human in outline but have poor facial features. Hands held in front of faces are inadequately rendered. In consequence we attempted a new approach.

Theory of computer-generated cartoons

The new approach was to formulate the rule for drawing cartoons in the three-dimensional space of the object rather than the two-dimensional space of the image. It seemed to us, as a matter of intuition, that the important surfaces of the face and hands were the ones which fell away sharply from the line of sight of the television camera (or the eye of an observer).

If we imagine straight lines drawn from the lens of a camera in all conceivable forward directions, some will pierce the surfaces of objects in the field of view, others will miss them altogether, but a small subset (Fig. 3.2) will just graze the surface. The basic postulate of the theory[6] states that a cartoon point (usually forming part of a cartoon line) should be drawn in the image plane wherever a line grazes the surface of the object in this way[15]. On any given scan line in the image (Fig. 3.2) there are only a small number of these points (indicated as A, B and C) which have to be identified.

It is necessary to pay attention to scale[16] in this definition; the correct degree of conceptual smoothing has to be applied to the physical microstructure of the human form, so that the cartoon has neither too much nor too little detail. It is also helpful to provide a relaxation of the rather strict criterion of lines being tangent to the surface, to allow slight penetration of the surface by the straight line; this accommodates features like the edges of noses. In engineering it is wise to build in tolerances.

Implications and implementations

Since in practice the cartoon extractor is required to work with images and not objects, it is necessary to analyse the varieties of illumination falling on smooth surfaces defined by the postulate. If light is reflected to the camera at such surfaces in a consistent way, producing a well-defined feature in the image, it may be possible to locate the surfaces by an operation on the image.

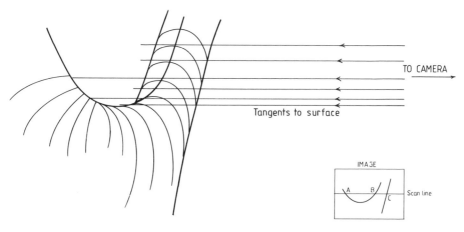

Fig. 3.2. The basic postulate in the proposed theory of cartoons identifies surfaces which are grazed by straight lines drawn from the camera. When the image of the object is scanned, the computer has to identify points A, B and C as cartoon points.

This analysis has been carried out, taking into account mutual illumination, that is light reflected from one surface to another before being reflected to the camera[6, 17]. It has been found that the image feature produced at a surface satisfying the postulate is a luminance *valley* when all local surfaces have the same reflectance (for example at the side of the nose or at the side of a finger held in front of the face); it is, however, a luminance step edge at an occluding contour seen against a background of different reflectance (for example, a hand held in front of a wall of greater or lesser lightness than skin). We have therefore argued that what is required is a feature detector with a primary response to luminance valleys, but possessing a secondary response to luminance edges.

Figure 3.3 gives a simplified portrayal of the type of detector required. Its action may be contrasted with that of the edge detector in Fig. 3.1. Like the edge detector, it searches for a particular pattern; in this case, it is a pattern consisting of a line of relatively dark elements in the image (represented by minus signs), surrounded by relatively light ones (the plus signs). This is what would commonly be called a valley in geographical terms. In practice the differences between the minus elements and the plus elements can be quite small.

Like edge detectors, valley detectors are defined on a window of image elements (5×5 elements in Fig. 3.3). The size of the window affects the ability of the detector to discriminate in favour of valleys and against other features (such as edges). The situation is rather like that of a radio receiver. Some radio

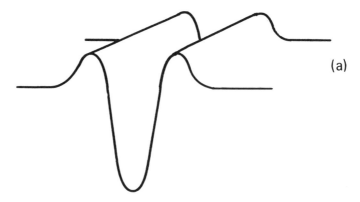

(a)

Fig. 3.3. (a) Luminance feature to which a valley detector is primarily sensitive. This may also be viewed as the required impulse response of a spatial filter, preceding a peak detector, which will be maximally sensitive to such a feature.

0	+	−	+	0
0	+	−	+	0
0	+	−	+	0
0	+	−	+	0
0	+	−	+	0

(b)

(b) Pattern searched for by the detector for a valley running north to south. The characteristic of the pattern is a column of slightly darker (−) elements seen against a surround of slightly lighter (+) elements. The elements marked 0 allow for some flexibility in interpretation.

receivers have sharper tuning than others, so that they can more easily reject unwanted radio stations with similar broadcasting frequencies to the desired station. The rejection of unwanted image features is carried out by detecting only those valleys whose depth is greater than a preset amount[18].

The 'tuning' of a valley detector gets sharper as the window size increases. Unless it is of infinite size, it will have some response to edges. So to produce a valley detector with a secondary response to edges, it is only necessary to make its window of finite size. This is fortunate since, as remarked earlier, the scale of the valley – that is, its width and length – must be matched to the size of the face or hand in the image for the best results.

In our actual implementation we have used certain refinements on the simplified valley detector given in Fig. 3.3. These are mainly to increase the speed, to discriminate against noise and to ensure that only the valley floor is identified. Figure 3.4 describes an actual 5×5 detector we have used[6, 17]. This was the one which generated the cartoons illustrated in the next section.

We are able to generate moving cartoons in real time from 64×64 element images at 6 frames/s using a 3×3 window and a 68000 microprocessor. We have also developed a simple parallel architecture which can process 256×256 images at 25 frames/s[19].

a	b	c	d	e
f	g	h	i	j
k	l	m	n	o
p	q	r	s	t
u	v	w	x	y

a — y are picture elements

T_1, T_2 are thresholds

To test for a vertical valley through m:

if $((1 - m) > T_1$ or $(n - m) > T_1)$

then

if $(f + k + p + j + o + t - 2(h + m + r)) > T_2$

and $(g + l + q + i + n + s - 2(h + m + r))$

$> (f + k + p + h + m + r - 2(g + l + q))$

and $(g + l + q + i + n + s - 2(h + m + r))$

$> (h + m + r + j + o + t - 2(i + n + s))$

then there is a valley through m.

Tests for a horizontal valley and for diagonal valleys have the same form, but the thresholds for the diagonal valleys are higher.

Fig. 3.4. Actual implementation of a 5×5 cartoon operator, comprising a valley detector as in Fig. 3.3, with elaborations.

Comparison of computer-drawn and human-drawn cartoons

Two examples of computer-drawn cartoons are shown in Figs. 3.6b and 3.7b, which were derived from the photographs shown in Fig. 3.5. These photographs were first converted into discrete electronic representations of 260×245 picture elements, each element having 64 grey levels. The electronic images were processed to produce the cartoons by use of the cartoon operator in Fig. 3.4. In addition, some uniform black shading was added for effect. This shading was produced by 'thresholding', that is, by identifying all the areas in the original grey-level images which were darker than a certain predetermined value. This is easily done electronically and does not add significantly to the amount of information which has to be transmitted.

To see how the computer's efforts compared with those of a human artist, we asked a professional cartoonist (Mr S. Wood, known widely as 'Woody') to emulate the computer. He too was given the photographs of the male and female subjects in Fig. 3.5. He was not shown the computer-drawn cartoons, nor any other examples of the computer's work, but the required style was described (as few lines as possible, with uniform black fill-in allowed). No indication was given as to where he should place his lines nor of the cartoon operation which the computer uses. The human cartoonist's renditions are shown in Figs. 3.6a and 3.7a. He also decided to caricature the two subjects, as shown in Fig. 3.8.

As non-artists, we were struck by the considerable similarity between the human-drawn and machine-drawn versions, while noting some differences.

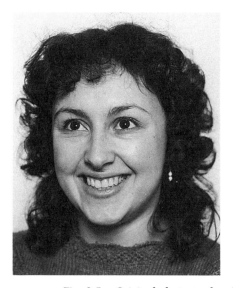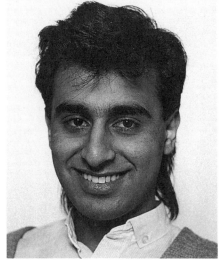

Fig. 3.5. Original photographs of (a) female and (b) male subjects.

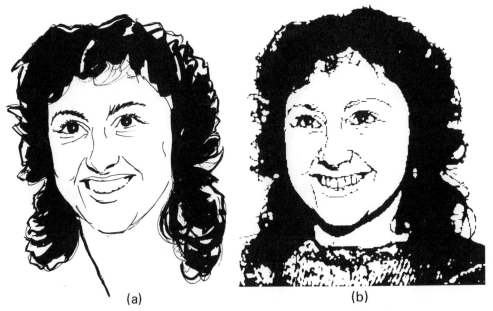

Fig. 3.6.   Comparison of (a) artist-drawn and (b) computer-generated cartoons
of the female subject.

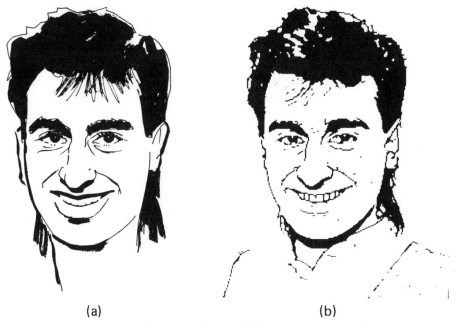

Fig. 3.7.   Comparison of (a) artist-drawn and (b) computer-generated cartoons
of the male subject.

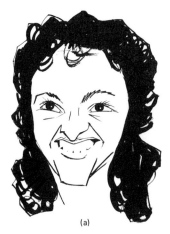
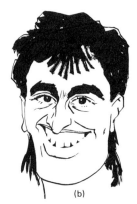

(a)   (b)

Fig. 3.8. Caricatures by the human artist.

The main feature lines around the eyes, mouth, nose and chin are remarkably alike, although the human artist does not show the same detail in the teeth. The black shading in the hair, in the corners of the mouth and in the eyebrows of the man is very similar. The number of lines used by the cartoonist and by the computer is about the same for the face, excluding the clothing; however, because of the relatively low sampling density used in the processing, the lines in the computer versions have a jagged appearance. There are differences, too, in higher-level interpretation of the photographs (of which the human but not the computer is capable) as to what is and what is not of importance. For example, the woman's earring and details of the clothing of both subjects have been omitted by the human cartoonist.

Mr Wood agreed that the computer cartoons were quite similar to his and that some of the line placements were remarkably good; however, he noted some further differences. In both subjects the computer had produced little rectangles in the rendition of the lower lids of the eyes, due to a tear causing a highlight in the original photograph. On the male subject, he thought there should be a shadow under the lower lip, smile lines at the side of the eyes and a small bifurcation in the line at the right of the mouth. In the cartoon of the female subject, the computer had erroneously run together the long and short lines to the left of the mouth. He felt that his own knowledge of human anatomy helped him in making these judgements.

We have not attempted to produce computer-generated caricatures. The variations in line which produce caricature have been discussed by Gombrich and Hochberg[20, 21].

Low-level processing in human vision

If a human cartoonist and a computer place their basic feature lines in roughly the same locations, might this be an indication that low-level processing in the visual system of the human cartoonist bears some correspondence to the cartoon operation used by the computer? It is interesting to note that the one-dimensional (cross-sectional) form of a valley detector (Fig. 3.3) is similar to the difference-of-Gaussian weighting function for the retinal receptive field at ganglion-cell level, while the two-dimensional form is similar to the weighting function of a cell in the visual cortex, where orientation becomes important[22, 23]. We did not model our valley detector on the human eye, but derived it from considerations of light falling on matt surfaces; in view of the correspondence between the two, could it be that the eye is particularly sensitive to surfaces identified by our postulate, that is, those which fall sharply away from the line of sight? These are clearly very important surfaces in the recognition of faces.

We note, further, the interest in Marr's idea of the 'raw primal sketch' as a first processing step in the representation of shape information in the human visual system[24]. Marr's concept is that this is produced by a spatial filter with a response similar to that of Fig. 3.3, followed by a detector of 'zero-crossings'. However, in a more recent version of this process suggested by Watt and Morgan[25] the detector of zero-crossings is replaced or supplemented by a detector of centroids. This is rather similar in its effect to our peak detector. We have also noted that scale is an important parameter in producing a recognizable cartoon. If the cartoon detector window is too small, unnecessary detail creeps in; if, on the other hand, it is too large, the shapes of the features are distorted. In human vision there are known to be several spatial filter channels operating at different scales[26].

To explore these ideas further, we carried out some experiments which involved electronic inversion of the tone scale of the images.

Inverting the cartoon

It is possible to represent a cartoon as black lines on a white background or as white lines on a black background. Our earliest cartoons[4] were in fact of the latter kind, but we noticed that when we inverted them electronically, turning black to white and white to black, they looked better. This is illustrated in Figs. 3.9–3.11; Fig. 3.9 shows an original photograph, Fig. 3.10 a black-on-white computer-generated cartoon derived from this photograph and Fig. 3.11 the white-on-black version.

Although there is exactly the same information in Figs. 3.10 and 3.11, Fig. 3.10 somehow looks more natural. Why is this? The result can be explained if

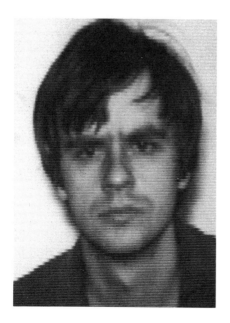

Fig. 3.9.   Original photograph.

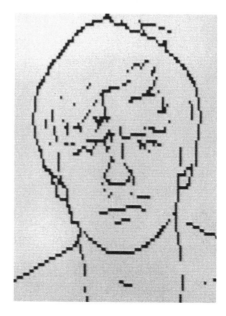

Fig. 3.10.   Black-on-white computer-generated cartoon derived from Fig. 3.9.

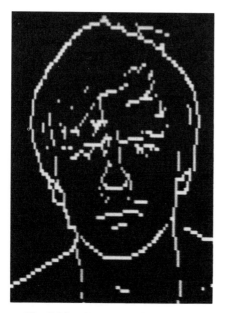

Fig. 3.11.   Inversion of Fig. 3.10.

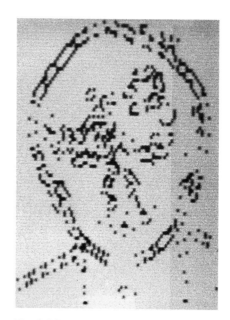

Fig. 3.12.   Computer-generated cartoon
using Fig. 3.11 as input.

we suppose that the early stages of human vision involve an operation similar to that of the cartoon operator, which has its primary sensitivity to valleys[27]. In a cartoon consisting of black lines on a white background, the luminance valleys in the original image are reproduced as luminance valleys in the cartoon; the depths of the valleys are not the same in the original and cartoon but their location is the same. The white-on-black inversion of this cartoon has its valleys turned into ridges. Such ridges are pointers to a different three-dimensional shape from that of a face, but by virtue of its flexibility and powers of high-level processing the human visual system is still capable of interpreting the cartoon as a face.

A black-on-white cartoon can be viewed as an image in which all the information except the valleys has been thrown away. But these valleys, according to our postulate, are very significant; they locate the bounding surfaces of smooth objects as they turn away from the line of sight. They are fundamental in gauging the size and shape of such objects.

Cartoons of cartoons

It is possible to take this experiment a step further. If the early stages of vision involve a mechanism like the cartoon operator, we can see what the output of this stage looks like by putting an image through the computer-cartooning process twice, that is by taking a cartoon of a cartoon. We can compare this double-processed image with the single-processed image or cartoon; this may give us some insight into differences between the way the eye processes a cartoon and the way it processes an ordinary image.

We took the black-on-white cartoon in Fig. 3.10 and used it as an input image for the cartoon detector. We found that it passed through the detector *unchanged*, that is the output was exactly the same as Fig. 3.10. On the other hand, when we took the white-on-black cartoon in Fig. 3.11 and passed that through the cartoon extractor, the different result shown in Fig. 3.12 was obtained. In a system using the valley detector which we have described, a black-on-white cartoon of an object thus has the interesting double property of passing through the system unaltered and of producing the same output as the original object from which it was derived. So the aim of a cartoonist may be to create a line drawing which produces the same or a similar early visual response to that of the object which it purports to represent.

Inverting the source image

If the human face-recognition system had its primary sensitivity to edges rather than to valleys, then a photographic negative should produce the same response in the early stages as the positive from which it is derived.

Inverting an image converts rising edges into falling edges (Fig. 3.1) or, equivalently, rotates the edge by 180°. A competent edge detector should find the edge location unchanged. On the other hand, if the human face-recognition system has its primary sensitivity to valleys, inverting the image will produce a different response to negatives from that to positives since the valleys are converted to ridges[28].

In Fig. 3.13 the original image of Fig. 3.9 has been inverted electronically to produce a negative. Observation indicates that it is more difficult to recognize the person concerned from the negative (though it has been suggested to us that this might be different with training).

In Fig. 3.14, we show the result of applying our cartoon operator to the inverted image of Fig. 3.13. Whereas the outlines of the head and shoulders are retained, the facial features are distorted. If we again suppose that the output of the cartooning operator is similar to the output of the early stage of the human mechanism for recognizing faces, then this output can be seen to be quite different for positive and negative images, with the positive input producing the recognizable cartoon.

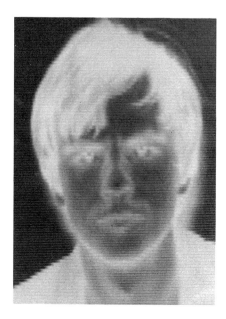

Fig. 3.13. Inversion of Fig. 3.9.

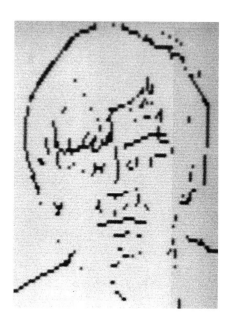

Fig. 3.14. Computer-generated cartoon using Fig. 3.13 as input.

Discussion and conclusions

We have developed a theory and ways for generating cartoons by computer. The theory states that cartoon lines should be placed wherever straight lines drawn from the television camera (or the eye of an observer) graze the surface of the human form. Analysis of the light falling on surfaces approximating skin have indicated that at such surfaces the luminance variation in the image has the shape of a valley when all local surfaces have the same luminance factor, for example at the side of the nose or at the edge of a finger held up in front of the palm of the hand. At other times, as at the skin-hair boundary or when a hand is held in front of a darker or lighter piece of clothing, a step edge of luminance occurs. What we have discovered experimentally is that a detector with a primary response to valleys and a lesser response to step edges is effective in delineating the main cartoon lines of faces and hands.

The cartoon operator which we have implemented has two component parts, the first an inverted 'Mexican-hat' filter with the required sensitivity to valleys and edges, and the second a peak detector. In practice the two are merged in the software algorithm, which has to have consideration for both speed and discrimination against noise. The working system we have produced can process still or moving grey-level images to produce the cartoons.

Using the computer-cartoonist, we have attempted to explore the nature of cartoons and the response which they set up in the human visual system. We found that when a human cartoonist was asked to draw cartoons in the style of the computer (as few lines as possible, with black fill-in), but without having seen the computer's efforts in advance, the results were remarkably similar to those of the computer. It is possible to fault the computer on some details, including its apparent knowledge of human anatomy (which was zero).

We have suggested that the degree of correspondence between the computer and the human cartoonist might be explicable if low-level processing in the human face-recognition system was similar to that used by our computer. We noted that both the filter and detection components of our cartoon extractor were similar to those being discussed in current theories of vision though they were derived from fundamental considerations of light falling on smooth surfaces and not as a model of vision. If our suggestion is correct, it provides an operational explanation for the type of early visual processing which is found in the human visual system, namely that it is good at picking out important surfaces of faces and hands in three-dimensional object space. These surfaces are ones which fall away sharply from the line of sight and which therefore either bound the object itself, or some protrusion or indentation on it. Such surfaces are important, as has been noted, for facial recognition. Their identification may also be useful for grasping; the surfaces of fingers or hands which are detected by the cartoon operator are those which would frequently be grasped by the fingers of another person, as in shaking hands.

Since our cartoon extractor has its primary sensitivity to valleys, we noted that a cartoon drawn with black lines on a white background can reproduce these valleys at the same spatial locations as the original; it is an equivalent image in so far as the cartoon-generating system is concerned. Its equivalence has been demonstrated by taking a cartoon of the cartoon; this process leaves it unchanged. We speculated that a black-on-white line drawing which is judged to be a good likeness of something may set up the same early response in the human visual system as the thing itself.

The idea of certain images being able to pass through an image-processing system unchanged (apart from a gain constant) recalls to mind the concept of the eigenvector. Strictly speaking, this is applicable in signal theory to linear systems only, but for such systems, at any rate, there is an established notion of a signal or vector which is only amplified or attenuated and not otherwise altered by passage through the system. A sine wave, for example, is an eigenvector of a linear amplifying system, since it always emerges as a sine wave. Extending this idea rather loosely to the non-linear cartooning system we have been discussing, a black-on-white cartoon could be said to be an *eigenimage* for this system. Eigenimages form a small subset of the totality of possible images, but they include many different black-on-white line drawings, some representing real objects and some not. The suggestion we have made is that a cartoon which is a good likeness of a person is an eigenimage for the early stage of the human face-recognition system, having the further property that it approximates or corresponds with the response produced by the actual, three-dimensional, person.

4

The tricks of colour

JOHN MOLLON

Figure 4.1 shows an image of the Newtonian spectrum that was prepared by one of the most vehement anti-Newtonians of the eighteenth century. It was published in 1752[1] and almost certainly it is the first image of the spectrum to have been printed in colours. It serves well to illustrate how a graphic artist can create an image of high quality without necessarily grasping the theory that underlies his craft.

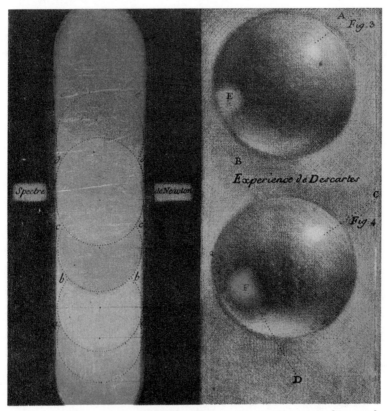

Fig. 4.1. A colour print published by Jacques Gautier D'Agoty in his popular science magazine '*Observations sur l'histoire naturelle*' in 1757 (reproduced by permission of the Syndics of Cambridge University Library).

The engraver and printer was one Gautier D'Agoty. Portalis and Béraldi[2] write of him:

> Jacques Gauthier [sic] D'Agoty, né à Marseille vers 1717, fut un de ces esprits à la fois intelligents, superficiels et inquiets, qui embrassant toutes choses à la fois, n'étreignent rien. Demi-savant et demi-artiste, il s'occupa de physique, d'anatomie, de botanique, de peinture et de gravure avec un égal insuccès.

This account gives perhaps too little credit to his artistic talent. Some of his anatomical plates – for example his extraordinary still life of the human viscera arranged on a table[3] – exhibit true flair and imagination in their composition. Many of his images lie between the surreal and the prurient; they disturb the modern eye, and we may suspect they still more disturbed his eighteenth-century contemporaries, who were not yet exposed to widespread colour printing.

But Gautier combined his successful colour printing with quite mistaken theorising about colour. He argued that Newton must be wrong in supposing that light could vary continuously in the physical property that corresponds to hue – the property we now know to be wavelength. Instead Gautier claimed that all colours were derived from three (blue, yellow and red), which were themselves derived from the interaction of white and black[4]. He found practical and daily confirmation of his theory in his mezzotint colour printing, achieved with blue, yellow and red plates, plus a black plate.

Although historical accounts of colour theory often suggest otherwise, the idea that all colours can be produced from three was already a commonplace by the middle of the eighteenth century[5]. In 1708, for example, we find a clear statement by the anonymous author of a treatise on painting in miniature[6]:

> Il n'y a proprement dit que trois Couleurs Primitives, lesquelles ne peuvent pas être composées par d'autres couleurs, mais dont toutes les autres peuvent être composées. Ces trois Couleurs sont le Jaune, le Rouge, et le Bleu. . .

As a second example, Fig. 4.2 shows part of a more elaborate statement published in 1740 by Père Castel[7], the Jesuit priest and *philosophe* who invented the 'clavecin oculaire', the first colour organ, and who was a foreign member of the Royal Society of London. It is easy to find many similar statements in the eighteenth-century, and even seventeenth-century, literature. Colour printing with three plates, first introduced by J.C. Le Blon early in the eighteenth century[8], provided empirical evidence that there were only three primitive colours. Le Blon even understood the difference between subtractive and additive mixing of colours, using the latter in his ill-fated scheme for weaving tapestries.

L'OPTIQUE

DES

COULEURS,

Fondée fur les fimples Obfervations, &
tournée fur-tout à la pratique de la
Peinture, de la Teinture & des autres
Arts Coloriftes.

Par le R. P. CASTEL, *Jefuite.*

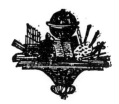

A PARIS,

Chez BRIASSON, rue Saint-Jacques,
à la Science.

M. DCC. XL.
Avec Approbation & Privilège du Roy.

122   L'OPTIQUE

VIIIes. OBSERVATIONS.

Sur la maniere de compofer toutes
les Couleurs avec les trois
primitives.

Démonftration de tous les dégrés
poffibles , harmoniques & pit-
torefques du Coloris.

PUifqu'il n'y a que trois couleurs fimples, dont le mélange
feul doit produire toutes les couleurs de la nature & de l'art, il s'agit
de voir quelles couleurs peuvent
refulter des mélanges divers, qu'on
peut faire de ces trois couleurs.

Tous les mélanges poffibles fe
reduifent d'abord en général à qua-
tre combinaifons. Car on ne peut
mêler, 1°. que le bleu avec le jaune : 2°. Le jaune avec le rouge.
3°. Le rouge avec le bleu. 4°. Les
trois enfemble.

Fig. 4.2.   Title page, and description of 'the means of producing all colours from
the three primitives', from *L'Optique des Couleurs* of Père Castel.

The miscategorisation of trichromacy

Of those eighteenth-century scientists who did experimental work on colour
mixing, or who had practical experience of colour printing, almost all were
led to conclude that there were only three kinds of light and that Newton was
wrong in holding that the physical variable underlying colour was a continuous one. They were, of course, committing a category error, assigning the
results of colour mixing to the wrong domain of knowledge. The fact that you
can, by additive or subtractive mixing, produce all colours from three, the fact
of trichromacy, is certainly true (with certain technical qualifications), but it
has its basis not in the physical nature of light but in the properties of our eye.
It is a fact of human physiology rather than a fact of physics. It is historically
instructive that the fact of trichromacy was known empirically, but
miscategorised, by artists, engravers and scientists for almost two centuries
before its true nature was understood – from about the second decade of the
seventeenth century until 1801. I believe that this miscategorisation of a fact

about human vision held back the understanding of physical optics more than has been appreciated by historians of science.

A general obstacle to the understanding of colour was the reluctance of the eighteenth-century mind to allow that there might be physical variations in the world that were not apparent to our senses. But the specific concept that was lacking was that of the narrowly tuned sensory transducer, the modern idea of a specialised receptor cell that converts external stimuli into the electrical signals that are the common coinage of the nervous system. The standard eighteenth-century view was that the vibrations of the air or of the ether were directly transmitted along the sensory nerves to the sensorium or sensory, the place where the soul has intercourse with the brain[9].

It was Thomas Young, celebrated for his contributions to wave optics and to the deciphering of the Rosetta Stone, who realised that the contradiction in the eighteenth-century literature could be resolved if trichromacy were taken to be a property of man, rather than a property of the physical world. Trichromacy is a limitation of our own colour vision, and one that arises, Young suggested, because there are just three classes of receptor cell in our eye[10]. Physically different lights will look the same to us provided that they stimulate the three receptor cells in the same ratios.

The receptor cells are the so-called cones, which lie in the retina of the eye and form the light-sensitive surface on which the optical image is focussed[11]. The curves of Fig. 4.3 show, for each type of cone, how the absorption of light varies with wavelength. The data are obtained by a technique called microspectrophotometry, in which a narrow beam of light is passed through individual cells from fresh human retinae (the tissue is obtained from eyes that have to be removed on account of cancer)[12]. Notice that the peak sensitivities of the three types of cone lie in the violet, the green and the yellow-green. I shall refer to the three types rather clumsily as short-wave, middle-wave and long-wave. Whatever its mnemonic convenience, the use of colour names for the different cone types has been one of the most pernicious obstacles to the proper understanding of colour vision.

It is important to emphasise that the cones themselves do not distinguish colours; the individual cones are colour blind. The electrical signal that comes out of the cone depends only on the total number of photons of light absorbed. At wavelengths at which a cone is not very sensitive, one needs more light to get the same signal from the cone than at a wavelength to which it is very sensitive; but there is nothing in the signal itself to distinguish the two wavelengths. What do vary with wavelength are the *ratios* of the signals from different cones. So, if the visual system is to know about colour, it must have the neural machinery to obtain these ratios. I shall give some description of

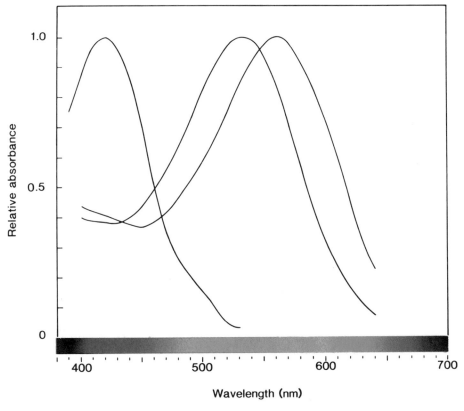

Fig. 4.3. The absorbance curves of the cone cells of the human retina. Each of the solid lines corresponds to one type of cone and shows how the absorption of light varies with wavelength (see note 12).

this neural machinery below, since colour vision offers a clear and very typical illustration of how nerves can analyse the storm of information that batters on our senses.

But before I come to the neural machinery, I should like to draw attention to several asymmetries among the three types of cone receptor, which have traditionally been thought of as equal members of a trichromatic scheme.

Five asymmetries of cone vision

1. The absorbance curves (Fig. 4.3) for the middle- and long-wave cones lie very close together in the spectrum, separated in wavelength by only 30 nm, whereas there is an interval of 100 nm between the wavelength at which the short-wave cones are most sensitive and the wavelength at which the middle-wave cones are most sensitive.

2. The short-wave cones are much rarer than the long- and middle-wave receptors, accounting for less than 5% of all cones in the human retina[12, 13].

3. Hereditary deficiencies of the short-wave cones are rare, but those of the middle- and long-wave cones are very common[14]. About 8% of men in our population exhibit some form of hereditary colour deficiency or colour anomaly: this minority in our midst live in different perceptual worlds, seeing colours as the same that are different for the normal person, and (in most cases) seeing colours as different that match for most of us. Almost invariably this hereditary change in colour vision arises from a change in either the long-wave cones or the middle-wave cones.

4. The rare genetic deficiencies of the short-wave cones, when they do occur, have the same incidence in men and women, whereas those of the middle- and long-wave cones are sex-linked, being much the more common in men than in women and showing the same pattern of inheritance as does haemophilia.

5. When our vision depends on the short-wave cones alone, we become very poor at resolving small intervals in either space or time. To demonstrate the poor resolution in *space*, one can make up a grating pattern from alternating bars of a blue and a green chosen to be of equal brightness and nearly identical in their effects on the middle- and long-wave cones. One's resolution of the grating then depends on the short-wave cones and one will have to come very close to the grating to distinguish the alternate bars – much closer than if the grating is made out of equally bright red and green bars[15]. Artists and graphic designers are aware of a distinction between 'soft' colours that melt into one another (a blue-green on a grey field) and 'hard' colours that do not (a red on a green field): the 'melting' in fact occurs when the boundary is one that is visible only to the short-wave cones[16]. It is also easy to show that our resolution in *time* is poor when we depend only on the short-wave cones. A blue and a red bar, both flickering at same rate, are presented on a bright yellow field. The yellow field serves to reduce the sensitivity of the middle- and long-wave cones, so that the blue bar is visible only by means of our short-wave cones. The red bar is primarily detected by the long-wave cones. If we slowly increase the rate of flicker of the two bars, we find that there is a range of flicker rates over which the blue bar appears steady and unflickering, while the flicker of the red bar is still clearly visible[17].

I have listed five asymmetries in our trichromatic system of cone vision. I should like to propose that these asymmetries – as well as other features of our vision – can be understood in terms of an evolutionary scheme. Our colour vision depends on two rather different sybsystems, one recently overlaid on the other. This view has long been suggested by the very asymmetries I've mentioned, but is now particularly supported by some molecular genetics published recently by Jeremy Nathans and his colleagues[18]. Nathans has managed to isolate the genes that specify the photosensitive molecules that are found in the cone cells (Fig. 4.4) of normal and of colour-anomalous people. And for the case of one normal observer, he has been able to work out the exact sequences of amino acids that make up the three different photopigment molecules.

All the photopigments are known to be rather similar protein molecules (Fig. 4.4). In each case the molecule seven times crosses the membrane of the receptor cell in which it is embedded. It forms a kind of palisade surrounding the derivative of vitamin A that gives the molecule its light-absorbing properties. What Nathans has found is, first, that 96% of the amino-acid

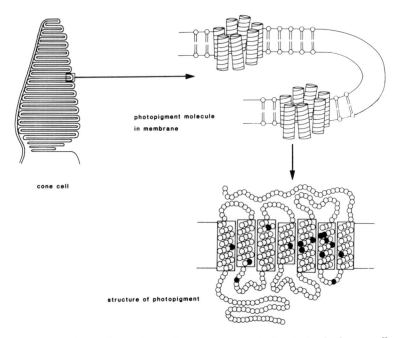

photopigment molecule
in membrane

cone cell

structure of photopigment

Fig. 4.4.   At the top left is shown the outer segment of an individual cone cell from the retina. Its multiply-infolded membrane contains molecules of photopigment (top right). The latter have a characteristic form, crossing the membrane seven times and clustering into a palisade around the derivative of vitamin A that gives the molecule its light-absorbing properties. At the bottom right is represented (after J. Nathans) the sequence of amino acids in the protein part of the photopigment, with the filled circles indicating those amino acids that differ between the long- and middle-wave pigments of the human retina.

sequence is similar for the middle- and long-wave pigments (Fig. 4.4 bottom right), whereas the short-wave pigment shows only a 43% identity with the middle- and long-wave pigments. The second salient finding was that the genes for the middle- and long-wave pigments lie very close together. (They are both, in fact, on the X-chromosome, as has long been inferred from the pattern of inheritance of colour blindness: a man, since he inherits only one X-chromosome, will always exhibit colour blindness if his mother passes on to him an aberrant gene, whereas a woman, having two X-chromosomes, must normally inherit the aberrant gene from both parents before she will be overtly colour blind.)

The extreme similarity and the juxtaposition of the middle- and long-wave genes strongly support the long-held suspicion that they evolved very recently by duplication from a single ancestral gene. It is this evidence that leads me to argue that our colour vision is really two subsystems, a very recent system overlaid on an ancient system[19].

The subsystems of colour vision

1. Widespread among mammals is an ancient, 'dichromatic', form of colour vision that depends on a comparison of the rates at which photons of light are absorbed in (i) a short-wave class of cones and (ii) a second class of cones with peak sensitivity that varies between species but always lies in the green to yellow region of the spectrum[20]. The results of this comparison are carried within the visual system by a special neural channel.

The concept of a 'neural channel' deserves some elaboration. The cornea and lens of the eye form an optical image on the array of receptor cells in the eye, but that image is not then transmitted passively to the brain. Rather, the array of receptor cells is examined in parallel by further stages of retinal nerve cells, which identify different attributes of the images, such as colour, motion and edges. So, what is sent to the brain is already a much-analysed version of the information in the optical image formed on the retina. The subsystems, which carry information about different attributes of the image, are commonly referred to as 'channels'.

The ancient subsystem of colour vision serves well to illustrate the concept of a channel, and the way in which sensory systems extract information. Fig. 4.5a represents, to the left, the array of receptor cells in a local region of the retina, and, to the right, a later, higher-order cell that draws input from this local region. The higher-order cell draws excitatory input from one type of cone, but is inhibited by another type. Typically, such cells are excited by short wavelengths and inhibited by long wavelengths. Thus this cell becomes sensitive to the ratio of absorptions in the different cone classes, rather than to the absolute level of light. There is no intensity of long-wave (red or yellow) light that will make the cell respond, since the inhibitory signal will always outweigh the excitatory.

The trick the visual system uses to extract information about colour is really the one main trick that sensory systems have for analysing the information in the physical image. In general terms, the trick is this: a higher-order cell is connected to two distinct subsets of cells at the preceding level and draws signals of opposite sign from the two subsets. It is the same trick, for example, that is used to extract information about edges in the image (see below).

When the first electrical records were obtained from higher-order cells of the kind shown in Fig. 4.5a, it was generally assumed that the antagonism of the inputs was there to allow 'opponent coding': it was thought that the cell signalled one colour by an increase in its response and the complementary colour by a decrease in its response. This is probably a mistaken way of looking at it. The inhibitory input from the second class of cones lends a *specificity* to the response of the higher-order cell[21]. A cone cell responds in the same way to all wavelengths – provided the light is intense enough – but the higher-order cell will give a positive response to only part of the spectrum.

Cells of the type shown in Fig. 4.5a draw their excitatory and inhibitory inputs from co-extensive, or nearly co-extensive, areas, and so they are insensitive to spatial detail, to variations in the illumination of adjacent areas[22]. Thus this ancient subsystem of colour vision carries almost pure chromatic information. It allowed our ancestors to distinguish browns and yellows from greys and whites, and blues from all of these. In other words, it allowed them – as it allows us – to estimate the direction in which the reflectance of a surface varies across the visible spectrum, and the steepness of that variation. A sign of the antiquity of such colour vision systems is the antagonism between long- and short-wave stimuli that can be recorded electrophysiologically in the pineal gland of the frog[23].

2. In the Old World monkeys, in the apes, and in man is found a second colour vision system that depends on a comparison of the rates at which photons of light are absorbed in the middle-wave cones and the long-wave cones. This system has evolved very recently through the duplication of an ancestral gene, and there does not seem to have evolved a special morpho-logical system to carry the second type of chromatic information. Rather, this type of colour vision is parasitic upon an existing neural channel that subserves the analysis of spatial details in the image. In all mammals one finds higher-order cells in the retina that draw inputs of opposite sign from distinct, concentric sub-regions of the array of receptor cells (Fig. 4.5b). A higher-

J. Mollon

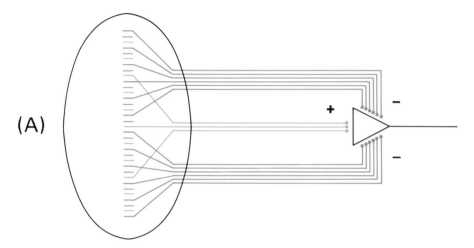

(A)

Fig. 4.5. (A)   The ancient colour system of the mammalian retina. To the left is
represented the array of cone cells in a local region of the retina. To the right is
represented a higher-order cell (a 'retinal ganglion cell') that draws excitatory
inputs from short-wave cones and inhibitory inputs from middle-wave cones. The
area circumscribed by the solid line to the left is called the 'receptive field' of the
ganglion cell: it is defined as the small region of receptor cells that have an
influence on the response of the ganglion cell.

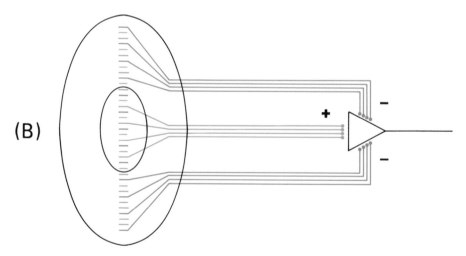

(B)

(B)   The second colour system, found in the primate retina. The retinal ganglion
cell on the right draws excitatory input from long-wave cones in the centre of the
receptive field and inhibitory input from middle-wave cones in a concentric
region. In other ganglion cells of this class it may be the middle-wave cones that
are excitatory and the long-wave ones that are inhibitory; and the excitatory
input may be drawn from the surround rather than the centre of the receptive
field. (After Wiesel and Hubel.)

order cell of this kind typically gives strong response when light falls exclusively on the sub-region from which it draws excitatory input, but the cell gives little or no response when the illumination is spatially homogeneous and also falls on the other sub-region, from which the cell draws inhibitory input. Thus the cell is responsive to local contrast in the retinal image, to the spots, edges and lines that carry the information in our visual world. In the retinae of Old World monkeys, and presumably in our own retinae, such higher-order cells usually draw their antagonistic inputs not only from spatially distinct regions but from different classes of cone: the cell is either excited by middle-wave cones and inhibited by long-wave cones, or *vice versa* (Fig. 4.5b). But, significantly, there is little evidence for an input from the short-wave cones to this kind of cell[20].

Now that we have considered the evolutionary history of our colour vision, we can guess why our discrimination is so odd when it depends only on the short-wave cones. Signals from these sparsely distributed cones reach us only over a neural channel that was not designed to carry precise spatial information. If we abut a green and a blue patch, the two being equally bright and chosen to produce identical absorptions in the long- and middle-wave cones, then our visual system cannot know the exact position of the edge between the two patches. And subjectively the colours melt into one another. For our ancestral colour vision system (Fig. 4.5a) was not designed to detect spatial contrast: it was able to rely on the fact that edges in the real world almost always offer to the eye a change of lightness as well as a change of colour and so can be detected by other neural channels. But if we abut a green and a red patch of equal brightness, then we do perceive a clear and well-localised edge. For the subsystem (Fig. 4.5b) that compares the absorptions in the long- and middle-wave cones is an ancient edge-detecting system, one that still has as its main job the analysis of fine detail and so continues to be sensitive to the exact position of a boundary. It is on this detail-discriminating system that our new dimension of colour vision is parasitic.

Recognising the colours of things

I have described the trick that the visual system uses to discover the wavelengths locally present at some point on the retina. But this alone will not give us accurate and reliable colour vision. What we have evolved to do is recognise the *spectral reflectances* of objects, that is, to recognise the permanent tendency of objects to reflect some wavelengths more than others. And to achieve this, our visual system must take into account the colour of the illumination. For the spectral composition of the light that reaches us from the object – the proportion of different wavelengths within it – depends not only on the permanent properties of the object's surface but also on the fluctuating tone of the illumination, which may change in colour from moment to moment. We enjoy a remarkable ability to make allowance for the colour of the illumination and to identify accurately the permanent colour of the object. A piece of white paper continues to look white as we pass from the red-rich light of a domestic tungsten bulb to the bluish illumination of northern daylight. 'Colour constancy' is the term traditionally used for this stability of our perception in the face of changes in the illumination[24].

Because, most of the time, our visual systems achieve colour constancy so effortlessly, direct demonstrations of the phenomenon are rather boring. It is more vividly demonstrated by the classical illusion of 'coloured shadows'[25]. Upon a screen we cast white light from one projector and pink light from a second, so that the screen appears to be flooded with a pinkish white illumination (Fig. 4.6, lower left). In the beam from the pink projector we now interpose a cardboard shape, which casts a corresponding shadow on the screen. In the area of this shadow, the screen is physically illuminated only by white light. But in fact the shadowed area looks clearly bluish green.

Such coloured shadows are usually spoken of as illusions, as tricks that the eye plays upon us; but like most illusions they serve to draw attention to the normal operations of our perceptual systems, operations that run so smoothly they go unnoticed most of the time. And the coloured shadows are an illusion only if we cast our account in terms of pink light and white light drawn from separate projectors. In fact, our visual system is making the most plausible interpretation of the stimuli presented. It assumes that the scene is lit by a single illuminant, one that is pinkish white in colour. In such an illumination, an area that does not reflect its fair share of the pink component of the illumination must be a greenish or bluish object. And that is how the shadowed area looks to us.

Figure 4.6 helps explain this point. To the left are shown two demonstrations that are normally treated as distinct – a demonstration of 'colour constancy' above, and a demonstration of a 'coloured shadow' below. The figure shows how the two demonstrations deliver the same actual stimulation to the eye (bottom right). In the case of the *coloured shadow*, the light reaching the eye from the tree-shaped area is white because the pink beam is obstructed. Graph (c) at the bottom right shows what is meant by saying the light is white: all wavelengths are present in equal amounts. In the case of *colour constancy*, the tree-shaped area is truly green: it reflects the middle wavelengths of the spectrum more than others (graph b). But when it is illuminated by a suitably chosen pinkish light (graph a), which is *deficient* in

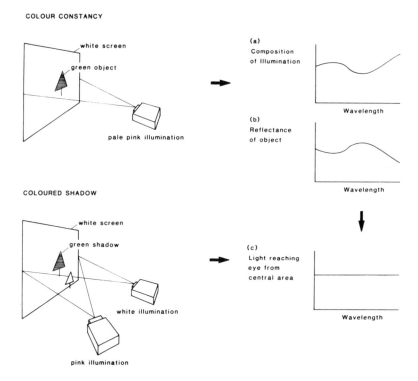

COLOUR CONSTANCY

white screen

green object

pale pink illumination

(a)
Composition
of Illumination

Wavelength

(b)
Reflectance
of object

Wavelength

COLOURED SHADOW

white screen

green shadow

white illumination

pink illumination

(c)
Light reaching
eye from
central area

Wavelength

Fig. 4.6. A coloured shadow as a demonstration of colour constancy. At the bottom left a white screen is illuminated by light from two projectors, one giving pink light and one giving white light. An opaque card in the pink beam casts a shadow on the screen. This area therefore reflects only white light to the eye (c), but it appears a quite vivid, bluish green. Above is shown how a truly green object would present the same stimulation to the eye if it were presented on a white ground in a pale pink illumination (top left). If we multiply the strength of the illumination at different wavelengths (graph a) by the proportion of light reflected from the object at each wavelength (graph b), then we derive (c) the relative intensity of different wavelengths reaching the eye from the central area. Graph (c) is identical in the case of 'colour constancy' and in the case of the 'coloured shadow'. It is also the case – and this is crucial – that the light reaching the eye from the surround is identical in the two cases.

the middle of the spectrum, then the net result is that white light is reflected to the eye (graph c). What we see, nevertheless, is a green tree, because our visual system can take account of the fact that the illumination is biassed in its colour – in, that is, the relative predominance of different wavelengths. The visual system takes its estimate of the illumination from the surrounding field. Compared to the assumed illuminant, the white light from the tree-shaped area is deficient in red light: it ought therefore to derive from a greenish or bluish surface, a surface that absorbs the red component of the light. In the case of this demonstration of 'colour constancy' we would say that our visual system is effortlessly recovering the true colours of objects, despite the biassed colour of the illuminant. In the case of the 'coloured shadow', we might speak of an illusion. But the stimulus for the eye, and the underlying process, is the same in the two cases.

How can the visual system achieve colour constancy, reconstructing the true colours of objects from the changing flux of wavelengths on the retina? Almost certainly it does it by playing its standard trick a second time, this time taking the ratio of cone signals found in a local region of the scene and comparing this ratio with the set of ratios found elsewhere in the field of view. So true colour vision depends on extracting a ratio of ratios.

The worlds of the colour blind, and of their mothers

I should like lastly to consider those who live in perceptual worlds that are different from those of the rest of us. I include here not only the 8% of men who exhibit some anomaly or deficiency of colour vision, but also the 16% of women who are carriers of colour blindness and who can be led to reveal themselves in subtle perceptual tests.

The work of Nathans and his collaborators (discussed above) has changed our views of how colour blindness arises. Most of us in this field of research thought that the various forms of red-green blindness arose from local errors in the genes for the long- and middle-wave photopigments – that is to say, from very circumscribed mutations of the sections of DNA that specify the sequence of amino acids which make up the photopigments. Instead it seems that colour deficiencies arise from a genetic phenomenon called 'unequal crossing-over', a genetic error that is encouraged by the juxtaposition, and extreme similarity, of the two genes. There is a stage in the formation of the ovum when corresponding chromosomes line themselves up, the matching strands of DNA aligning themselves at one end and working along in something of the manner of a zip fastener (Fig. 4.7A). But if one carelessly closes a zip fastener, an error of alignment sometimes occurs, with a few teeth on one side forming a little loop. In an analogous way, the middle-wave gene on one chromosome may appose itself not to its fellow gene on the second chromosome, but to the (very similar) long-wave gene on the second chromosome (Fig. 4.7B1). The slack on each chromosome will form a little loop, rather as in the case of our zip fastener.

Now, at this stage, when the two chromosomes come together, sections of the DNA of one chromosome are exchanged with corresponding sections of DNA from the second chromosome (Fig. 4.7B2). This is the process called

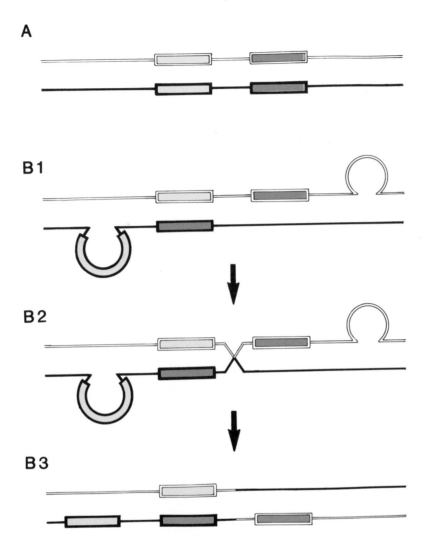

A

B1

B2

B3

Fig. 4.7.   Unequal crossing-over as an explanation of the origin of dichromatic colour vision.

(A)   The normal case, where corresponding sections of two X-chromosomes are correctly aligned. The yellow boxes represent the gene for the long-wave pigment and the green boxes represent the gene for the middle-wave pigment. Between the genes lie sections of DNA that do not code for proteins.

(B1)   A case where the two chromosomes have become locally misaligned, so that the middle-wave gene on one is apposed to the long-wave gene on the other.

(B2)   A crossing over occurs – DNA is exchanged between the two chromosomes – and the breakpoint lies to the right of the misaligned pair of genes.

(B3)   After the crossing over, one chromosome carries two middle-wave genes and the other carries none. A man who inherits the latter chromosome will exhibit the form of colour blindness called 'deuteranopia'.

'crossing-over'. If the break-point of the DNA occurs between the long-wave and middle-wave genes of one chromosome and if the genes have been misaligned, then one chromosome will lose its middle-wave gene and the other chromosome will end up with two (see Fig. 4.7B3). A man who inherits the former chromosome will lack the middle-wave pigment and exhibit the relatively severe form of colour blindness called 'dichromacy', whereas many of us with normal colour vision are carrying around extra copies of the middle-wave gene – which our forebears have unwittingly purloined from the colour blind. If, at crossing-over, the break-point occurs in the middle of two misaligned genes, then hybrid genes may be formed and these may produce hybrid photopigments with sensitivity curves different from those in Fig. 4.3. Men who inherit a hybrid gene may exhibit the milder and most common form of colour deficiency called 'anomalous trichromacy', in which one of the curves of Fig. 4.3 is displaced in its spectral position.

But what of the mothers of colour-deficient men? For some time there has been evidence for subtle anomalies in the vision of heterozygous carriers of colour-deficiency, that is, in women who have one normal X-chromosome and one that is abnormal in the region of the genes for the photopigments[26]. Consider a woman whose son exhibits either a lack of the long-wave pigment or an alteration in its sensitivity. Although her *matching* of colours is likely to be quite normal, the relative luminosities of different colours will be changed, so that red colours will look dimmer to her than to other women. This subtle change in the vision of carriers is analogous to the somewhat slower blood clotting that has been shown in carriers of haemophilia. In collaboration with J. Ellis and J. Watson, I have recently used the 'OSCAR' test of colour vision[27] to examine a group of carriers of colour deficiency. The OSCAR test measures the relative luminosities of a green light and a red light. The green and red lights are flickered out of phase and the subject is asked to adjust the depth of flicker of one so as to cancel out the flicker of the other. Subjectively, it is a matter of minimising the flicker that is seen. We tested mothers at the same time as their sons. We also tested a group of normal mothers and sons; these control subjects were all friends or neighbours of members of the first group. Figure 4.8 plots the OSCAR setting of each mother against the setting of her son: there is a very clear correlation between the two. The OSCAR test does not allow us to identify with certainty all women who are carriers; but Fig. 4.8 shows that the two groups of carriers are statistically distinct from the group of normal mothers.

The reason that visual abnormalities express themselves in carriers of colour deficiency is the phenomenon of 'X-chromosome inactivation': although a woman has two X-chromosomes, one or other of them is inacti-

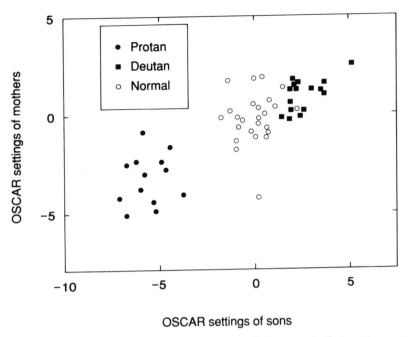

Fig. 4.8.   The relationship between mothers and their sons in their settings on the OSCAR test, a test that measures the relative luminosity of red and green light. Conventionally the 3 groups of mothers would all be held to have normal colour vision, but as groups they differ in their setting according to the type of colour vision exhibited by their sons. The 'protan' sons are those who exhibit an abnormality of the long-wave cones, the 'deutan' sons those who exhibit an abnormality of the middle-wave cones.

vated in any particular cell of her body[28]. So, if a woman is a carrier of anomalous trichromacy, there will be four types of cone cell in her retina – the three types of normal vision plus the anomalous type that her son may inherit. An interesting possibility now presents itself. We might have been wrong in assuming that carriers of anomalous trichromacy merely share a little in the disability of their sons. If there are four kinds of cone in their retinae, is it possible that the carriers are tetrachromatic, enjoying an extra dimension of colour discrimination? Since some 12% of women are carriers of anomalous trichromacy, there would be a sizeable group amongst us whose colour vision was as superior to that of the normal man as his is to that of a dichromat[29]. But would visual scientists not long ago have detected a tetrachromatic minority? The truth is that the necessary experiments have never been done. Instruments for research on colour are traditionally built with three variables. If a tetrachromatic carrier said that it was difficult to get a perfect match, a male experimenter would seldom think to offer her a fourth variable; he would accept the best match she could make and would remind himself that carriers of colour blindness are known to share in the disability of their sons.

If tetrachromatic women do exist, then a further possibility arises. Tetrachromacy may offer a biological advantage – the tetrachromat may, for example, be able to distinguish some property of complexions that is invisible to the rest of us and thus she might better choose a potential mate or better detect malaise in her infants. If the carrier did enjoy an advantage of this kind, then it might well be her advantage that maintained the high incidence of colour anomaly in the male population[30].

Conclusions

We do not all share the same world. It is certain that the tints of nature and of art look different to 8% of men; and that the relative luminosities of different colours are altered for a large minority of women. But there is also the possibility that some of these same women enjoy an additional dimension of hue discrimination, one that is unsuspected by the rest of us. Our colour vision has not yet yielded up all its secrets[31].

PART 2

Movement

NICHOLAS HUMPHREY

I once saw a photograph – it may have been taken by Man Ray – that showed a man holding up a placard on which was written *Une trentième d'une seconde de ma vie* (a thirtieth of a second of my life). It might have been titled – though I do not think it was – 'Still life, with man'. The term 'still life' derives from the Dutch *still-leven*, and denotes simply a motionless (*still*) aspect of nature (*leven*). But stillness and life do not belong together. Paradoxically, the term is the exact equivalent of the French term *nature morte*.

All of which is to say that this section of the book, on Movement, requires no introduction. To move is to live, and to live is to move. Not surprisingly, to detect the *image* of movement is the first task of all sensory systems; and to reach an *understanding* of movement is a primary goal of all later perceptual analysis.

I shall pick out just one of the chapters here. Sir Kenneth MacMillan and his colleague Monica Parker are makers of movement, not writers about it. In their ballets they use the forms of dance to convey – without use or need of verbal intermediary – the emotions of life. Yet the problem they address in Chapter 5 is the problem of how to preserve the *information* contained in these dances in written form.

As Miss Parker shows, it is possible to make a 'freeze-frame' analysis of a flowing dance. In principle at least, the information in the dance can be transcribed exactly into information on the page. Yet what interests me is not so much what is preserved in such a transcription as what is lost: for what is lost is, in one sense, the whole point of the ballet, namely its power to *please*. Quite simply, the written score is not and never could be an object of delight. A critic claimed of the fourth movement of Schubert's string quintet 'The very notes on the page look beautiful'; but the – somewhat puzzling – thing is that he was wrong.

"So what," you may say, "No one ever assumed the mental experience of a sensory event depends solely upon its information content." And yet isn't this precisely what, as brain scientists and psychologists, we *do* tend to assume? Both in this section, and elsewhere in the book, you will find the understanding of images being treated as if it were indeed an exercise in information processing – and nothing more.

A month after the conference I came across Sir Kenneth MacMillan sitting alone in the lobby of a New York hotel. "How are you?" I said. . . "Nicely, thank you. . . Look, I've been thinking about that meeting we were at. Tell me, do you people think that individual brain cells *understand* things?" It was a good question, and one that we should keep in mind.

5

Benesh: the notation of dance

MONICA PARKER AND KENNETH MACMILLAN

Dance notation

The 20th century has seen a dramatic development of the means to notate movement in all its complex detail and the advent of video recording techniques. Each now makes a vital, but distinctly different, contribution to the world of dance that can be likened to the diverse benefits of the written score and the sound recording to the world of music.

The dance notation systems that were devised prior to the 20th century have proved incapable of development beyond the range of 'steps' which they originally described. For example, the system invented by Raoul-Augur Feuillet (1675–1710) identified floor patterns and codified the steps of the time (Fig. 5.1). However, body, head and arm movements were not included because these, and the manner of performance, were well known to the Ballet Masters.

A more recent system known as the Stepanov Dance Notation (Fig. 5.2), which was devised by Vladimir Ivanovitch Stepanov (1866–96), provided choreographic scripts of sections of established classics such as *Sleeping Beauty*, *Swan Lake* and *Nutcracker*, but did not cope with developments in the art of choreography. According to the Soviet Choreographer Fedor Lopukhov – 'The imperfection and poverty of his notation became more evident when attempts were made to record the works of Fokine and Gorsky'[1].

Benesh Movement Notation

Benesh Movement Notation, the creation of artist, musician and mathematician Rudolf Benesh and his wife Joan, a former dancer with the Sadler's Wells Ballet (Fig. 5.3), has played a significant role in the documentation of dance. This system was conceived by Rudolf Benesh as a 'creative tool . . . a means of communication and dissemination of ideas'[2].

Whilst Joan's desire to write down specific choreography served as the catalyst, the system itself was developed so that it could be applied to all forms

81

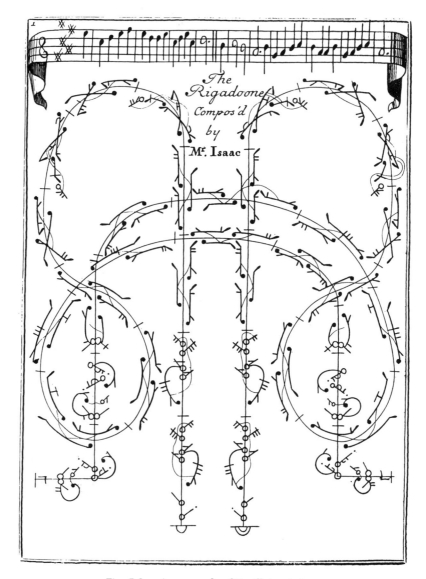

Fig. 5.1.   An example of Feuillet notation.

of movement. By using an 'alphabet' of signs that can be combined to form
the 'words' and 'sentences' of any movement, rather than limiting its descriptive capability to a number of 'well-known phrases or sayings', the system has
avoided the pitfalls of the past and happily encompassed the many changes in
choreographic style that have occurred in the intervening years.

In 1955, the year of its launching, Benesh Notation was introduced to the
professional dance world with the announcement by Dame Ninette de Valois,
Founder Director of the Sadler's Wells Ballet, of its adoption for company use.

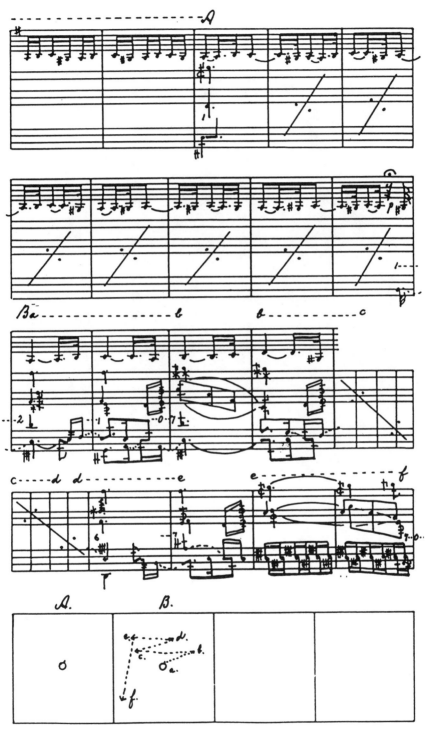

Fig. 5.2. Vladimir Stepanov wrote his choreographic instructions underneath the musical score. This excerpt is from Aurora's variation in Act 1 of *La belle au bois dormant* by Petipa, 1890.

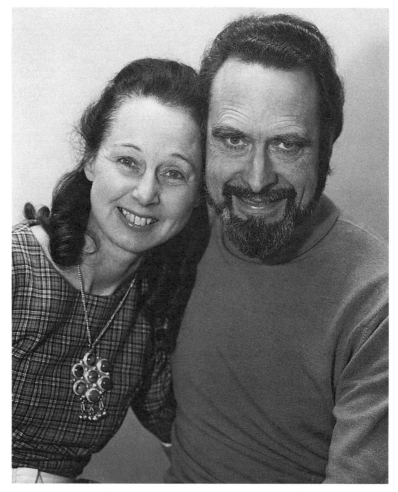

Fig. 5.3. Joan and Rudolf Benesh. Reproduced by kind permission of Helen
Seymer.

Aspects of the system

The Beneshes realised that there was a danger of sheer volume of information
swamping pertinent data, and that a practical system had to convey only
relevant information, as concisely as possible. Variation in perception and
conventions of diverse movement fields also had to be accommodated. Thus,
visual representation of movement was their primary concern. They chose
the five-line music stave on which to convey 'pictures' of movement; the
stave lines provide a framework that coincides naturally with the visually
distinct features of the human body (Fig. 5.4).

Three graphically distinct signs are used to plot the location of hands and

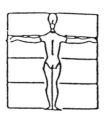

- height of the top of the head

- height of shoulders

- height of waist

- height of knees

- floor

Fig. 5.4.   The Benesh body matrix.

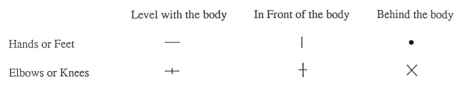

Fig. 5.5.   Basic signs of the Benesh system.

feet in the three dimensions. From these emanate a further group of signs which represent bent elbows and knees (see Fig. 5.5).

Figure 5.6 shows how the positions of arms and legs are recorded in the Benesh system. Each recording gives the same basic information to the reader whether he be a soccer player, gymnast, ballet dancer or physiotherapist. However each reader will interpret the information according to their own experience and expectation. If example Fig. 5.6A were read by a classical ballet dancer, first position of the feet would be assumed, because the dancer would be conditioned to stand in full turn-out (heels together with 180° between the tips of the toes). But this ballet dancer would consider the position of the arms to be unclassical, since they are shown in a straight line with the shoulders, and classical technique dictates that the arms should curve. These conventions in classical ballet mean that it is redundant to notate technical details of turn-out and arm position when compiling choreographic scores of classical ballet.

A dance syllabus, however, requires detail to specify the particular style or technique. Take as an example the *cou de pied* position. The generic definition is a position with one foot in contact with the 'neck' of the other foot. The instruction to adopt *cou de pied* with the right foot in front will be understood by a classically trained dancer who will assume the position appropriate to the context of the instruction. These examples of various *cou de pied* (Fig. 5.8) illustrate the flexibility of the system, allowing as much or as little information as required to be written.

Plotting extremities

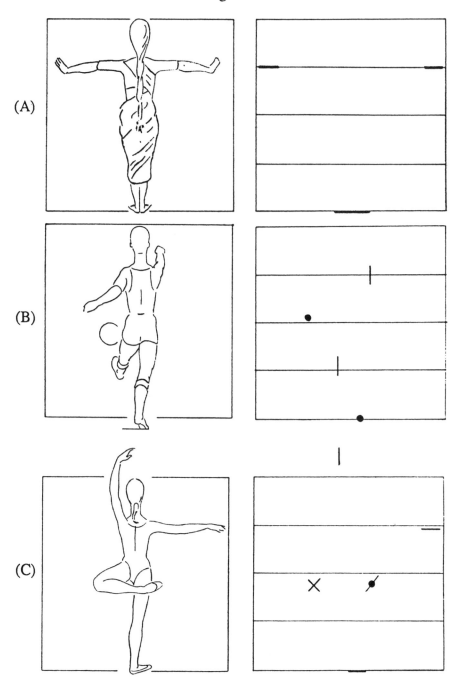

Fig. 5.6. The Benesh system for plotting the relationship of extremities to the body. A: Classical Indian dancer. B: Soccer player. C: Classical ballet dancer.

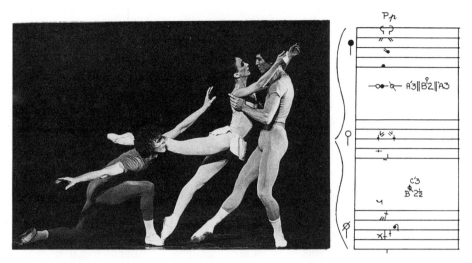

Fig. 5.7. A moment from *Das Lied von der Erde*. The photograph is reproduced by kind permission of Leslie E. Spatt. To the side is the Benesh Notation which records the choreographic detail of the Messenger of Death (Egon Madsen) in physical contact with the Woman; the Woman (Marcia Haydée) falling towards the Man; the Man (Richard Cragun) supporting the Woman[3].

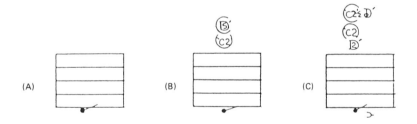

Fig. 5.8. Different representations of the *cou de pied* position. A: The generic position. No detail of contact or foot position is given. B: A Cecchetti *cou de pied*. The right side of the right heel (⑮) is touching the front of the left ankle (©2). C: A Bournonville *cou de pied*. The right foot touches the left leg below the calf (©2½) with the right heel (𝔻ʹ) at the side and the toes of the right foot (𝔻ʹ) touching behind the left ankle (©2). The right foot is turned out to 90° and is fully stretched (>).

The addition of 'movement lines', which trace the paths made by the extremities, turn the static figure into a moving image (Fig. 5.9). Movements of the head and body are shown by signs drawn in the spaces of the stave (Fig. 5.10).

This simple group of signs forms the basis for a vocabulary of some 355 descriptive options and is typical of the Benesh system's use of a limited 'alphabet' which is capable of great manipulation. For an example, see Fig. 5.11. (Note that 'bends' are again represented by a form of a cross. See Fig. 5.5.)

Another striking example of this approach is the capability of just nine signs and a short horizontal dash to describe over 230 different stage locations. These are written below the stave, together with details about the direction in which the performer is facing, turning or travelling to give the relationship of action to the performing area (Fig. 5.12).

Benesh Rhythm Notation provides a means of identifying the rhythmic structure of movement. It is compatible with music notation as well as existing in silent isolation.

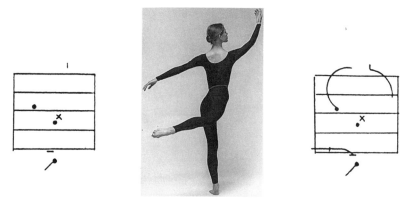

Fig. 5.9. The added 'movement lines' show that the dancer stepped forward from her previous position while moving her left arm in a wide arc from overhead and raising her right arm from the side. The photograph is by Chris Cheetham, reproduced by kind permission of the Benesh Institute.

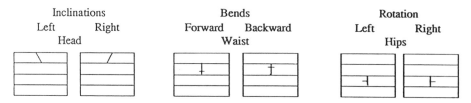

Fig. 5.10. The Benesh Notation for head and body movements.

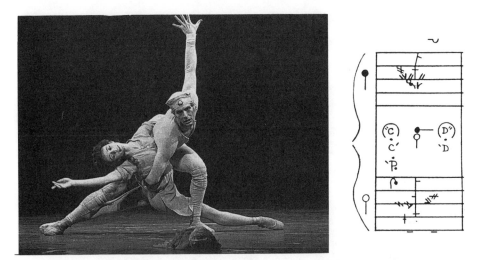

Fig. 5.11. The Benesh Notation of this photograph, which is reproduced by kind permission of Leslie E. Spatt, includes detail of the tilt, bend and rotations of dancers Alessandra Ferri and Wayne Eagling in a *pas de deux* from *Different Drummer*[4].

Location

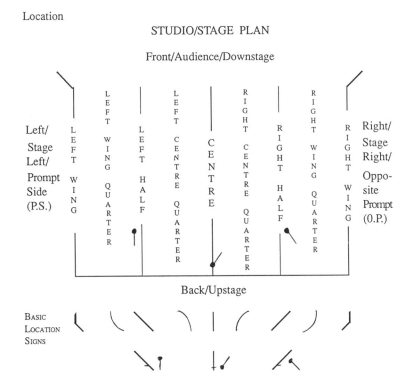

STUDIO/STAGE PLAN

Front/Audience/Downstage

Back/Upstage

BASIC LOCATION SIGNS

Fig. 5.12. The system for recording stage locations using the Benesh method.

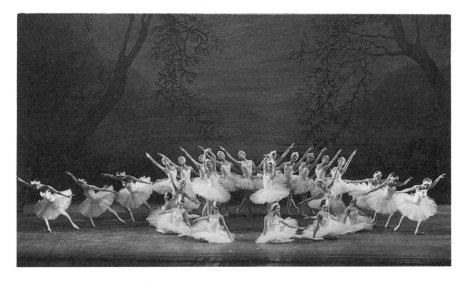

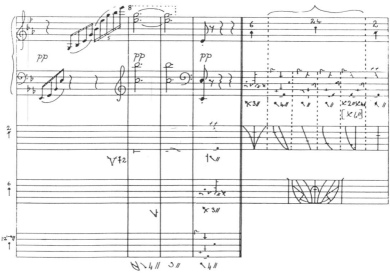

Fig. 5.13. This grouping is from *Swan Lake* Act IV; photograph reproduced by kind permission of Stuart Robinson. The Benesh Notation excerpt includes the music score and gives a summary of the locations of the dancers[5].

The Beneshes understood that musicians and dancers do not perceive music, and hence timing, in the same way. The musician needs to know the duration of a note; the dancer reacts to a pulse.

The sign ϕ represents the pulse or main beat of a rhythm. Divisions of the main beat are represented by a series of sub-beats: half beat ＋ , third beats ＼ ／, quarter beats ＼ ／, etc. as required (Fig. 5.14).

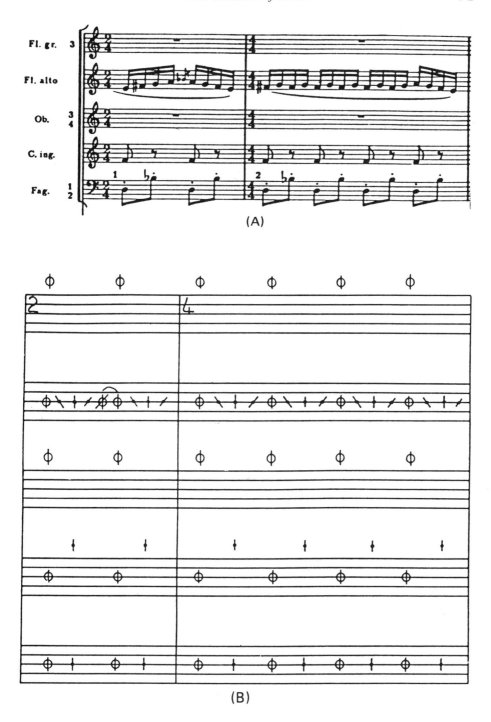

Fig. 5.14.   A: Part of the music score of the *Rite of Spring,* B: Benesh rhythm
notation for the music.

Notation and video recording

The simplest and most efficient method of recording movement would appear to many to be that of video taping. Many dance companies video their repertoires for archive purposes. However, these tapes, and the tapes made for public broadcast, are rarely satisfactory for dance reconstruction purposes.

The primary failure of the video tape is that it is a record of a particular performance and thus contains idiosyncracies of individual performers and, probably, performers' errors. As Professor N. Goodman[6] stresses, the score 'has the logically prior office of identifying a work'.

Often it is impossible to 'see' in a video recording the required information. An instance occurred during the reconstruction in 1983 for the Royal Ballet of *Requiem* (originally created for the Stuttgart Ballet in 1976) where the viewing of the video frustrated the reconstruction process. A particularly complex section for six people was described to the dancers in the studio. A

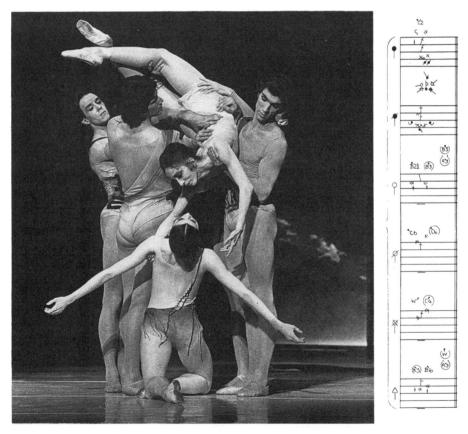

Fig. 5.15.   Marcia Haydée, Birgit Keil and partners in *Requiem*. Reproduced by kind permission of Leslie E. Spatt. To the side is the Benesh Notation.

visit to the video room was made in the expectation that a viewing of the required manoeuvres would facilitate execution. A performance was observed and, although all the information was ostensibly there, no-one could identify *how* to perform the choreography. So back to the notated score for the mechanics of the operation (Fig. 5.15).

Whilst technological advances will overcome certain problems currently afflicting video recording – for example, expense, poor lighting, perspective distortion, obscured movement – it is not a medium capable of development as the ultimate recording device but its use, in conjunction with a score, can be extremely helpful. However, to quote Professor Goodman[6] again, 'a score has as a primary function the authoritative identification of a work from performance to performance'. Given a necessity of choice, it is thus more practicable to consult the notated record rather than the moving image.

6

Three stages in the classification of body movements by visual neurons

DAVID PERRETT, M. HARRIES, A.J. MISTLIN AND
A.J. CHITTY

Introduction: an internal visual encyclopaedia

One way to determine how images are understood by the brain is to record the electrical signals of individual brain cells that are produced when an image is being processed. Such techniques have provided much information relating to the initial steps of visual processing in the cerebral cortex where images appear to be 'broken down' into elementary components, with individual cells signalling the value of simple attributes such as orientation, colour and movement of each point in the image[1].

In early visual processing information about any object in the image exists only as an unstructured array of components, much as a car exists as disassembled parts at the start of a factory production line. Further processing is necessary for the meaning of the image to be recognised from the components. Recordings from one region of the monkey brain (cortex within the temporal lobe) indicate that such a synthesis of visual information does take place for biologically important objects. In this brain area studies from our laboratory and others[2] have begun to uncover a vast visual encyclopaedia. The media on which entries are made in this encyclopaedia are the brain cells themselves – for individual nerve cells (neurons) respond selectively when the monkey looks at particular types of objects, movements and events. The encyclopaedia considered in this article seems to be a specialist volume being predominantly concerned with the analysis of bodies and their movements. Volumes for other types of objects have not yet been discovered, perhaps because so little of the cortex has been studied.

Our laboratory has attempted to catalogue the contents of this visual encyclopaedia and to define the information required to gain access to each entry. We present here an overview of our research which poses two questions, 'What is analysed?' and 'How is it analysed?'. We will restrict our

94

discussion to the processing of the dynamic appearance of bodies rather than their static form.

What kind of neuronal responses do we study? Figure 6.1 shows the electrical signals recorded from one cell in the temporal cortex. When the monkey sees a person walking from the left of the laboratory to the right the cell increases its activity. Note, however, that the cell only responds to the movement when the person faces in the same direction as he moves (i.e. faces right and moves right). Other directions of walking, towards or away from the observing monkey or to the left were ineffective in producing responses for

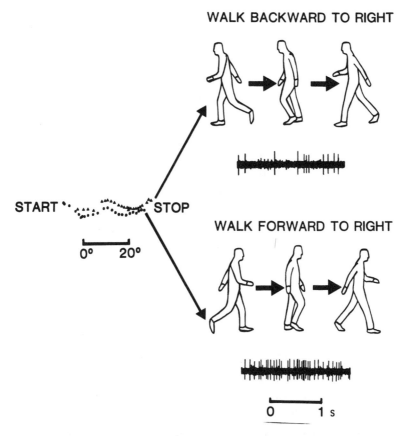

Fig. 6.1. Neuronal responses to the sight of walking. Right: The outline figures of the body illustrate three successive frames of a person walking from the left to the right of the laboratory. Beneath each 'movie' sequence is an oscilloscope trace of the electrical activity of one neuron evoked by the stimuli. Note that the cell is more responsive when the body faces the right and moves right.
Left: Similarity of eye movements (irrespective of body view) as they followed the person walking to the right. Eye positions recorded every 60 ms during the trial with the left profile [▲] and right profile [●].

this cell. The cell was also unresponsive to the movement of a variety of
stimuli other than a body (e.g. large boxes, bars etc.). This cell is thus selective
for a single combination of body view and direction of movement.

These data indicate the extraordinary selectivity of temporal lobe neurons.
Arousal or behavioural responses (such as eye movements) cannot account
for the cell's selective activity since these are the same for the stimuli which
provoke no neuronal responses.

Breaking down complex movements into simple components

Having given an example of cellular sensitivity to a complex motion pattern
we can now explore the general principles that appear to be used in the
cataloguing and analysis of such movements. The visual system could tackle
the analysis of complex movements in the same way as a physicist describes
the behaviour of a moving object: by resolving the complex movements into
simple independent components (i.e. vectors or degrees of freedom). Our
studies indicate that the most basic division in the analysis of body movement
is that between translation and rotation. Of course, for movement patterns as
complicated as walking there is normally both a translation from one place to
another and rotations of individual limbs (articulations) but in principle it is
possible to describe these components separately and this appears to happen
in the temporal cortex.

Translation: an intuitive arrangement of principal directions?

After studying several hundreds of cells sensitive to motion in the temporal
cortex[3] we have tentatively concluded that there are six categories of cells
sensitive to translation, each type being selective for one direction of
movement. This appears to be the case both for cells that are selective for body
movements and for those that only care about type of motion, not what is
moving. These six directions correspond to movements along the three
Cartesian axes – x, y and z (see Fig. 6.2A). This conclusion is supported both
by the finding of many cells responding best[4] to directions on or close to the
three axes and by the absence of units responding best to intermediary
directions. Interestingly, we have names for each of these directions (up,
down, left, right, towards and away) but not for other directions. In the same
brain region we have found cells which respond selectively to the sight of
particular static views of the face or head but not to other objects[5]. Like the
motion system there appear to be six categories of cell each selective for one
orthogonal view (front and back, left and right sides, top and underside). Thus
information about body view and direction of motion appears to be segregated
into channels of processing which use the same three-axes system.

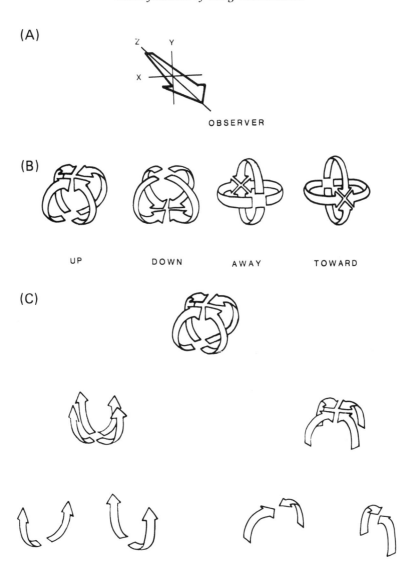

Fig. 6.2.   Coordinate axes for analysis of translation and rotation. A: The three Cartesian axes are illustrated relative to the position of an observer. B: Four types of cell sensitive to articulation (up, down, away from and towards an observer) whose directional selectivity relative to the observer corresponds to the Cartesian axes above. C: Sensitivity to articulation in each major class appears to derive from cells sensitive to movement over a limited angular range. Thus for rotation up, one subtype of cell responds to articulations only up to the horizontal and a second subtype responds only to articulations above the horizontal. These can be further subdivided into subtypes with an even more limited working range which responds to rotations with a component in depth or a component in the fronto-parallel plane.

Articulation: stick figure elements

Some cells are unresponsive to translation alone but do respond to the articulation of component limbs. From preliminary studies the vast majority of such cells can be categorised into four basic types[6]. These types are selective for rotation in one of four directions: up, down, towards and away from the observer (see Fig. 6.2B). For a long time the absence of cells responsive to rotations left and right was worrying. But if a limb is regarded as a stick which is fixed at one end, with the other free to move through any angle, then there is no direction of movement which is not represented by one of the four spheres of motion illustrated in Fig. 6.2B.

In reality a limb has a complex surface with prominent musculature which makes visible another type of articulation, rotation, around its long axis. We do not know how this is visually encoded. Perhaps in the monkey brain a body is treated only as a simple stick figure. This seems likely because we find (see later) that the details of surface pattern of a limb do not matter – they need not be visible as long as the points of articulation are defined. It is also significant that in the approach of artificial intelligence to visual recognition several investigators[7] have found it very useful to treat complex images as a series of 'generalized cones' (elements which are radially symmetrical about their long axes, stick figures by any other name).

For each group of cells which respond to articulation we find subtypes that respond to one direction of rotation but only through 90 or 180 degrees (i.e. one-quarter or one-half of the full sphere). Again we find only subtypes whose responses start and stop as rotations pass through places formed by the principal axes. The sensitivity to one type of articulation irrespective of starting position, e.g. up, Fig. 6.2C, could be constructed by pooling the outputs of appropriate subtypes.

Routes of understanding using different categories of dynamic information

The movement of a small number of lights attached to points of articulation of a human actor (whose outline is invisible to the observer) is sufficient to support the perception of a person and to allow us to recognise the person's actions, sex and even identity. Indeed the perception of these displays which G. Johansson has termed 'biological motion' is both compelling and immediate[8]. In everyday situations visual information is available both from the biological motion and from the static pattern of contours at each instant. We have used Johansson's technique of attaching lights (known as patch lights) to the joints to investigate whether particular neuronal types can rely on dynamic information alone.

Translation

It is possible to arrange experimentally for a body to be translated from A to B without articulating. This can be achieved simply by moving a projected slide of a person or a three-dimensional body on a trolley.

Figure 6.3 illustrates the selectivity of one cell (the same as illustrated in Fig. 6.1) for the right profile view of a body translating, without articulation, to the right. Additional testing revealed that under patch light conditions this cell did not discriminate between left and right body views (for a body walking to the right) or a control object with attached patch lights moving to the right [$F = 0.25$; df 2, 28; $P < 0.05$]. Half of the cells responsive during normal movement, which includes articulation, continue to be selective for body form as the body is moved on a trolley, i.e. translation without articulation. However, these cells are generally unresponsive under biological motion conditions when only the patch lights are visible. They cannot make use of dynamic information arising from limb articulations alone.

Internal articulation

We found that about 40% of cells selective for body movements continued to respond under patch light conditions. Figure 6.4, for example, illustrates the responses of one cell selective for arm movements made towards the monkey. This cell is less responsive to movements of a rigid stick, or to arm movements away from the monkey under normal and patch light conditions. This cell appears to respond to a specific articulation (reaching) performed by the upper and lower arm, this articulation being absent when a rigid stick is moved towards the monkey.

We have found that many of the cells which are unresponsive during patch light conditions show selective responses to body movements if additional minimal contour information is provided in the form of a stripe joining points of articulation. Thus there are two populations of cells activated by articulation, one population able to interpolate the existence of rigid interconnections between points of articulation, and a second that requires the rigid interconnections to be defined explicitly by a linking contour.

Segregation and integration of processing

From the description so far it appears that coding of different types of dynamic information is performed by different cells. Why should this be? Johansson has suggested that in analysing complex movements, such as arm movements, one refers the elbow movement to the shoulder and the wrist movement to the elbow. Each component (torso, upper arm, lower arm) in this

D. Perrett et al.

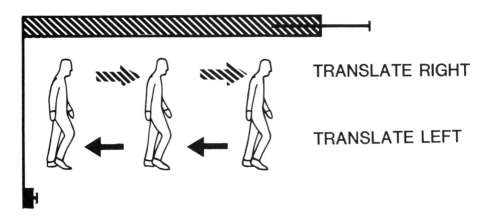

RIGHT PROFILE

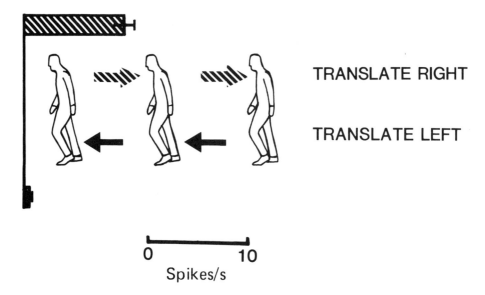

LEFT PROFILE

Fig. 6.3. Selectivity for form through translation. The outline figures illustrate stages during the translation of a body (on a trolley) in the directions indicated by the arrows. The histogram bars illustrate the response (mean ± 1 s.e. for five trials) for different directions of translation and different views of the body. Spontaneous activity for the cell = 3.6 ± 0.9. The cell responds significantly faster for the right profile view of the body translating to the right than to other conditions ($P < 0.05$ each comparison Newman Keuls; overall effect of conditions, $F = 31.2$; df 4,16; $P < 0.01$).

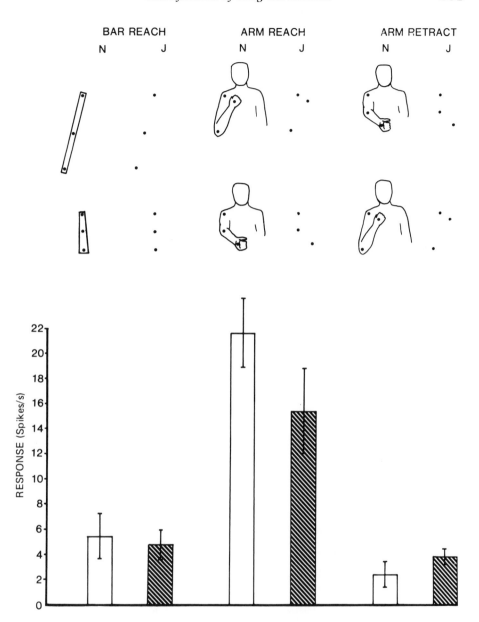

Fig. 6.4. Sensitivity to limb articulation. The upper and lower rows illustrate the start and finish positions of moving stimuli presented to the monkey under normal lighting (N) and low lighting conditions (J) where only luminous patch lights attached to the surface of the stimuli are visible. Lower, histogram of the responses (mean ± 1 s.e. for ten trials) of one cell to the stimuli illustrated above. The cell responds significantly faster (P < 0.01 each comparison) to an arm reaching towards the monkey than to the movement of a stick, arm retraction and spontaneous activity (2.1 ± 0.6) both under normal ($F = 25.6$; df 3,27; P < 0.01) and low lighting conditions ($F = 11.6$; df 3,27; P < 0.01).

hierarchical scheme forms a frame of reference for the next, linked component. Thus the fact that the torso (principal axis of the body[7]) translates to the right allows one to define the movement of the proximal limb as an articulation relative to this frame.

The channels of information do not necessarily remain separate. There are many indications of a convergence of information (see later). Further we have found evidence[9] that the sensitivity of individual cells to one attribute of the body (e.g. frontal body view) is often derived independently through both static and dynamic information.

Different frames of reference

Descriptions of movements from the observer's point of view

The visual coding described above (which accounts for the major proportion of the cells we have studied) is conducted using the viewer as the frame of reference (i.e. all movements are defined relative to the viewer). The neuronal responses can be classified as representing high level viewer-centred descriptions because the responses generalise across distance from the observer to the moving subject and retinal position – the subject can be straight ahead or to one side while the observer looks forward.

Descriptions from the point of view of the moving object

In physics and computational science people often try to describe internal articulations using a coordinate system centred on the moving body itself. Such descriptions are referred to as object-centred[7, 10].

Object-centred descriptions of body movement are more difficult to derive from the visual image but they do have an important place in our understanding of what somebody is doing. Consider a scene in which we see an actor turning his head to look over his left shoulder. This is an object-centred description and it holds for any vantage point of an observer. One would need several viewer-centred descriptions of the type we have described (covering different vantage points of the observer) to give the same information.

A minority of cells that we have studied in the macaque temporal cortex appear to code body movements using the actor's moving body itself as a frame of reference[6]. Figure 6.5 illustrates one such cell that is responsive to arm movements. When the monkey observed the front view of the actor all the arm movements effective in eliciting a response were directed towards the observing monkey. (This was true both for vertical and for horizontal rotations, though only horizontal arm movements are depicted.) The response pattern, however, is completely reversed when the monkey observed the back

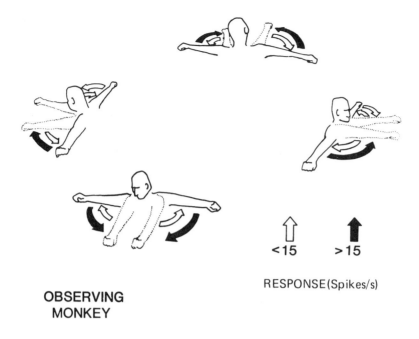

RESPONSE(Spikes/s)

⇧ <15   ⬆ >15

**OBSERVING
MONKEY**

Fig. 6.5. Object-centred coding of arm movement. Neuronal responses to different directions of arm rotation and to different views of an actor. The direction of
rotation of a laterally extended arm is indicated by the direction of the arrowhead.
The monkey's vantage point is indicated at the base of the figure. The directional
selectivity relative to the monkey changes for different views of the actor. For the
front view of the body, movements of either arm towards the monkey were
significantly (P < 0.01 each comparison) greater than spontaneous activity
(1.2 ± 0.5) and movements away ($F = 43.0$; df 4, 21; P < 0.01).
For the back view of the body, movements of either arm away from the monkey
were significantly (P < 0.01 each comparison) greater than movements towards
and spontaneous activity ($F = 13.0$; df 4,21, P < 0.01). The directional sensitivity
relative to the actor's body remains constant since the cell always responds to
movements which bring the arm in front of the actor's chest.

view of the actor's body; for this view the effective arm movements were
directed away from the monkey.

Thus attempts to describe the directional preference of this cell using the
observing monkey as the frame of reference are complicated because the
pattern changes for each view of the actor's body. One can, however, easily
understand this pattern of responses if one relates the arm movements to the
position of the main body axis during each movement. The cell responds
selectively to arm movements which bring the hand in front of the chest. This

description holds for each of the views. (Note that for the side views movements of the arm furthest from the monkey are partially occluded – which
probably accounts for low responses to the movements from these starting
positions.)

Perhaps the nervous system achieves object-centred encoding by selecting
and combining the appropriate viewer-centred descriptions of articulation
for each particular body view. More evidence for viewer-centred descriptions
providing a stepping stone for making object-centred descriptions has been
obtained in experiments on other forms of static and dynamic information
processing[5].

Actions

A different type of description to those just described is needed for understanding actions. The descriptions which use frameworks based on the viewer or
the object being observed are adequate for telling one what an object is and
how it is moving but they tell one little or nothing about what it is doing in the
environment.

Object-centred descriptions and goal-centred descriptions: the difference

To understand what a person is doing (and to get an idea of why they are
doing it) one needs to be able to describe the relationship between the
movements of the person and the object or goal of these movements. We have
termed descriptions which make this type of information explicit 'goal-
centred descriptions'. The contrast between goal- and object-centred descriptions can be illustrated using an example of choreographic notation for
dance. A choreographer could use a set of instructions centred on each
dancer in turn (these would be object-centred descriptions or instructions)
and could take the form: to Mikhail (currently lying prostrate and oriented to
front of stage) 'Raise head slowly' and to Markella (currently at the rear of the
stage facing stage left) 'Turn head to look over left shoulder'. Alternatively the
choreographer could give a single instruction to all members of the dance
troupe 'Move the head slowly to face the audience'. Such an instruction is
economic (since it does not depend on the individual dancers current positions or previous moves) and more importantly it makes explicit the goal
(end-point) of their head movements.

The coding of actions in temporal cortex

Whole body movements as actions We came to realise that goal-centred analysis was central to understanding a great deal of visual encoding in temporal
cortex. This was initially apparent when studying a population of neurons in

an area called TEa[3] which was involved in the coding of hand movements[11]. More recently we have discovered that other populations of cells coding movements of the whole body or just the face are also best understood by considering coding in terms of goal-centred descriptions.

Consider for example the responses of the cell illustrated in Fig. 6.6A and Fig. 6.6B, which responds to whole body movements (walking). This cell responded to a person walking from different starting positions when the direction of walking led the person to the threshold of the laboratory door. Directions of walking that did not take the person straight to this door were less effective in provoking a response from the cell.

The selectivity of the cell for this direction of walking was the same even when the monkey's vantage point and orientation in the room had been changed (see Fig. 6.6B). One cannot describe all the effective directions of walking using the viewer as a frame of reference because what is effective in one situation (e.g. walking to a position 4 m in front of and 2 m to the right of

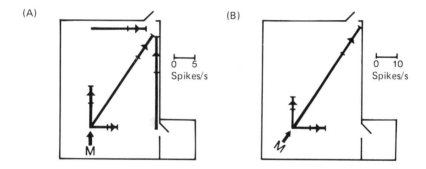

Fig. 6.6. Goal-centred coding of whole body movement. A: Neuronal response to the sight of an actor walking in different directions in the laboratory. The length of each line represents the magnitude of neuronal response (mean ± 1 s.e. for five trials) for one direction of movement. The external boundary of the figure gives the plan view of the laboratory with an indication of the position of the external door and an internal door to a small preparation room. The direction of walking is given by the filled arrowheads and the starting position by the origin of the lines. The vantage point and orientation of the monkey (M) is given by the short arrow at the base of the figure. From a starting position close to the monkey movement towards the external door produces a significantly larger response (P < 0.05 each comparison) than the other two directions of movement (F = 16.6, df 2, 8; P < 0.01). B: The same conventions as in A but the monkey's orientation (short arrow) in the room was modified. The triggering level, which is used to isolate a single cell's response, was changed slightly to prevent the slowly changing activity of background cells influencing the results. With the monkey's vantage point changed the cell still gave a significantly larger response (P < 0.01 each comparison) to movement towards the external door than to other directions (F = 19.8; df 2, 8; P < 0.01.)

the viewer) is changed for the second situation (e.g. walking to a position 4 m in front and 1 m to the left of the viewer). Similarly one cannot use the walking person as a frame of reference (object-centred description) as the person always walked forward in the same direction that they were facing (following their nose). Only those movements directed towards the door provoked a response. One can only begin to make sense of the cell's responses if one considers the relationship between the direction of the person's movements and the position of the external door to the laboratory.

The coding of actions of the hand: perceptions of causality In area TEa of temporal cortex we have discovered large numbers of cells which appear to be involved in the encoding of actions of the hand (e.g. picking, tearing, manipulating). Here we note how these cells respond when one action is directed towards a particular goal and is effective in achieving it, but do not respond to the component actions and motions when there is no causal connection between them.

With a suitably restricted view of the world – either on a video film or for live movements behind a screen aperture (such as a 'Punch and Judy' show box – it is possible to arrange for hand movements and object movements to be contiguous or separated in space or time. For example, hand and cup in view, hand is retracted and after a short delay the cup moves (as if by itself) along the same trajectory as the hand. As the discrepancy between hand movements and object movements widens, the perceptual impression of this scene moves from a state where the hand appears to cause the object to move, through a state where the impression of causality is weakened and the hand appears magically to control the object, to a state where the hands' and objects' movements are completely unrelated[12]. Using these viewing situations we find invariably that cells tuned to hand actions are less responsive when the movements of the hand and objects are spatially separated and appear not to be causally related. This neuronal sensitivity to causality is a direct consequence of the coding of the movements of the hand *relative* to the movements of the object (a goal-centred analysis). The degree to which these movements are related (i.e. are contiguous) is a direct index of the probability that the hand movements and the object movements are causally related.

Linking the understanding of an event to a behavioural reaction

The event of a person going to the laboratory door (as previously described) is evidently understood by monkeys because such an event can in certain circumstances provoke 'isolation' calls from the monkey. In different circumstances the same action can provoke 'threats'. Generally the particular emotion or behavioural reaction evoked by the sight of an action is highly variable. Throughout our studies we find neuronal responses related to what the monkey sees rather than to how it reacts. We therefore see the temporal cortex as providing a detailed visual understanding of events in the world, and not directly causing motor or emotional reactions to the events. The richness and subtlety of any animal behaviour must derive from their ability to react in different ways to a given sensory event depending on many other circumstances. The temporal cortex projects to a large number of brain structures and through these connections the visual comprehension of one action or body movement could subsequently influence systems controlling diverse reactions from eye movements to hormonal changes.

Achieving goals by a variety of means

The responses of the temporal cortex cell illustrated in Fig. 6.6A and B serve to document one important property of goal-centred encoding, i.e. these goals can be achieved by a variety of means; this is a well-known fact in the domain of motor control. Some of the neural mechanisms involved in the control of hand movements are thought to operate as a 'command system' controlling an action such as reaching to a particular target irrespective of the starting position of the hand relative to the target[13]. Thus in the parietal cortex the production of movement is coded not in terms of muscles but in terms of goals.

Understanding actions: the realm of vision, not just linguistics

It is a remarkable omission that such goal-centred descriptions have been generally absent from computational and psychological models of vision. This is perhaps because psychologists have generally treated the understanding of actions as something beyond the realm of vision and more in the sphere of linguistics or semantics. Understanding of actions is seen as requiring logical inference based on previous experience. This attitude ignores the fact that the database and processing from which a comprehension of actions can be made, can be purely visual and does not necessitate the use of language.

Conclusion

We have suggested that there are three ways in which body movements are classified by nerve cells in the temporal lobe. By referring the movements to three different frames of reference, the viewer, the object viewed or the goal of an action, in this classification a comprehensive understanding of the nature and intention of movement can be derived.

7

What does gesture add to the spoken word?

PETER BULL

Introduction

Non-verbal communication has often been regarded as acting in opposition to speech: thus, in the popular literature on 'body language', it is claimed that words may conceal feelings, but the body never lies[1]. However, what I wish to emphasize in this paper is the close relationship which exists between body movement and speech. The studies which I shall discuss here have been based on two situations: informal conversation and public speaking. In general, the results of this research show that body movement is related to speech in terms both of vocal stress and of speech content. I shall begin by discussing some detailed examples of my work on body movement in informal conversation; then I shall turn to the use of hand gesture in political speeches.

Conversation

Vocal stress in spoken English is communicated through changes in pitch, loudness and duration, of which changes in pitch are undoubtedly the most important[2]. Spoken English can also be divided into what are called phonemic clauses or tone groups, a group of words averaging about five in length in which there is one primary or tonic stress, on which the major pitch movement within the tone group occurs.

My own observations suggest that body movement is a fourth factor that must be taken into account in the communication of stress. In one study[3], I had videotapes made of pairs of students in conversation with one another, discussing controversial issues such as their attitudes towards euthanasia and abortion. Six of the conversations were then transcribed and scored for primary or tonic stress. Gesture associated with tonic stress was also scored using a system which I have developed for this purpose, called the Body Movement Scoring System[4]. This system takes as its basic unit of analysis the single movement act; hence, the system is dynamic, not static and so it describes gestures as a series of movements rather than as a series of positions.

Movements which involve contact with an object or part of the body are treated differently from those which do not involve any such contact. Body-contact and object-contact acts are coded in terms of the way the contact is made (e.g. touching, grasping. scratching), the part of the body which makes contact, and the object or part of the body with which contact is made. Any change in any one of these three elements is regarded as starting a new movement act. Non-contact movements are described in terms of the various movements which are possible from each of the major joints of the body, e.g. the forearm can flex, extend, rotate inwards, rotate outwards or perform these movements in combination. The basic unit of analysis for non-contact acts is movement along one axis; if the axis is changed, then a new movement act is scored.

Highly detailed observations of body movement can be made from a videotape or film record using this procedure (regardless of whether the observations are obtained in a social psychology laboratory or in naturalistic settings). By focusing on physical description alone, the task of the observer is made more objective; he does not have to make decisions about the meaning or the functions of particular movements, only to describe them in terms of the appropriate parameters for contact and non-contact movements. By classifying non-contact acts into the different movements which are possible from each of the major joints of the body, and by classifying contact acts in terms of the way the contact is made, the observer is also provided with a finite but comprehensive range of possible movements. Thus, the system has the advantages both of objectivity and of comprehensiveness.

In the study of students in conversation, this system was used to categorize body movements related to tonic stress; these were selected for each subject from the first 15 of such movements occurring in the first, second and final third of the conversation. For the 12 subjects so observed, a mean 90.5% of the tonic stresses within the segments of tape scored were accompanied by body movement (total number of tonic stresses within the segments of tape scored = 277). The results also showed that it was not just movements of the hands and arms which accompany tonic stress, but movements of all parts of the body. Of 540 movements observed in relation to tonic stress, movements for different parts of the body were as follows: head 35%, trunk 15%, hands/arms 34% and legs/feet 16%.

These results are interesting for two additional reasons. Firstly, the fact that most tonic stresses are accompanied by body movement suggests that body movement constitutes a fourth component (in addition to pitch, loud-ness and duration) of the way in which stress is communicated in speech. Secondly, body movement was most commonly related to stress in the form of repeated movements, such as nodding the head, or extending and flexing the forearm, where the apex of the movement coincides with the tonic stress. Hence, it may be possible for a person to use forms of body movement that are idiosyncratic in terms of their visual appearance, but which communicate emphasis quite clearly through their temporal relationship to tonic stress. A number of researchers have distinguished between 'speech-related' and 'non speech-related' movements[5] without specifying exactly what it means to say that a movement is speech-related. These findings suggest that what leads to a movement being perceived as speech-related is its relationship to vocal stress.

Political speeches

More recently, I have attempted to extend this work to a study of the use of hand gesture in political speeches[6]. I chose hand gesture because it may be a particularly important form of non-verbal communication in public speaking. Usually the speaker is separated from his audience by a considerable physical distance, so that hand gesture is probably especially significant because of its greater visibility than, say, facial expression or gaze; during television presentations, in contrast, a speaker's facial expression and gaze can be observed in much greater detail and hence may play a correspondingly more important role.

The first purpose of the study was to investigate whether hand gesture and vocal stress would be synchronized in the same way as demonstrated in informal conversation. The second was to investigate the relationship between hand gesture and rhetorical devices used to evoke applause. In a number of publications, Atkinson[7] has argued that a limited range of rhetorical devices such as contrasts (e.g. 'There's something criminally insane about a government which puts war before peace') and three-part lists (e.g. 'Soviet marxism is ideologically, politically and morally bankrupt') are consistently effective in evoking applause from audiences. He has also proposed that skilled use of these devices is characteristic of 'charismatic' speakers and that such devices are often to be found in those passages of political speeches which are selected for presentation in the news media[7].

More recently, Heritage and Greatbatch[8] have carried out an extensive analysis of 476 speeches delivered to the British Conservative, Labour and Liberal Party Conferences in 1981, representing all the speeches televized from those three conferences. They investigated seven basic rhetorical formats: contrasts, lists, puzzle-solution, headline-punchline, combinations, position-taking and pursuits.

Contrasts and lists have already been illustrated with reference to the work of Atkinson described above. In the puzzle-solution device, the speaker begins by posing some kind of problem for the audience, and then offers as the solution to the puzzle the statement which he wishes to get across. In the headline-punchline format, the speaker states that he is going to make a declaration, pledge or announcement, and then proceeds to make it. In position-taking, the speaker first describes a state of affairs towards which he might be expected to take a strongly evaluative stance, and then explicitly either praises or condemns this state of affairs. If an audience fails to respond to a particular message, speakers may actively pursue applause by, for example, re-completing the previous point; this is referred to as a pursuit. Finally, all the devices discussed above may be combined together in various forms, which Heritage and Greatbatch refer to simply as combinations.

These seven basic rhetorical formats were found to be associated with more than two-thirds of all the sustained applause which occurred during the 476 speeches analysed by Heritage and Greatbatch. Of these seven formats, the contrast and the list were by far the most effective: contrasts were associated with no less than 33.2% of the incidences of applause, lists with 12.6%. Heritage and Greatbatch's data thus provide impressive quantitative support for Atkinson's observations, since contrasts and lists were the two rhetorical formats originally identified by Atkinson as significant in the generation of applause.

An obvious criticism of all this research is that it fails to take into account the role of speech content. Heritage and Greatbatch are well aware of this problem, and have carried out a number of content analyses in relation to rhetorical formatting. For example, in an analysis of two debates at the Conservative and Labour Party Conferences, they looked at one particular class of statements the audience might be expected to applaud, which they called 'external attacks': statements critical of outgroups such as other political parties, which should evoke unambiguous agreement amongst the party conference participants. Their results showed that whereas 71% of external attacks expressed in one of the seven rhetorical formats were applauded, only 29% of those not expressed in these formats were applauded.

Atkinson[7] also discussed the role of intonation, timing and gesture in the delivery of political messages, arguing that non-verbal behaviour can be used to signal additional information to the audience that this is a point where applause is expected. Heritage and Greatbatch carried out a quantitative analysis of the extent to which vocal and non-vocal stress may influence the likelihood of a message being applauded. A sample of speeches formulated in terms of one of the seven basic rhetorical formats was coded in terms of its degree of 'stress'. This was evaluated by taking note of whether the speaker was gazing at the audience at or near the completion point of the message, whether the message was delivered more loudly than surrounding speech passages, or with greater pitch or stress variation, or with some kind of rhythmic shift or accompanied by the use of gestures. In the absence of any of these features, the message was coded 'no stress'. One of these features was treated as sufficient for an 'intermediate stress' coding, while the presence of two or more features resulted in a coding of 'full stress'. Results showed that well over half of the 'fully stressed' messages were applauded, only a quarter of the 'intermediate' messages attracted a similar response and this figure fell to less than 5% in the case of the 'unstressed' messages. Thus, Heritage and Greatbatch's results clearly suggest that the manner in which a message is delivered plays a substantial role in influencing audience applause.

Heritage and Greatbatch have provided impressive statistical support from a wide sample of political speeches for Atkinson's observations concerning the role of rhetorical devices in evoking applause. But the demands of sampling a large number of speeches means that in their analysis of 'stressed' and 'unstressed' messages they could not provide a detailed examination of the way in which vocal and non-verbal features of stress are organized. The alternative is to make a few detailed case studies and investigate the way in which gesture is organized in relation to speech. This was the approach adopted here, based on the detailed analysis of three speeches from a Labour Party rally which took place at St George's Hall, Bradford on May 28th, 1983.

The three speakers were Arthur Scargill (President, National Union of Mineworkers), Pat Wall (Labour Party candidate, Bradford North, West Yorkshire) and Martin Leathley (Labour Party candidate, Shipley, West Yorkshire). Pat Wall has a reputation both as a public speaker and is also well known through his association with Militant Tendency (a left-wing group in the Labour Party). Martin Leathley is unknown in the national political context; at the time of the 1983 General Election, he was a schoolteacher and a local councillor, contesting a Conservative seat which was held by a substantial majority. Neither of these candidates was in fact returned to Parliament in the 1983 General Election. The third speech selected for analysis was by Arthur Scargill, who acquired a national reputation during the miners' strikes of 1973 and 1974, and who also has a reputation as a highly effective public speaker. This speech was chosen because it evoked a great deal of applause and because in the speech Arthur Scargill made extensive use both of gesture and of the rhetorical devices described by Atkinson, Heritage and Greatbatch. Thus, the three speeches can be seen as representing a continuum: one speaker a national figure with a high reputation for oratory, the second speaker less well known, but with something of a political reputation, the third speaker a local councillor unknown in the national political context. To avoid introducing too many other variables into the analysis, the speakers were from the same political party and the speeches were delivered at the same public meeting.

The speeches by Pat Wall and Martin Leathley were transcribed to investigate the relationship between hand gesture and intonation. The results showed that 65.5% of Pat Wall's gestures and 49% of Martin Leathley's were directly related to vocal stress, in the sense that the movement is synchronized to occur at the same time as vocal stress. But not all of the remaining hand gestures can be regarded as unrelated to vocal stress. Some can be regarded as preparatory movements, in which, for example, the speaker flexes his forearm before extending it to coincide with the stressed word. Other movements can be seen to terminate a clause, where the speaker extends his forearm after a sequence of stress-related movements. A third category consists of movements in a repeated sequence of gestures, where the apex of the movement does not always coincide with the vocal stress; for example, in a sequence of five repeated forearm movements, two may not actually coincide directly with the vocal stress. If gestures indirectly related to vocal stress are included in the total of stress-related movements, the proportion of gestures related to vocal stress rises to 87.5% for Pat Wall and 59% for Martin Leathley. Thus, the majority of the hand movements of both speakers were related directly or indirectly to vocal stress; where hand movements were not related to stress, they typically took the form of contact movements, where the speaker adjusts the position of his hand on the rostrum. These results were clearly consistent with the close relationship between body movement and vocal stress found in the previous study of informal conversation[3].

The other major function of hand gesture which was investigated in this study was its relationship to the elicitation and control of applause; the speech by Arthur Scargill was analysed for this purpose. Applause was categorized into 'sustained' and 'isolated' applause: sustained applause refers to clapping from a substantial proportion of the audience, isolated applause to claps from just one or two people. The importance of this distinction is that if rhetorical formatting is effective in signalling to the audience when applause is appropriate, then it should be associated with sustained rather than isolated applause. The results showed that 22 out of the 33 the incidences of sustained applause occurred in response to rhetorical formatting, whereas only two out of 18 incidences of isolated applause occurred in response to rhetorical formatting. Thus, the overall pattern of results supported the proposition that rhetorical formatting is effective in arousing audience applause.

Nevertheless, it could still be argued that audience applause occurs in response to the content rather than the form of political speeches. Thus, a further content analysis was carried out of the types of statements used by Arthur Scargill in his speech. The results of these content analyses were clearly consistent with the argument that rhetorical formatting is effective in evoking applause. A large proportion of Arthur Scargill's speech is made up of external attacks (58% of the total number of speech acts): 86% of formatted external attacks received sustained applause in contrast to only 13% of non-formatted external attacks. The remaining types of speech act typically received more sustained applause when rhetorically formatted, whereas isolated applause typically occurred more frequently in response to non-formatted than formatted types of speech act.

The demonstration that rhetorical formatting in this speech was clearly associated with sustained applause was then used as the basis for an analysis of Arthur Scargill's use of hand gesture in relation to audience applause. The three most commonly occurring rhetorical formats employed in the speech were contrasts, three-part lists and the headline-punchline. Within this headline-punchline format, the speaker proposes to make a declaration, pledge or announcement and then makes it; thus, it is totally explicit that here is an appropriate place for the audience to applaud.

Of the ten contrasts which occur during the course of the speech, eight were followed by sustained applause. In the case of contrasts, Arthur Scargill made use of a particularly interesting device, that of ambidextrous gesturing, illustrating one part of the contrast with one hand, the other part of the contrast with the other hand (see Figs. 7.1, 7.2). However, this should not be seen as a device which is simply confined to illustrating contrasts. Switching from one hand to the other is a characteristic feature of Arthur Scargill's speaking style; in fact, in this speech it occurred on no less than 80 occasions. Contrasts typically involve a transition from one syntactic clause to another, and an examination of the speech as a whole shows that the majority (62.5%) of the hand switches occurred at clause boundaries. Thus, it seems that the use of ambidextrous gesturing to illustrate contrasts is merely a special case of the way in which Arthur Scargill makes use of this device to mark out syntax.

With regard to three-part lists, Scargill used nine of which six were followed by sustained applause. In every case, the three items in a list were marked out by carefully synchronized gestures. Where a three-part list comprises three words, each word is stressed vocally and accompanied with a single hand gesture (see, for example, Fig. 7.3); where a three-part list includes a phrase or clause with more than one vocal stress, then a repeated

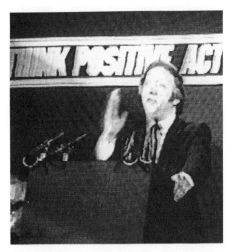

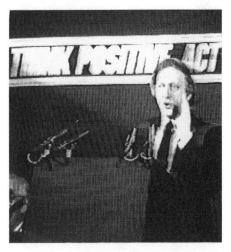

'Of course our nation is facing the most crucial election not since 1945. . .'

'. . . but the most crucial election in Britain's history.'

Fig. 7.1. Use of ambidextrous gesturing in relation to a contrast.

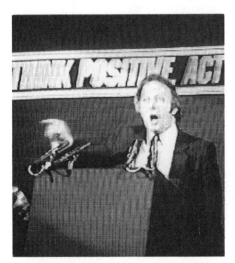

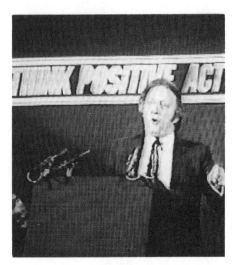

'There's something criminally insane about a government that puts war. . .'

'. . . before peace.'

Fig. 7.2. Another example of ambidextrous gesturing in relation to a contrast.

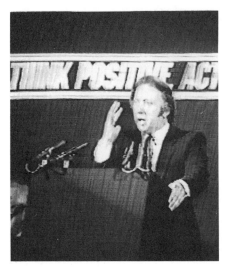
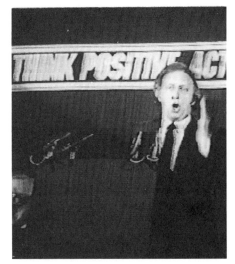

'We are facing an economic. . .'   'social. . .'

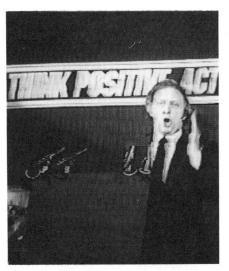

'. . . and political crisis unparallelled in the
history of our nation.'

Fig. 7.3.   Gesturing in relation to a three-part list.

movement is usually employed picking out two or more vocal stresses and
terminating at the end of the list item, a new gesture starting on the next item.
He typically uses non-contact gestures to accompany three-part lists, but on
one occasion actually smacked one hand on the other on the stressed word in
each of the three phrases which made up the list (see Fig. 7.4).

The third common rhetorical device which Scargill uses to evoke applause

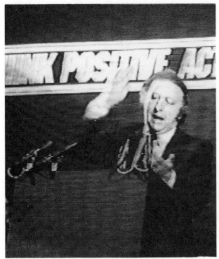
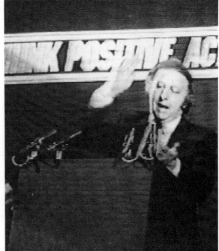
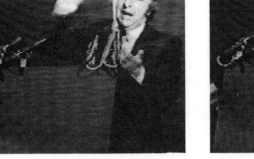

'We want an end to Cruise. . .'   '. . . an end to Trident. . .'

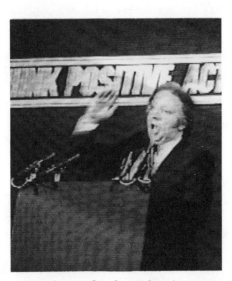

'. . . and end to Polaris.'

Fig. 7.4. Another example of gesture in relation to a three-part list.

is the headline-punchline device. Scargill used this format on seven occasions during the course of the speech, each time receiving sustained applause. On three occasions, the final part of the punchline was presented with a gesture using both hands (see Figs. 7.5, 7.6). Although bilateral gestures were used frequently throughout the speech, they were only used on one other occasion in relation to a rhetorically formatted statement. In association with the

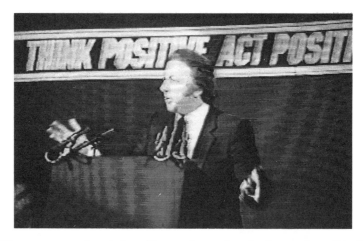

'All I want to say to those lads and lasses who say that they're members of the NUJ
is that those people who were guarding the concentration camps also pleaded
that they had no alternative.'

Fig. 7.5.   Bilateral gesture in relation to a headline-punchline device. (Gesture
occurs on 'no alternative')

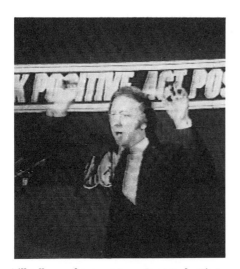
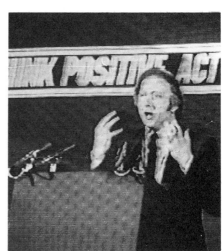

'I'll tell you the most important task: it's to   '. . . the Press.'
say to the Lord Matthews, it's to say to the
Lord Rothermeres, it's to say to the Rupert
Murdochs that the first obligation of a new
Labour government will be to take into com-
mon ownership. . .'

Fig. 7.6.   Another example of a bilateral gesture in relation to a headline-
punchline device. (Bilateral gesture begins on 'will be taken into common
ownership'.)

headline-punchline device, they seem to have had the effect of bringing the punchline to a climax, highlighting the fact that here was an appropriate point in the speech for the audience to applaud.

If Scargill's hand gestures are closely intertwined with rhetorical devices which have the effect of arousing applause, they also constitute a significant part of the way in which he attempts to control applause. Thus, he consistently talked through the 18 incidences of isolated applause; on four of these occasions, he also held up his hand to suppress the applause, either with hand or index finger outstretched. In the 33 incidences of sustained applause, he always started speaking before the applause ends, and on eight occasions he used gesture to try and control the applause. A further analysis of all 12 occasions on which he used gesture to control applause shows that on two-thirds of them, he used such a gesture just before a point in the speech where applause might have been considered appropriate, in that he was about to present a statement in one of the rhetorical formats discussed above (see Fig. 7.7).

Thus, Arthur Scargill creates the impression of overwhelming popularity, continually struggling to make his message audible both by speaking into the applause and by using gesture to restrain it. At the same time, he whips up applause by presenting his speech in the kind of rhetorical formats which Atkinson and Heritage have shown are highly effective in evoking it, the structure of these devices being highlighted by the carefully synchronized use of hand gesture. In fact, Arthur Scargill actually seems to conduct his

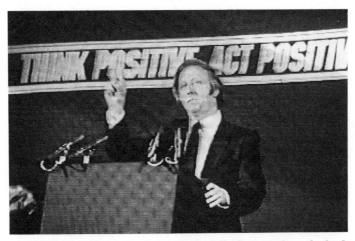

'We've had a number of speeches here tonight including one from the leader of our party and the next prime minister about the important tasks. . .'

Fig. 7.7. Use of gesture as an applause suppressor. (Applause-suppressing gesture occurs after 'important tasks'.) This applause-suppressing gesture is followed by the rhetorical device illustrated in Fig. 7.6.

audience: his gestures not only accompany rhetorical devices which evoke applause but also curtail the applause once it has been aroused – even to the extent of indicating to the audience the points at which they should, or should not, applaud.

Conclusions

The findings from the two studies reported in this chapter were obtained in two very different situations, but they both provide strong support for a close relationship between body movement and vocal stress. In addition, gesture also appears to be related to syntax, picking out clause structure (in the case of Arthur Scargill's use of ambidextrous gesturing). As a by-product of this relationship to syntax, gesture provides information about the structure of rhetorical devices used to evoke applause, hence providing further information to the audience that here is an appropriate point where they may express their solidarity with a political speaker.

Why do speakers supplement the spoken word in this way through gesture? One advantage of conveying information through a number of different channels is that if a listener misses the information from one source, it is always possible to obtain it from another. For example, if a listener misses information about stress from intonation, it is possible to obtain that information from gesture. The implication of this view is that gesture essentially plays a secondary role, supplementing information which is already available in speech.

However, it can also be argued that gesture conveys a distinctive type of information in its own right. Gestures related to speech are certainly intended to be communicative. For example, gesture is used more frequently face-to-face than when talking over an intercom[9]. Gesture is also a part of the turn-taking system in conversation: it may be used as an attempt-suppressing signal to prevent someone else taking the turn[10], while ceasing to gesture also acts as a turn-yielding cue[11].

These findings can all be taken as supporting the view that gesture is intended to be communicative; but the use of gesture in conversational turn-taking also suggests a further proposition: that gesture indicates a *wish* to communicate. This proposition has some intriguing corollaries. Gesture may be used when a person is interested in communicating to another person or group of people: for example, Mehrabian and Williams[12] found that people attempting to be persuasive used significantly more gesture than when asked to present a message in neutral fashion. Conversely, an absence of gesture may indicate a lack of desire to communicate. Thus, people suffering from depression used significantly fewer gestures on admission to hospital than on discharge[13]; an obvious explanation for this is that they simply do not wish to communicate.

The notion that the use of gesture conveys a wish to communicate is also supported by the association of gesture with vocal stress and with rhetorical devices used to evoke applause: these are points the speaker regards as of especial importance and hence particularly wants to communicate. In a more general sense, whether or not a speaker uses speech-related gesture may contribute to the overall effect of whether he appears to be interested and concerned about what he is saying; for a political speaker, the use of speech-related gesture may not only highlight particular aspects of the speech which he regards as important, but also contribute to an overall impression of enthusiasm, interest and commitment to the cause which he espouses.

The view of gesture as an accompaniment to speech I propose here is essentially twofold: it picks out significant features of the spoken message such as stress and syntax, and it also conveys general information about the speaker's degree of communicative motivation. According to this view, gesture is not simply secondary to speech; it also conveys distinctive information about the speaker's level of commitment to the process of communication itself.

8

Visual processing of moving images

ANTHONY MOVSHON

Practically everything of any interest in the visual world moves. Even when objects in the world do not move, their images on the retina do, because the eyes and head are never entirely still. It is therefore not surprising that for more than a century, a growing body of evidence has accumulated which suggests that the visual system has a special sensitivity to moving images. More recently it has become clear that special neural subsystems exist for the visual processing of movement.

It is not obvious that the visual system needs to have a special system to analyse motion. Detecting movement in an image involves only a comparison of the positions of objects recorded at different times. The visual system is exquisitely sensitive to spatial position, and can resolve events separated in time by only a few hundredths of a second. By comparing the remembered location of an object with its present one – making *separate* measurements of space and time – one should be able to extract the motion information. This would not need any special piece of visual hardware, but could be accomplished with whatever elements were needed to analyse static images. Nonetheless, the existence of special visual mechanisms designed to detect the *linked* spatio-temporal changes that constitute motion is now well established, and there can now be no doubt that motion is indeed a fundamental visual dimension.

Perceptual evidence

A number of compelling perceptual phenomena point to the existence of brain mechanisms specifically designed to analyse the motion of visual targets. The two most important of these are the *motion after-effect* (sometimes known as the *waterfall effect*) and the various phenomena of *apparent motion*.

The *motion after-effect* occurs after prolonged viewing of a moving stimulus, such as a waterfall or, as in the case of the first modern report by Purkinje[1] in 1825, a cavalry parade. Stationary objects appear to move backwards, and the apparent speeds of slowly-moving objects are comparably distorted.

Interestingly, despite the clear sense of *motion* that the after-effect gives, the apparent *position* of objects is quite unaffected. This paradoxical percept of motion without a consequent change in position is conveniently explained if motion and position are separate sensory dimensions, signalled by separate underlying processes. The distortions of motion perception result from some specific form of *fatigue* in motion-sensing elements. Separate mechanisms responsible for the sense of position seem to be unaffected by adaptation to motion, although they are susceptible to other kinds of after-effect.

The motion after-effect can be shown to depend on processes central to the point at which signals from the two eyes are combined. If a moving scene is inspected through one eye, the after-effect is strongly expressed when a stationary scene is viewed through the other eye, even when signals from the adapted eye are abolished temporarily by pressure blinding[2]. This is in good agreement with physiological evidence (discussed below) that visual motion processing in such higher mammals as primates is performed largely by binocularly innervated neurons in the cerebral cortex.

Apparent motion is the term commonly used to describe the sense of visual motion that accompanies successive presentations of appropriately displaced static images. Everyday examples of apparent motion include cinema and television images, which consist of series of static frames. Apparent motion is commonly studied with less complex stimuli, often consisting of just two frames of a display. Studies[3] reveal that movement can be seen in response to two stationary flashes if these are properly placed in space and time. Most conditions that produce two-flash motion probably excite a 'long-range process', which is not the same one normally activated by smooth 'real' motion. Nevertheless, the fact that stationary images can produce a percept of 'pure' motion was important early evidence that a special motion-detecting system must exist. Apparent motion is now commonly studied with multi-flash targets, which make clear the relation between apparent-motion displays and 'sampled motion'. Imagine a smoothly moving target illuminated intermittently – each moment of illumination *samples* the continuous spatio-temporal progression of the moving target.

Spatio-temporal filtering

A common framework for understanding much of the data on early visual processing is based on analysing the behavior of simple linear spatio-temporal filters. The success of this approach is probably due to the fact that much of the early visual pathway acts approximately linearly, at least with respect to its relay of signals concerning spatio-temporal contrast. A rough idea of how this kind of explanation works for simple phenomena of apparent or sampled motion is shown in Fig. 8.1. The left panel of the figure (1A) shows a simple space-time representation of a moving object. The ordinate represents one dimension of space, the abscissa, time. The solid line ('smooth motion') represents the natural case of a target moving at a constant velocity and having a continuous representation in space and time. The trajectories of targets moving at different velocities would be given by lines of different slope. The parallel dotted line (sampled motion) represents a multi-flash presentation of a moving target. The two representations reveal the similarity between the targets. For example, it is clear that given dense enough samples, the visual system could not distinguish the two motions.

The right panel of this figure shows a simple representation of a motion detector based on linear spatio-temporal filters[4]. This detector acts by combining signals over space and time, weighted by a function simply represented by the positive and negative zones in the figure. It is intuitively clear that the detector will respond well to motions that have a trajectory in space-time matching the 'orientation' or slope of the detector, like those represented in Fig. 8.1A. Other motions (slower, faster, in the opposite direction) will cross both positive and negative regions and produce smaller responses or none at all. Notice also that the detector will respond similarly to the two kinds of motion shown in Fig. 8.1A, because several of the flashes in the spatio-

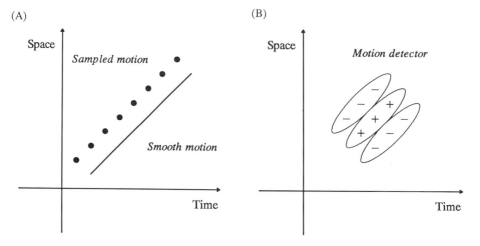

Fig. 8.1. A: Space-time representations of the trajectories of objects in smooth and sampled motion. B: Diagrammatic representation of the spatio-temporal receptive field of a simple linear filter that would respond preferentially to targets moving with the direction and velocity of those shown in A. Targets moving at different velocities would not 'fit' the positive zone of the receptive field of this filter.

temporal train will fall within the zone of space-time that the motion detector weights positively. If the sampling were to become very coarse, the motion detector would no longer respond selectively to a particular speed and direction. This failure would correspond to the failure of widely separated flashes to give rise to any sensation of 'good' or 'smooth' motion.

Notice that this explanation for the phenomena of apparent motion works only if the visual system contains many filters like that represented in Fig. 8.1B, each having a different preference for direction and speed. If there were no distinctive motion analysers, elements in the visual pathway would not have any 'orientation preference' in space-time, and they would respond to each flash of a series without regard to the implicit speed and direction of the signal of which it formed a part.

Neurobiological evidence

In the last two decades, electrophysiologists have measured the responses of the neural elements that comprise the mechanisms of motion analysis in the visual pathway, revealing the existence of neurons that are selectively sensitive to the speed and direction of image motion. The more recent focus of this kind of work on the visual system of primates has revealed the existence of a specific *motion pathway* in the cerebral cortex.

Basic elements of motion detection

The most important early observations on visual motion processing in the nervous system were made by Horace Barlow and his colleagues in the early 1960s[5]. These documented the existence of neurons in rabbits that were selectively sensitive to the speed and direction of retinal image motion. In these neurons it may not be possible to predict the speed and direction preferences from a knowledge of the spatial and temporal structure of their receptive fields, as suggested in the notional motion detector of Fig. 8.1B, but nonetheless the salient properties of directionally selective neurons can be captured by a simple generic scheme like that shown in Fig. 8.2. The key elements of this scheme, and of any scheme of motion analysis, are the acquisition of two (or more) *temporal* intervals. Fig. 8.2A presents the two spatial samples by the two offset 'Mexican hat' functions, which resemble the sensitivity profiles of several common types of visual neurons; the separation between these profiles is Δx. Figure 8.2B illustrates a simple schematic circuit to compare the outputs of the spatial sensors, represented by the boxes '1' and '2'. The output of the first sensor is passed through a time-delay element (Δt), and then compared in some way ('C') with the undelayed output of the second. If the comparison operator seeks a conjunction between signals that

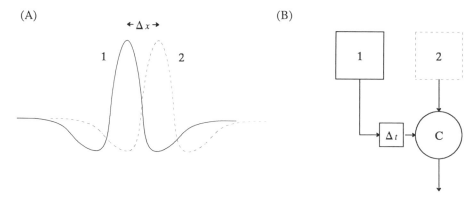

Fig. 8.2.   A generic scheme for creating direction selective neurons. (A) Two spatial sensors separated from one another by some distance Δx. (B) A simple circuit to combine signals from the spatial sensors with a time delay Δt introduced for one of the sensors. Depending on the nature of the comparison operation symbolized by C, the motion analyser would prefer motion from 1→2 or from 2→1.

arrive from its two inputs, the output of C will be *large* when targets move in the direction 1→2 – the delayed signals from sensor 1 will arrive in synchrony with the signals from sensor 2. If, on the other hand, the comparison operator *vetoes* responses when the signals occur at the same time, the output will be *small* when targets move in the direction 1→2 – the delayed signals from sensor 1 will prevent the relay of signals from sensor 2. Both kinds of model receive support from data on the response properties of real neurons[5, 6]. Variants of this model in which the underlying operations are linear can result in space-time receptive fields similar to that in Fig. 8.1B. If, however, the comparison operator is nonlinear, the directional selectivity of the neuron may be unpredictable from a map of the receptive field, as is the case for neurons in the rabbit's retina.

Visual pathways in primates

In primates, motion analysis is not explicitly performed by neurons in the retina. Instead, it turns out that two main groups of retinal neurons feed into pathways that can be traced directly to higher levels of processing in the cerebral cortex. These pathways form two distinctive segments of the cortical visual system[7, 8]. One of these pathways is responsible for the analysis of motion.

The early stages of the primate retinocortical visual pathways are shown in diagrammatic form in Fig. 8.3. (See p.11 for an anatomical drawing of the primate visual pathway.) The pathway begins in the retina, where two

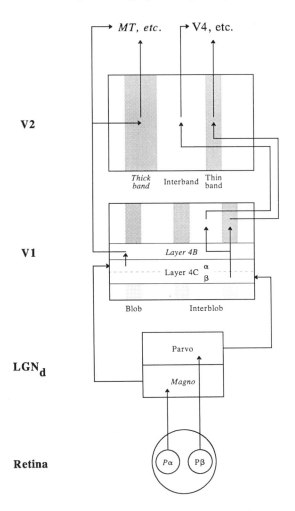

Fig. 8.3. The principal connections of the early portions of the primate retino-cortical visual pathways. Components of the system labelled in *italics* are thought to belong to the motion pathway. Both blob and inter-blob zones in the upper layers receive their major visual input from layer 4Cβ, while layer 4B receives its input from 4Cα. Signals from all three compartments of V1 (blob, inter-blob, layer 4B) are relayed to extrastriate cortical regions, including the second visual area (V2), which can also be subdivided by staining for CO. It shows a very distinctive pattern of alternating thick and thin bands of CO-rich cortex interdigitated with lighter-staining 'interbands'. The projections from V1 to V2 are largely segregated according to the compartments defined by these bands. The CO-rich blobs of V1 project to the thin CO-rich bands in V2; the inter-blob cortex of V1 projects to the interband cortex of V2; and *layer 4B* of V1 sends its output to the thick CO-rich bands of V2. The thin bands and interbands of V2 send their output to a collection of ventrally placed cortical areas, of which the most prominent is the fourth visual complex, V4. The thick bands of V2 send their output to more dorsally placed areas, primarily an area in the superior temporal sulcus called MT or V5[9].

distinctive groups of retinal ganglion cells can be identified that have projections to the forebrain. These neurons, Pα and Pβ cells, project respectively to the *magnocellular* and *parvocellular* divisions of the lateral geniculate nucleus in the thalamus (LGNd), the main relay nucleus carrying visual signals from the retina to the cerebral cortex. These separate divisions of the LGNd project separately to the primary visual receiving area of the cerebral cortex, the striate cortex, V1 (also called Area 17). Here, they terminate in separate but adjacent portions of the cortical layer 4: parvocellular neurons project to layer 4Cβ, and magnocellular neurons project to layer 4Cα. They, in their turn, send connections to other neurons that in turn relay signals to the second visual area (V2) and elsewhere.

An anatomical subdivision of V1 can be made by staining it to detect the presence of the respiratory-chain enzyme cytochrome oxidase (CO). This enzyme is concentrated in CO-rich 'blobs' which are dense in upper layers and weak in the deeper layers: between these blobs lies CO-poor 'inter-blob' cortex. Cells in blob and 'inter-blob' cortex have different characteristics because they receive different inputs, and they send their outputs to different destinations, resulting in the segregation of pathways shown diagrammatically in Fig. 8.3 and described in more detail in the legend[9].

The functional significance of these two divisions of the cortical visual system is now becoming clear. One pathway, which one may summarize as

Retinal Pα $\rightarrow$ LGN Magno $\rightarrow$ V1 layer 4Cβ
$\rightarrow$ layer 4B $\rightarrow$ V2 thick band $\rightarrow$ MT

appears to be particularly devoted to analysing signals about motion. The names of elements of this pathway are shown in italics in Fig. 8.3. The other pathway

Retinal Pβ $\rightarrow$ LGN Parvo $\rightarrow$ V1 layer 4Cβ $\rightarrow$ V1
blobs/inter-blobs $\rightarrow$ V2 bands/interbands $\rightarrow$ V4

appears to be more concerned with the analysis of the form and colour of visual images, and less with their motion. The evidence for this distinction between the functional pathways or 'streams' is derived in part from analyses of the behavior of visual receptive fields in different areas[10] and partly from analyses of the effects of lesions of different cortical areas on visual behavior[7].

The pathways whose roots may be found in these two early streams of visual processing do not end with the projections of V1 and V2. They can in fact be traced extensively on functional and neuroanatomical grounds through the cerebral cortical visual system of the monkey. Figure 8.4A shows two lateral views of the cerebral cortex of a macaque monkey. In each view, a portion of the cortex that is normally buried in folds (or *sulci*) is revealed by artificially opening one or more sulci. All of the areas traced out and identified on the cortical surface in the figure are known to have visual functions; they

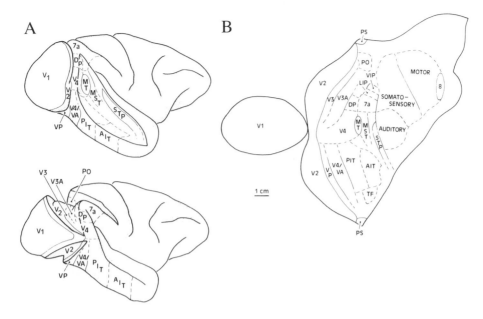

Fig. 8.4.   Two sketches of lateral views of the right hemisphere of the cerebral cortex of a macaque monkey, showing the approximate locations of visual areas.[8] Many visual areas are partly or wholly buried in cortical folds or *sulci*. In the upper of sketch A, the superior temporal sulcus has been unfolded to reveal the positions of areas MT, MST and STP. In the lower sketch, the lunate, intraparietal, parieto-occipital and inferior occipital sulci have been unfolded to reveal the positions of areas V2, V3, VP, V3a and PO. B: A completely unfolded and flattened representation of the locations of different areas in the right cerebral cortex of a macaque monkey. Visual cortex occupies the left (posterior) portion of the map, and comprises roughly half of the cortex. The abbreviations used for the names of areas in this figure and in Fig. 8.5 are based partly on beliefs about the serial order of visual processing (V1, V2, V3, V3a, V4), partly on old architectural maps of the cerebral cortex (7a, 8, TF), and partly on geographical location in the cerebral cortex. For names of this last kind, the abbreviations are as follows: PO-parieto-occipital area, DP-dorsal prelunate area, VIP-ventral intraparietal area, LIP-lateral intraparietal area, MT-middle temporal area, MST-medial superior temporal area, STP-superior temporal polysensory area, VP-ventral posterior area, VA-ventral anterior area, PIT-posterior inferior temporal area, AIT-anterior inferior temporal area, PS-prostriate area. To make matters even more confusing, three of these 'geographical' names – MT, VP and VA – are derived from the positions of the areas in the brain of the owl monkey, which is rather different from the brain of the macaque. The figures are reproduced, with permission, from the *Annual Review of Neuroscience*, Volume 10, © 1987 by Annual Reviews Inc.

can be divided into a dorsal group terminating in the posterior portion of the parietal lobe, and a ventral group terminating in the inferior portions of the temporal lobe.

Because the cerebral cortical mantle has the form of an intricately folded sheet, it is helpful to produce an unfolded and flattened representation of the distribution of areas along the surface of the cortex[11]. This has been done in Fig. 8.4B, which shows such an unfolded flattened map. Apart from cuts around V1 and along the medial surface of the cerebral hemisphere the map is uninterrupted and represents the locations and sizes of cortical zones with minimal visual distortion. The named visual areas seen in Fig. 8.4A can be located again in this figure, which also makes it clear that these areas occupy more than half the area of the cerebral cortex.

It is possible, using anatomical techniques, to chart the interconnections among these cortical areas, and to assign the areas to distinct positions in a cortical *hierarchy*. This is done first by establishing which areas communicate with which others. It turns out that all cortico-cortical connections are reciprocal, meaning that if cells in area A send projections to area B, then cells in area B also project to area A. However, the precise anatomical structure of the two projections is usually asymmetrical, so that it is almost always possible to assign one of the projections as an 'upward' or feed-forward' projection, and to identify the other as a 'downward' or 'feedback' projection[10]. Because of this asymmetry, one may construct a hierarchical chart of cortical areas like that shown in Fig. 8.5, which summarizes the most important and best-known of the interconnections of the visual cortical areas marked out in Fig. 8.4. The areas at the bottom of the figure form the roots of both cortical visual pathways. The higher areas on the left side represent the motion pathway; the higher areas on the right represent the form/colour pathway. Solid and dashed lines represent interconnections among the areas. The solid lines show connections *within* a pathway, while the dashed lines show connections *between* the pathways. The areas shown in light stippling are partly involved with the motion pathway; the heavily stippled areas are entirely involved with motion processing.

Neurophysiology of the primate motion pathway

Connectional anatomy of the kind laid out in the preceding section can demonstrate that the structural substrate exists for a particular kind of function. Functional evidence in support of the idea of a 'motion pathway' can, however, only be obtained from functional analyses of neural activity. Looking 'back' down the pathway from its termination in the parietal lobe,

MOTION PATHWAY   **FORM/COLOUR PATHWAY**

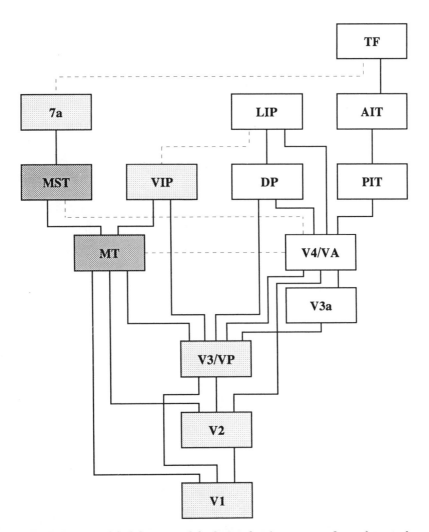

Fig. 8.5.   A simplified diagram of the hierarchical structure of visual cortical connections in the macaque monkey. Connections among areas are always reciprocal, with the upward connections being of the 'forward' type. The connection between MT and V4 complex is of unusual form, and is represented as horizontal (neither 'feed-forward' nor 'feed-back'). Areas related to the motion pathway are stippled, with lighter stippling representing areas only partly or inferentially belonging to that pathway, and darker stippling reserved for MT and MST, the two key areas of the pathway. The unstippled areas on the right-hand side are portions of the 'form/colour' pathway. The dashed lines represent interconnections between the 'motion' and the 'form/colour' pathways; solid lines represent connections within the pathways.

and examining the functional properties of the neurons it contains, provides the necessary evidence.

From a functional point of view, two striking features of visual receptive fields change over the early stages of the motion pathway: the spatial organization of the receptive fields, and the selectivity of the receptive fields for motion. Figure 8.6 shows an outline summary of the process. For the present purpose, we may consider the early stages of the pathway (see Fig. 8.3), from the retinal Pα ganglion cells, through magnocellular LGN cells to layer 4Cα of V1, to be functionally homogeneous. Neurons at all these levels of the pathway have receptive fields on the retina that are circularly symmetric and concentrically organized. These consist of a central region in which light either excites or inhibits the cell's activity, surrounded by a larger annular zone in which light has an effect opposite to that which it has in the centre of the receptive field. Because of this spatial structure, these neurons have a certain selectivity to spatial patterns: they respond better to spatially structured targets than to uniform fields of light[12]. But their symmetric receptive field organization means that they do not respond differentially to different directions of movement; these points are summarized in Fig. 8.6A. On the left is shown a map of the receptive field of a concentric neuron of the 'on-centre' type, with its annular inhibitory surround. On the right is a schematic polar diagram of the influence of the direction of motion of a bar target on the neuron's response. The angular coordinate of the plot represents direction of motion (always at right angles to the bar's orientation), while the radial coordinate represents the magnitude of the neural response. Only small variations in response with direction of motion are observed for neurons at this level of the system.

Within layer 4C of V1, the first major signal transformation in this pathway becomes evident with the onset of *orientation selectivity*, schematically illustrated in Fig. 8.6B. The receptive fields of the 'simple' cells of layer 4C are divided, like those of neurons at earlier stages, into separate excitatory and inhibitory regions. These regions, however, are arranged in parallel stripes, and this arrangement gives the neurons a preference for a particular orientation of a bar target[13]. This orientation preference is expressed in the polar response diagram on the right: the two oppositely directed response peaks show that the response is optimal for a particular orientation, in either of its two possible directions of motion.

Until this level of the pathway, there is no special evidence for motion selectivity. Neurons in both the 'motion' and 'form/colour' pathway are organized in fundamentally the same ways. However, there are already hints at this level that the motion pathway is specialized for relaying motion signals:

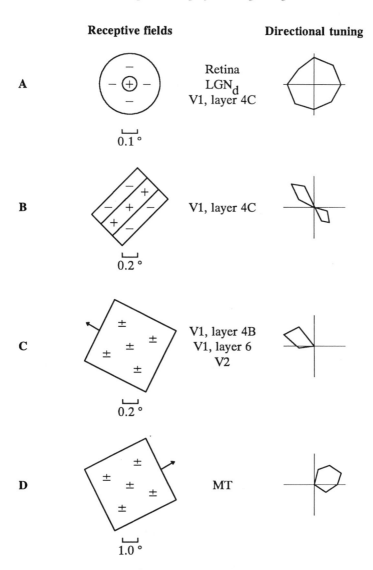

Fig. 8.6. Schematic representations of the spatial structure of visual receptive fields (left) and their directional selectivity (right), as seen at different levels of the motion pathway. The spatial scales under the receptive fields shown at the left are appropriate for neurons representing the center of gaze; in the periphery, these dimensions would be larger. The polar diagrams on the right schematically illustrate typical responses to variation in the direction of motion of a bar target that is always oriented at right angles to its direction of motion. The angular coordinate of the plot indicates the direction of motion, and the radial coordinate indicates the magnitude of response. Note that for the bottom three pairs of illustrations, the particular directional preference shown is arbitrary – different neurons in each region would prefer different directions of motion dispersed more or less uniformly around the clock. Note also that the spatial scale of the receptive field maps on the left changes for different parts of the figure.

neurons in the motion pathway are more sensitive to stimuli that vary rapidly in time and are less sensitive to fine spatial detail and colour[14].

In layer 4B of V1 a second major signal transformation takes place, with the onset of *directional selectivity*. Most directionally selective neurons in V1 have receptive fields of the 'complex' type. These receptive fields are relatively large and apparently uniform, as shown in Fig. 8.6C. They seem to be excited everywhere by either light or dark targets, hence the '±' symbols in the receptive field map. As indicated by the arrow on the left and the polar response diagram on the right, these neurons are also often direction-selective: they respond better or solely to one direction of motion of an optimally oriented bar target, and less well or not at all to the other. In addition to layer 4B, neurons having this character are found in layer 6 of V1, and in the thick CO bands of V2. While these neurons have a complex receptive field structure and directional selectivity, they are typically insensitive to stimulus colour. They are often activated similarly by targets delivered to either eye, which suggests that they may be involved in the inter-ocular transfer of motion after-effects mentioned above.

In the middle temporal area (MT), the most obvious transformation of the motion signal involves its integration over space. This is shown in Fig. 8.6D by the considerably larger size of the receptive field of the MT neurons. Also, in MT, the precision of the selectivity for direction of motion that the neurons exhibit is typically less than in V1, hence the somewhat 'fatter' example tuning curve. Like the neurons in V1 and V2 that project to them, neurons in MT are frequently binocular and are usually insensitive to stimulus colour[15].

MT and the aperture problem

The description above does not capture one of the most significant features of the organization of visual signals in and beyond MT, the way in which local motion signals are integrated to provide information about the motion of complex objects and patterns. This is often termed the 'aperture problem' because it becomes obvious when considering measurements of motion made through finite apertures. Figure 8.7A illustrates the problem by considering the motion of two diamond figures, one moving down and one moving to the right. Although the global motion of these figures is quite different, a local measurement of motion made in the circular apertures drawn on the lower right-hand border of each diamond would yield the *same* value in each case. The local motion of a border is usually seen as being orthogonal to the border, as shown by the arrows linked to the circular apertures of measurement. In the graph below, the angle of a vector represents direction of motion and its length represents speed. The local measurement of motion made in each of the apertures is not sufficient to define the motion of the whole object – there is an *ambiguity* concerning the motion measured locally. The true motion of the border consists of the measurable component *orthogonal* to the border and some unmeasurable and therefore locally unknown component *parallel* to

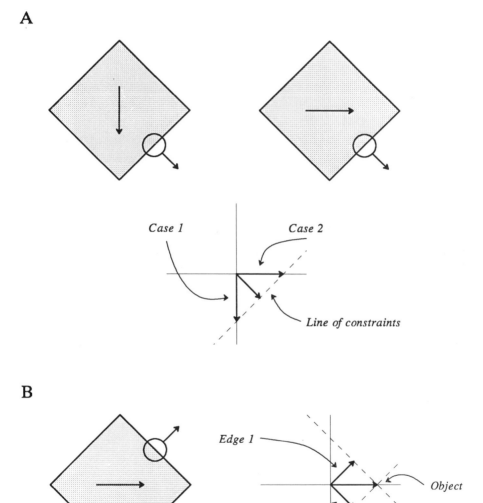

Fig. 8.7. The aperture problem. A: Two diamonds, one moving downward and one moving rightward, showing that locally measured motions (circles) do not unambiguously reflect the overall motions of objects. B: A formal solution to the aperture problem based on using the intersection of the contraints set up by local measurements to resolve their ambiguity.

the border. The measurable component is represented on the figure by the oblique vector directed down and to the right, and the unmeasurable component is represented by the dashed line orthogonal to it. The motion of the local border thus does not specify object motion completely, but imposes the *constraint* that the motion of the object containing the border must fall somewhere along the dashed line. The true motions in the two cases illustrated (the vertical and horizontal vectors) both correspond to different points along this 'line of constraints'.

The existence of these constraints makes possible a simple formal solution to this class of problem, if measurements made over two or more contours are combined[16]. The form of this solution is shown in Fig. 8.7B. Measurements made along the upper right border of the figure ('edge 1') provide one line of constraints; measurements made along the lower right border ('edge 2') provide a second line of constraints; the intersection of these two lines ('object') is the only motion consistent with the two constraints, and must therefore yield the motion of the object.

The neural implementation of this model requires that some set of directionally selective neurons should integrate signals from several local measurements of motion. Because of the larger spatial scale of MT receptive fields (Fig. 8.6), and the fact that MT receives directionally selective inputs from V1 and V2, it is natural to suppose that MT might be the site of this integration. It turns out that this is indeed the case. MT contains two distinct kinds of directionally selective neurons. *Component direction selective* neurons, like neurons in V1, provide signals about the local motions of individual contours or orientations. *Pattern direction selective* neurons, found only in MT, carry more fully integrated information about motion that emerges from the combination of signals about motion from several different contours or orientations[17]. These neurons provide motion signals that are invariant with the orientation of the contours that move, and represent a level of abstraction of motion information not seen at lower levels of the pathway.

Higher functions of the motion pathway

Our knowledge of the functional characteristics of neurons in the portions of the motion pathway beyond MT is relatively sketchy. Even the anatomy is not yet fully understood, and it is likely that areas such as MST, 7a and VIP will ultimately prove to have complex functions related to several different aspects of motion processing. For example, some neurons in areas MST and 7a have been shown to respond to complex patterns of motion and not to the simple rigid motion of objects across the field. Brad Motter and Vernon Mountcastle[18] have shown a pattern of directional responsiveness in parietal neurons that could suit them to analysis of the patterns of optic flow produced by locomotion through the environment. More recently others[19] have reported several complex patterns of response in MST neurons, including preferences for rotations both in the fronto-parallel plane and in depth, as well as for optic flow patterns of the kind suggested by Motter and Mountcastle. Still other data suggest a role for the higher areas of the motion pathway in the control of smooth pursuit eye movements[20]. Signals concerning motion must also be involved in such basic perceptual tasks as the segmentation of complex images[21]. It is clear that further analyses of this complex and important neural system cannot fail to yield new insights into the way that the brain processes visual images.

Conclusions

Neurons at successively higher stations in that part of the visual pathway responsible for analysing motion have a progression of properties that are beginning to make functional sense. This might be crudely summarized thus: first, these neurons have special sensitivity to rapid changes of luminance; second, they acquire selective sensitivity to local velocity and direction of motion; third, they abstract the direction of motion of objects, rather than edges or lines. Beyond this, there are hints of neurons having selective sensitivity for rotations and optic flow. Although much remains to be done to understand the anatomy, physiology and functional organization of the motion system in cerebral cortex, the glimpse we have is beginning to show how motion perception is organized.[22]

PART 3

Narration

MEL CALMAN

Mel Calman was the Chairman of the session on Narration.

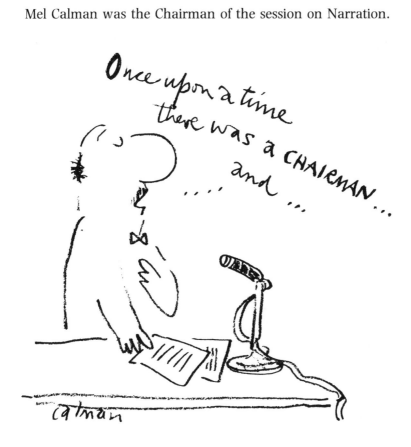

9

Narration with Words

DAVID LODGE

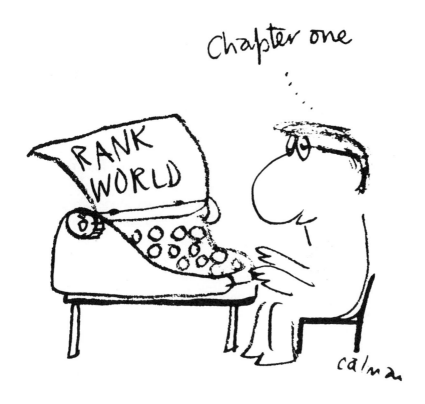

I shall be mainly concerned in this paper with literary narrative, especially prose fiction, which is the area in which I have some professional competence. But it would be appropriate to the occasion, I think, to begin with some remarks about narrative in general.

The nature of narrative

Narrative (or narration) is one of the fundamental sense-making operations of the mind, and would appear to be both peculiar to and universal throughout humanity. At least, I am not aware that animals can tell stories, though

141

they can communicate with each other and with humans; and I am not aware that any human community has been discovered, however primitive, that does not have its repertory of stories – myths, legends and folk-tales.

Narrative in my terms is more than the report of a single discrete event. Narrative is concerned with *process*, that is, with change in a given state of affairs, or it converts problems and contradictions in human experience into process in order to understand or cope with them. The anthropologist Claude Lévi-Strauss[1] famously demonstrated that the Oedipus legend, of which analogues are to be found in South American Indian culture, originates from the difficulty primitive men experienced in reconciling their belief that human beings sprang from the earth, like the crops, with their empirical observation that they are born from sexual union. The knowledge gained from or organised in narrative differs from the propositional knowledge in which science and philosophy are interested. The meaning of a narrative cannot be adequately encapsulated in a single proposition, like, say, the meaning of a scientific experiment. It has to be experienced in time, as process. Hence the essentially iterative nature of narrative and narration – for example, the readiness of primitive or archaic peoples to hear the same stories recited again and again, or the pleasure sophisticated modern readers take in re-reading classic novels, or seeing the plays of Shakespeare performed repeatedly.

A narrative cannot be reduced to a proposition, but it must have a point, and it must have some kind of unity. The most basic kind of narrative is the chronicle. A happened and then B happened and then C happened, and so on. But we expect A, B and C to have something in common – they happened in the same place, or to the same people or person – otherwise we should not be much interested in D, in knowing what happened next. Wanting to know what happened next is the basic narrative appetite, and it usually depends on the narration privileging some persons involved in the events over others – we call these privileged persons the hero or heroine. We shall be still more interested in the sequence of events if they are connected by causality – B happened because of A and C because of B. If you start with C and work back to A you have the basic structure of a mystery story. If you start with B, work back to A and then go forward to C, you have the basic structure of the classical epic. In short, although narrative depends on the concept of chronological sequence for intelligibility, it need not follow that sequence.

Narrative, then, obtains and holds the interest of its audience by raising questions in their minds about the process it describes and delaying the answers to these questions – questions like 'and then?' or 'why?'. As each question is answered, another must be left unanswered, or a new one raised, for when all the questions are answered the narrative must end. Narrative describes a series of events which are continually opening and closing possibilities for the characters and thus contributing to the ultimate resolution of some overarching question, such as, will the hero/heroine find true love, conquer evil, solve the mystery etc. When this question is answered in a way that is both unexpected and plausible we have the effect Aristotle called *peripeteia* or reversal, which satisfies what Frank Kermode[2] has called the 'credulity' and the 'scepticism' of the audience – our desire to find an intelligible order in life, and our experience that it is disorderly and unpredictable.

Narrative is not necessarily or exclusively mediated through language. There are forms of narrative that are partly or wholly non-verbal: drama, film, dance, strip cartoon etc. (M. Parker and K. Macmillan discuss the Benesh notation of dance on pp.81–93 and Jonathan Miller the grammar of movie editing on pp.180–194.) Narrative is a kind of language of its own that translates readily from one natural language to another and from one medium to another. The story of 'Cinderella' has essentially the same meaning whether read in Perault's *Contes de ma mère l'oye*, or *The Oxford Book of Fairy Tales* or told to a child on its parent's knee or presented as a film or pantomime or ballet. Modern literary narratives like novels do not translate quite so easily because they contain more than merely narrative; they contain information which may be tied to a particular language community or which cannot be adequately represented in a nonverbal medium. Nevertheless because narrative is their basic structural principle of cohesion, novels translate more easily than, say, lyric poems.

Verbal narrative

The difference between oral and written narrative and the difference between fictional and non-fictional narrative are fascinating questions which I shall have to pass over in order to address myself to the question of what is specific to verbal narrative. One of the earliest and still one of the most pertinent discussions of this subject is to be found in Book 3 of Plato's *Republic*. There, Socrates[3] distinguishes between two ways of representing action in verbal discourse. Either the writer describes the action in his own words (*diegesis*) or in the words of his characters (*mimesis*). Drama, in which the author does not speak in his own voice, is all mimesis. The dithyramb (a kind of hymn describing the actions of a god) is all diegesis. The epic, which is the ancestor of our novel, is according to Plato, a mixed form. It alternates mimesis and diegesis, author's voice and characters' voices. Socrates illustrates the point from the opening of Homer's *Iliad*, where Chryses appeals to the Achaeans to let him ransom his daughter:

> You know that as far as the lines,
>> *He prayed the Achaeans all*
>> *But chiefly the two rulers of the people,*
>> *Both sons of Atreus*
>
> the poet himself speaks, he never tries to turn our thoughts from himself or to suggest that anyone else is speaking; but after this he speaks as if he himself was Chryses, and tries his best to make us think that the priest, an old man, is speaking, and not Homer.

Plato here put his finger on an obvious but easily overlooked fact about narrating with words, namely that words can only *imitate* other words, a speech act can only imitate another speech act. Language refers to the world not by imitation but by employing a conventional code. The implication, pertinent to this book, is that the most iconic component of a literary narrative is its least visual. In semiotics an icon is a sign in which the signifier bears a factual resemblance to the signified, such as a picture or a diagram. An index is a sign in which the signifier is connected with the signified by contiguity or causality (e.g. smoke is an index of fire, a Rolls Royce is an index of wealth), and a symbol is a sign in which the signifier is linked to the signified arbitrarily, by cultural convention. Language is a symbolic system, but when we quote speech our language is, at a second level, iconic[4].

Plato's distinction is sometimes stated in terms of 'telling' and 'showing'. A picture shows us something about the world, a story tells us something about the world. But insofar as a story incorporates the quoted speech of characters, it shows rather than tells. (Conversely, insofar as a picture encourages us to infer a *before* and an *after* of the moment it presents, it tells rather than shows.) This showing in narrative, this imitation of speech *in* speech, is of course, stylised and conventionalised. Dialogue in a written text necessarily lacks most of the intonational expressiveness of real speech, and its grammar and punctuation are quite different from real speech, which is almost unintelligible when faithfully transcribed. Nevertheless the difference between mimesis and diegesis, showing and telling, is real and important, and a typology of literary narrative can be based on how they are combined or which is dominant in any given text. Roughly speaking, mimesis gives us the sense of reality in fiction, the illusion of access to the reality of personal experience, and diegesis conveys the contextualising information and framework of values which provide thematic unity and coherence.

The Homeric epic on which Plato drew for illustration alternates the two modes more or less evenly. We have a passage of authorial description – of the preparations for battle, for example – then some speeches by the warriors, then an authorial description of the fighting, and so on. This alternation of authorial description and characters' verbal interaction remains the woof and warp of literary narration to this day. A novel or short story that consists exclusively of authorial narration or exclusively of dialogue will strike us as deviant, experimental and probably rather alienating. But there are more ways of combining mimesis and diegesis, author's voice and characters' voices, than through simple alternation.

One obvious variation is to let one or more of the characters tell the story, in the form of an autobiography or confession, or in journal entries, or correspondence. The rise of the novel in England in the 18th century was marked by several developments of this kind – Daniel Defoe's pseudoautobiographical novels like *Robinson Crusoe*, for example, or Samuel Richardson's enormously popular epistolary novels, *Pamela* and *Clarissa*. It remains a very common narrative technique in 20th century fiction. In such narrative, the diegesis is in effect simultaneously a mimesis of the character who narrates. For example, in Martin Amis's *Money*[5] we get a representation of Los Angeles that is simultaneously a representation of John Self's speech, and thus of his character:

> You come out of the hotel, the Vraimont. Over boiling Watts the downtown skyline carries a smear of God's green snot. You walk left, you walk right, you are a bank rat on a busy river. This restaurant serves no drink, this one serves no meat, this one serves no heterosexuals. You can get your chimp shampooed, you can get your dick tatooed, but can you get lunch? And should you see a sign on the far side of the street flashing BEEF-BOOZE-NO STRINGS, then you can forget it. The only way to get across the street is to be born there. All the ped-Xing signs say DON'T WALK, all of them, all the time. That is the message, the content of Los Angeles: don't walk. Stay inside. Don't walk. Drive. Don't walk. Run!

Another important way of combining mimesis and diegesis is indirect or reported speech, for this allows features of the author's discourse and the characters' discourse to be combined within the same sentence, especially when the device known as free indirect speech is employed. This is often used in 19th and 20th century fiction to represent thought. In earlier narrative thought is represented either by authorial report or by the rather artificial device of the character uttering his thoughts aloud, as in a dramatic soliloquy. A modern variation of the latter is the interior monologue. Free indirect style is a flexible compromise between author's speech and character's speech: by reporting the character's thoughts in the third person, past tense, but keeping to the vocabulary of the character, and omitting the tags, *he*

thought, she wondered etc., an effect of intimate access to the character's inner
self is produced, without relinquishing the task of narrating to the character.
The author retains a covert control of the narrative. The opening of Virginia
Woolf's *Mrs Dalloway*[6], for example, begins with an authorial or diegetic
narrative statement, 'Mrs Dalloway said she would buy the flowers herself',
and immediately moves into the heroine's stream of consciousness, her
thoughts and memories, by means of indirect speech, mostly in free style:

> Mrs Dalloway said she would buy the flowers herself. For Lucy had her
> work cut out for her. The doors would be taken off their hinges;
> Rumpelmayer's men were coming. And then, thought Clarissa
> Dalloway, what a morning – fresh as if issued to children on a beach.
>   What a lark! What a plunge! For so it had always seemed to her when
> with a little squeak of the hinges, which she could hear now, she had
> burst open the French windows, and plunged at Bourton into the open
> air. How fresh, how calm, stiller than this of course, the air was in the
> early morning; like the flap of a wave, the kiss of a wave; chill and sharp
> and yet (for a girl of eighteen as she then was) solemn, feeling as she did,
> standing there at the open window, that something awful was about to
> happen. . .

Finally, there is a kind of narrative discourse which is neither author's
speech nor the imitation of a character's speech nor a fusion of the two, but an
imitation of or allusion to another discourse, spoken or written, that has no
source within the text itself. The Russian literary theorist Mikhail Bakhtin[7]
called this 'doubly-oriented discourse', since it refers simultaneously to
something in the world and to another discourse about that thing. The most
obvious example is the use of parody in narrative. In *Joseph Andrews* (1742),
for example, Henry Fielding[8] renders absurd the attempt of the ill-favoured,
middle-aged Mrs Slipslop to engage the handsome young footman Joseph in
lovemaking, by describing it in language borrowed from classical and neo-
classical epic poetry:

> As when a hungry tigress, who long has traversed the woods in fruitless
> search, sees within the reach of her claws a lamb, she prepares to leap on
> her prey; or as a voracious pike, of immense size, surveys through the
> liquid element a roach or gudgeon, which cannot escape her jaws, opens
> them wide to swallow the little fish; so did Mrs Slipslop prepare to lay her
> violent amorous hands on the poor Joseph. . .

To judge these similes primarily by their visual appropriateness would be to
miss the point.

Point of view in narration

I have suggested that literary narrative is composed of different types of discourse, combined, alternated and fused in various ways. It is through the manipulation of these discourses that the novelist controls what is known as 'point of view' in criticism of the novel. The term is a somewhat vague and misleading one. It is a visual metaphor, but the phenomenon it refers to is not wholly a matter of visible appearances. Point of view is the position from which the action of a story is perceived and presented. This is a crucially important decision by the writer. For example, a story of adultery will affect us quite differently, and will have a different meaning, according to whether it is presented primarily or exclusively from the point of view of the guilty party, the innocent party, or the third party; but point of view here implies emotional, moral, psychological as well as visual experience – perhaps the visual is least important. Furthermore, in literary narrative, every seeing is a saying – what is visually perceived is mediated to us through the non-visual (i.e. non-iconic) medium of words. The adultery story might be told in the first person by one of the characters in a mode of persuasive special pleading, or told by the narrator from the same character's perceptual point of view but in a coolly ironic style that prevents the reader's sympathetic identification with the character.

It may seem that I am denying or minimising the importance of the visual image in literary narrative. In a sense this is true. The construction and reception of narrative depend on the concepts of time and causality, neither of which are essentially visual. Narrative organises time, the visual image organises space. When space is described in a narrative text – as in the description of a landscape, a street or a person's physical appearance – the narrative *qua* narrative stops, because the chronological progress of the action is arrested.

Does this mean that visual images play no significant part in our experience of literary narrative? No, of course not, because literary narratives of any sophistication contain more than just narrative, more than just the opening and closing of possibilities for the characters. The 19th and 20th century novel in particular is notable for the amount of description it contains of the visible world. In the 18th century novel descriptions of landscape, townscape, people's physical appearance, dress etc, are either conspicuous by their absence or highly conventionalised. From Sir Walter Scott onwards, however, novelists became lavish in detailed descriptions of such things. This was probably due firstly to the romantic movement, which stressed the creative nature of human perception in its apprehension of the natural world,

and secondly to the development of sociology and anthropology with their
awareness of the influence of environment on human behaviour. Reading
the 19th and 20th century novel, one is constantly required to *visualise* the
action, by responding to the verbal cues of the text. 'My task which I am
trying to achieve', Joseph Conrad[9] wrote at the turn of the last century, 'is, by
the power of the written word to make you hear, to make you feel – it is, before
all, to make you *see*.'

Description in narrative

How does the novelist make us see? Partly by appealing to the reader's
knowledge of the way pictorial art organises and structures space. The 19th
century novel is full of painterly descriptions of landscape. Thomas Hardy
often refers to specific painters or schools of painting to convey the visual
effect he has in mind. At the beginning of *The Woodlanders*[10], for instance, the
barber Percombe observes the country girl Marty South making spars for
thatching in her woodland hut by the light of a fire. He has come to buy her
beautiful chestnut hair:

> In her present beholder's mind the scene formed by the girlish spar-maker
> composed itself into an impression-picture of extremest type, wherein the
> girl's hair alone, as the focus of observation, was depicted with intensity
> and distinctness, while her face, shoulders, hands and figure in general
> were a blurred mass of unimportant detail lost in haze and obscurity.

More recently novelists have been influenced by the cinema in their presentation of physical space. When Christopher Isherwood says 'I am a camera' at
the beginning of *Goodbye to Berlin*, it was evidently a movie camera he was
thinking of. In another place[11] he wrote:

> I [have] always been fascinated by films . . . I was, and still am, endlessly
> interested in the outward appearance of people, their infinitely various
> ways of eating a sausage, opening a paper parcel, lighting a cigarette. The
> cinema puts people under a microscope . . . if you are a novelist and want
> to watch your scene taking place visibly before you, it is simplest to
> project it on to an imaginary screen. A practised cinema-goer will be able
> to do this quite easily.

Interestingly enough, 19th century novelists often anticipated the techniques of the cinema in tracking their characters through space and height-
ening the perception of that space. This suggests that there is a deep

structural similarity between prose narration and film narration. Hardy is full of cinematic effects – aerial shots, zoom effects, telescopic views. Or consider this passage from George Eliot's first story[12], '*The Sad Misfortunes of Amos Barton*', about a country curate, first published in 1857:

> Look at him as he winds through the little churchyard. The silver light that falls aslant on church and tomb, enables you to see his slim, black figure, made all the slimmer by tight pantaloons, as it flits past the pale gravestones. He walks with a quick step, and is now rapping with sharp decision at the vicarage door. It is opened without delay by the nurse, cook and housemaid all at once – that is to say by the robust maid of all work, Nanny; and as Mr Barton hangs up his hat in the passage, you see that a narrow face of no particular complexion – even the smallpox that has attacked it seems to have been of a mongrel, indefinite kind – with features of no particular shape, and an eye of no particular expression, is surmounted by a slope of baldness gently rising from brow to crown. You judge him to be about forty. . .

Change George Eliot's 'you' to 'we' and the passage would read very much like a film scenario. The description breaks down readily into a sequence of cinematic shots: *high-angle crane shot of Barton walking through churchyard; cut to door of vicarage opened by Nanny; close-up of Barton's face as he hangs up his hat*, and so on. In a way, the passage needs the cinema for its full realisation. The charmless but human ordinariness of Barton's face is something the cinema can convey easily and effectively, whereas George Eliot can only gesture towards it by means of negatives: *no particular complexion, no particular shape*. . . Barton's appearance is evoked for us in remarkably few particulars – his slimness, his pantaloons (a period touch, for George Eliot's readers as well as ourselves, since the story is set some thirty years before the time of writing), his quick and decisive movements, his smallpox scars (another period touch perhaps) and baldness.

All perception and representation is necessarily selective, but this is especially true of verbal description. 'No author worth his salt will ever attempt to set the *whole* picture before his reader's eyes', says Wolfgang Iser[13]. 'It is the unwritten part [of the text] that gives us the opportunity to picture things; indeed without the element of indeterminacy, the gaps in the text, we should not be able to use our imaginations.' Conversely, the more detailed a verbal description, the more difficulty the reader is likely to experience in synthesising the details into a composite image, because what would be simultaneously present in space is experienced sequentially in the linear medium of language. Flaubert[14] exploits this face in his famous description of Charles Bovary's cap:

> His was one of those composite pieces of headgear in which you may trace features of bearskin, lancer-cap and bowler, night-cap and otterskin: one of those pathetic objects that are deeply expressive in their dumb ugliness, like an idiot's face. An oval splayed out with whale-bone, it started off with three pompons; these were followed by lozenges of velvet and rabbit's fur alternately, separated by a red band, and after that came a kind of bag ending in a polygon of cardboard with intricate braiding on it; and from this there hung down like a tassel, at the end of a long, too slender cord, a little sheaf of gold threads.

I quote from the translation of Alan Russell in the Penguin edition. One might quibble with parts of the translation, but in truth the description is as difficult to translate as it would be to draw. Flaubert has given us more detail than we can accommodate in a single mental image. He has narrativised the hat – the description proceeds by a series of verbs and adverbial phrases of time – *it started off, these were followed by, after that came, ending in* – but when we come to the last detail we have forgotten the precise nature and disposition of the earlier details. Flaubert thus mimes the absurd heterogeneity and meaningless vulgarity of the cap by his incomprehensible description of it. The significance of the cap is conveyed not by its detailed specification, but by the metaphorical trope which compares it cruelly to an idiot's face.

Metaphoric and metonymic description in narrative

Description in verbal narrative is always a kind of troping. The report of brute, literal facts that signify nothing but themselves have no place in literary narrative. A trope is a figurative expression, a non-logical way of referring to something which has the effect of defamiliarising it, making it more vivid or emotionally loaded or thematically relevant than it would be in a simple literal reference. According to Renaissance rhetoricians, the four master tropes were metaphor, metonymy, synecdoche and irony. Modern linguistics and poetics, notably in the person of the late Roman Jakobson, have put irony, which is a matter of interpretation and cannot be described linguistically, to one side and opposed metaphor to metonymy as the two master tropes, synecdoche being a subclass of metonymy, as simile is a subclass of metaphor. Metaphor and metonymy are in fact manipulations of two processes that are basic to language, and perhaps to all perception and representation – selection and combination[15]. To construct a literal sentence like 'Ship crossed the sea', we select the words we need from the paradigms of the language and combine them according to the syntactical rules of the language – in English, subject-verb-object. A figurative transformation of this sentence might be, 'Keels ploughed the deep'. In substituting *ploughed* for crossed, we have produced a metaphor based on a perceived similarity between two things otherwise different – the movement of a ship through the water and the movement of a plough through the earth. In substituting *keels* for *ships*, we have used synecdoche – part standing for whole; in substituting *deep* for *sea* we have used metonymy – an attribute of the thing standing for the thing itself. Metaphor is derived from similarity; metonymy and synecdoche from contiguity. As soon as discourse deviates from strictly literal, denotative reference, it will tend to do so either in the form of metaphor and simile, or in the form of metonymy and synecdoche. Likewise, discourse tends to link one topic to another either according to similarity or contiguity, and types of discourses can be characterised according to which principle is dominant.

Description of the perceptual world in literary narratives tends to follow the metonymic path, since narrative itself is metonymic in structure, tracing a chain of events that are contiguous in space-time. Realistic fiction in particular evokes the appearance and quality of persons or places by a selection of synecdochic or metonymic details which stand as it were for the totality of items that would have been present in actuality. We see this exemplified, for instance, in George Eliot's description of Amos Barton – his pantaloons, his baldness, his smallpox scars. Metaphor is, however, often used in descriptive passages in order to convey a particular emotional or thematic colouring. The metaphorical expressions in the passage from Martin Amis's *Money* (e.g. 'You are a bank rat on a busy river') or Virginia Woolf's *Mrs Dalloway* ('like the flap of a wave, the kiss of a wave') are as expressive of the characters' sensibilities as they are of the things referred to. In the Virginia Woolf passage it is notable that the discourse actually *proceeds* by a series of metaphorical associations, associations of similarity. For this reason she is often called a poetic or lyric novelist.

Even in realistic narrative, however, the metonymic and synecdochic details, by the very fact of being selected, call attention to themselves, and begin to generate additional meaning by the process of connotation and by their interaction with each other. Connotation is the process by which one signified acts as the signifier of another signified, and it can itself be either metonymic – based on contiguity – or metaphoric – based on similarity. Consider the opening paragraph of Graham Greene's *The Heart of the Matter*[16]:

> Wilson sat on the balcony of the Bedford Hotel with his bald pink knees
> thrust against the ironwork. It was Sunday and the Cathedral bell
> clanged for matins. On the other side of Bond Street, in the windows of the
> High School, sat the young negresses in dark blue gym smocks engaged
> on the interminable task of trying to wave their wirespring hair. Wilson
> stroked his very young moustache and dreamed, waiting for his gin and
> bitters.

The basic technique of this passage is metonymic and synecdochic. There are
some vivid visual images, but they are highly selective, only a fraction of the
totality that would have been there in actuality. The hotel is represented
simply by its ironwork balcony and its very ordinary name. Wilson is
represented simply by his very ordinary name, his knees and his moustache.
The young negresses are represented by their gym smocks and wirespring
hair. The town is represented by the Cathedral, the High School, the name
Bond Street. There is, of course, some incongruity among these metonymic
and synecdochic details – the names and institutions all belong to England,
but the negresses and Wilson's pink knees (implying that he is wearing
shorts) to the tropics. The narrative is, in fact, set in West Africa, though we
are made to infer this before we are explicitly informed of it. The work of
inference emphasises the contrasts and contradictions of colonialism, the
superimposition of European values and institutions on African culture, and
the rather sad emulation of European culture by the Africans. Hair becomes a
kind of leitmotif in the communication of this theme. The epithets *bald* applied
to Wilson's knees and *young* applied to his moustache are faintly metaphorical, since we do not expect knees to be covered with hair, or customarily refer
to a moustache by its age. (Compare Amos Barton's baldness, a literal
metonymic index of his age and careworn existence.) Wilson's lack of or
difficulty in growing hair symbolises his callowness, weakness, out-of-
placeness metaphorically as well as metonymically, and is thus contrasted
with the negresses' wirespring hair which symbolises the instinctual vitality
and energy they are trying to tame. In the image of Wilson's bald pink knees
thrust against the ironwork of the balcony we have another metaphorical
symbol of the repression of instinct by the colonial ethos. The linguistically
invisible but all-pervasive trope in this passage is irony.

The passage shows how deceptive the term 'point of view' is. To say that it
is written from Wilson's point of view would be understandable but misleading. Another Russian theorist, Boris Uspensky[17], has proposed that there are
four planes in every narrative statement – the spatio-temporal, the psychological (i.e. whether subjective or objective), the phraseological and the
ideological, and that these planes may be distributed between the narrator

and the character in any combination. The spatio-temporal perspective of Greene's opening paragraph is certainly Wilson's. But Wilson is not so much the subject of this passage as one of its objects. He is described from outside, without access to his inner thoughts, such as we read in the passages by Martin Amis and Virginia Woolf. The phraseology of the passage is the authorial narrator's – Wilson would not think of his knees as 'bald' and his moustache as 'young' – and the ideological implications of the passage – that colonialism sets culture and nature at war – are also the authorial narrator's, not Wilson's.

Graham Greene is often described as a cinematic novelist, and has indeed written several highly successful film scenarios; but other people's adaptations of his novels for the screen have rarely been successful, and the reason may be that much of the meaning of his novels, as of most novels, is untranslatable into visual images. The motion picture camera could show us Wilson's knees thrust against the ironwork balcony, but could not describe them as 'bald', with all the connotations and cross-references within the passage that word sets off.

Conclusion

It is the multilayeredness, the polysemy inherent in language that makes it such a resourceful medium for description in narrative. The cinema, and other visual arts, can do more immediate justice to the visible world, but cannot match the power of language to *mean*.

10

Animal language

JOHN KREBS

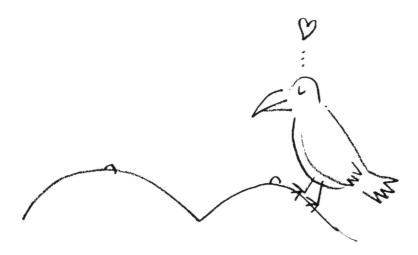

Introduction

Those of you who have watched animals will have seen, heard, smelled, or felt animals communicating – robins singing in the back garden, dogs scent-marking a lampost, peacocks showing off their extraordinary tails (Fig. 10.1). These are conspicuous acts of communication; more subtle are the electric signals generated by some species of fish that live in muddy water where visibility is low, and the rhythms of vibration tapped out by certain male spiders before they step on to the web of the predatory female. The fact that animals communicate to one another, usually but not invariably to members of their own species, in a great variety of ways, by means of special behaviour patterns or structures (called *signals* or *displays*), is familiar enough to need no elaboration. But if we wish to look at the nature of animal communication in more detail, we need to ask questions both about the structure of animal language – is there a vocabulary, grammar and so on, and the function of animal language – what kinds of messages are communicated when animals sing, wave, or vibrate at each other?

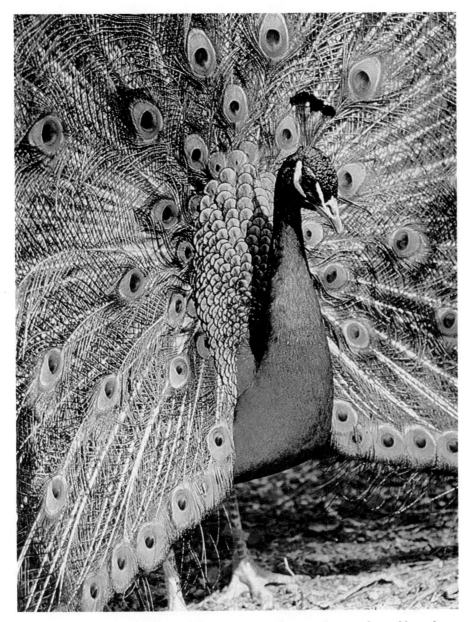

Fig. 10.1. The elaborate tail display of the male peacock poses the problem of
how and why elaborate signals used by animals evolve.

Finding out what signals mean: bird song

Rather than try to answer these questions in abstract terms, I am going to
start off by describing how one might go about investigating the function of

animal language by taking a particular example, bird song. What do birds say to each other when they sing?

First, a bit of background. Birds make lots of different sounds, but the term 'song', refers only to the loud, complex sounds made, primarily by males, during certain times of year, especially the breeding season. Song, as defined in these terms, is distinct from sounds such as alarm calls given when the bird is fleeing from a predator, and the begging calls of nestlings. The fact that song is a male vocalisation produced in the breeding season has suggested to many observers of bird behaviour that song serves two functions: it may repel other males, or it may attract a mate. These suggestions arise because males of many bird species are highly territorial in the breeding season and they often obtain a mate at the same time. I am going to describe an experiment that looks at the first of these putative functions; it asks whether song is part of an individual's battery of defences against intruders into its territory. How can we test this idea?

Studies of the song of a common garden and woodland bird, the great tit have helped to solve this problem. Pairs of great tits in deciduous woodland live in and defend a territory of about 1 hectare in the spring – from February until June in southern England. Simply by watching where individuals forage, sing and fight with neighbours, one can easily establish the territorial boundaries of a pair of birds. (To aid identification of individuals, each bird is marked with a little coloured plastic leg ring.) By doing this one discovers that in early February, when territories are set up, suitable breeding habitat rapidly fills up and space, like student housing in Oxford, is in short supply. Some individuals are excluded altogether. These birds either settle for a territory in a suboptimal habitat (for example farmland) or they are chased from territory to territory in the good, woodland, habitats. In either case they are constantly on the lookout for a vacancy: when a territory-owning pair dies, disappears, or is removed by an experimenter, replacements immediately move in. It is rather like the situation on a crowded beach in the summer: when you leave your prime spot on the beach for a few minutes someone else will soon put their towel down in 'your' spot. Territorial replacements in the great tit do not take place quite so rapidly, but often the new pair turns up within a few hours and starts to defend the empty area. This shows that intruders must test frequently to see if the former owner has disappeared.

The fact that there is continual pressure on territories from intruders provides a chance to ask whether the song of the territory-owning males is part of their armoury of defence, whether it actually acts as a 'keep out' signal to deter potential invaders. The experimental procedure is very simple: by removing birds from their territories and occupying the empty spaces with loudspeakers broadcasting great tit song, one can find out whether or not song will keep out intruders. Once the territory boundaries in a study area have been measured by following the individually colour-ringed birds around, and plotting their movements on a large-scale map, the study area is divided into three sections designated 'no sound', 'song', and 'control sound'. Then on one morning in the early spring, all the birds in the study area are captured and removed from their territories. In the 'no sound' area, territories are left silent; in the 'song' area a set of loudspeakers broadcasts the song of the bird that has just been removed, mimicking the natural pattern of singing in different parts of the territory at different times; in the third area a 'control' sound of similar volume and duration to tit song is played. This sound was a two-note phrase played on a tin whistle. Having set the experiment in motion, the whole area was monitored continuously from dawn until dusk every day to see where and when the newcomers settled. The result was that they settled first in the silent and sound control areas, and only after a delay of about three days did they gradually creep into the song-occupied area. In other words, song does indeed act as a deterrent: it is a form of 'keep out' signal[1].

The general point illustrated by this example is that animal signals usually convey simple messages about immediate events: 'keep out', 'I am a male', 'I am individual A' and so on. The song of the great tit is a relatively simple, two-note sound, but even very elaborate signals like the peacock's tail we saw earlier appear to operate in essentially the same way. But if this is all there is to animal language, how can we account for the apparent complexity and elaboration of many signals?

Complexity

Complexity and elaboration are striking in many kinds of animal signals: for example the display of the argus pheasant and the song of the nightingale. What is the complexity for? The answer lies in understanding how animal signals have evolved, how they started off and how they have been modified through evolutionary time by the Darwinian process of evolution by natural selection. In order to explain what I mean I have to go back to some basic definitions.

In a communicatory interaction there are two roles, *actor* and *reactor*. An individual may play either role at different points in a sequence of interactions, but it is always one or the other. Very often the actor and reactor do not share a common interest[2] in the outcome of the interaction. For example with the great tits I described earlier, the territory owner probably gains more benefit (measured in the Darwinian units of 'fitness' – survival and reproduction) when the intruder retreats from a song than does the intruder itself. In fact we could *define* signals as behaviour patterns used by actors to manipulate the behaviour of reactors to the advantage of the actor. Given such an asymmetry of benefit, one might well ask why reactors take any notice of signals at all. Why are they susceptible to manipulation? To understand this, we have to think back through evolutionary time to how signals might have originated. Imagine that in some ancestral state there was no communication at all. Even in this state animals must have interacted with one another in ways such that the behaviour of one individual, A, had effects on the survival of another, B. (For example a large A might have moved towards a small B and squashed it flat!) At this stage, any ability, however slight, of B to anticipate the future actions of A would be beneficial to B and therefore be favoured during the course of evolution. (An example from human behaviour of this kind of advantageous anticipation is seen in the boxing ring. High-speed film analysis of Muhammed Ali's left jab showed that about half of his jabs were of shorter duration than the human visual reaction time, but nevertheless his opponents managed to avoid most of them – they must have taken evasive action before the jab started[3]. In this human example the ability to anticipate is learned during the career of an individual boxer, but when I talk about animal signals and anticipation, I am talking about an ability that evolves over generations by the genetic analogue of learning, natural selection.)

Natural selection for the ability to anticipate the actions of others sets the stage for the evolution of signals. Imagine a hypothetical sequence of evolution of tooth baring as a threat display in dogs[4]. The sequence might have involved the following steps. (1) (a) A and B interact by A biting B, (b) B evolves the ability to anticipate the ensuing bite of A by noting that A's teeth are bared. B takes evasive action by retreating and escaping injury. This is to B's advantage. (2) Because B always takes evasive action from bared teeth, tooth baring is in effect a threat signal in the early stages of its evolution. The stage is now set for A to turn the situation to *its* advantage: it can force B to take evasive action simply by the threat signal of bared teeth. A now manipulates B's behaviour in a way that is advantageous to A but not necessarily to B. *Note that the susceptibility of B to being manipulated stems from the fact that the signal originated because of the advantage gained by B from responding.* (3) We can take the hypothetical sequence of evolution a stage further, and in doing so we reach the point of explaining how complexity and elaboration of signals came about. Given that the signal is used by A to manipulate the behaviour of B, we would expect 'sales-resistance' to evolve; B should ignore the manipulative signal, or at least become less sensitive to it.

The evolutionary counterploy to this is for A to increase the persuasive power of the signal by, for example, exaggeration, elaboration, repetition and any other device that might overcome sales-resistance. In short an *evolutionary arms race* between sales-resistance and persuasion develops. This is the explanation of how animal signals become elaborated. More elaborate signals do not necessarily carry more elaborate messages, they are simply more persuasive. One can draw an analogy with advertising. TV commercials go to extraordinary lengths and complexities to persuade viewers to wear Levi jeans, to drink Guinness or spread butter. The message is simple and could be stated in two or three words; all the rest is pure persuasion. Both animal signals and human advertisements are products of persuasion, sales-resistance, and arms races, and in both cases elaboration of the display has nothing to do with elaboration of the message. (It is worth emphasising again that a major difference between arms race in human and animal advertising is that the latter takes place over evolutionary time and the former within a lifetime.)

The analogy with advertising is not only useful in explaining how elaboration can come about through an arms race between sales-resistance and persuasion, it also brings home the message that persuasion is powerful. You can be persuaded by the psychological manipulation of advertisements to do things that are against your interests because they can kill you: smoke

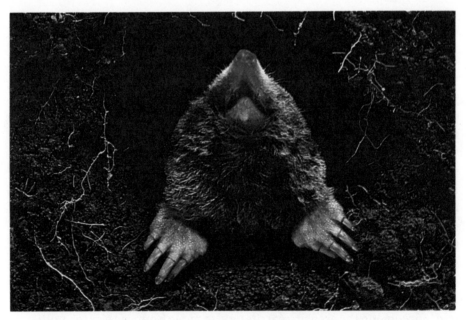

Fig. 10.2. Advertisements (in contrast to animal signals) often bear little iconic resemblance to the goods they advertise. In this sense they are more arbitrary than the advertising signals of animals. This picture advertises British Gas.

cigarettes, lie in the sun or drink a lot of alcohol, so you should not be surprised to see individuals of other species succumbing to similar manipulative signals from their fellows. The fact that manipulator and victim are roles that can be played by the same individual at different times does not detract from the argument. Although I know of no evidence on the matter, I would be surprised to find that those who design advertisements are less susceptible to manipulation by advertisements than is the rest of the population.

One important point of difference between animal signals and advertisements lies in the arbitrariness of the latter. It is often difficult to tell just by looking at an advertisement what the product is. Here are some examples to make the point. Fish to advertise office equipment, a tap for cigarettes, a mole for gas (Fig. 10.2), fingers for milk, music for a computer data base. Of course these images are in a sense not totally arbitrary – someone has thought out very carefully what kind of visual image will conjure up the right response in the reader – but they are less closely tied to 'real' message than are animal signals. Because of their evolutionary origins, animal signals, however distorted or exaggerated they become through the evolutionary arms race, must have started off as actions that predicted something of the actor's future behaviour: in this sense they are not arbitrary (for further discussion see Margaret Deuchar 'Are the signs of language arbitrary?' p.168).

Evidence for the role of elaboration

Although one cannot test the hypothetical evolutionary pathway that I outlined in the previous section, one can ask whether or not exaggeration and elaboration increases the effectiveness of present day signals as persuaders. Referring back to the example with which I started, the song of the great tit, it appears that complexity does indeed enhance the effectiveness of the signal. Although the basic song of the great tit is very simple, each male has a repertoire of different 'song types'. The different types are used by the male interchangeably – they do not appear to carry different kinds of message. However, when territories occupied by loudspeakers playing a repertoire of songs are compared with territories occupied by a single song, it is found that the intruders are more effectively deterred by a repertoire than by a single song. Complexity *per se* seems to enhance the effectiveness of the signal. Perhaps intruders find a repertoire of song types more intimidating than a single song because the repertoire persuades the listener that more than one bird is occupying the area[5]. Great tits tend to move from one tree to another as they switch song types, a ploy that to the human observer enhances the deception. This idea has been termed the 'Beau Geste' effect, after the hero of

P.C. Wren's novel of the same name who defended a fortress single-handed by simulating the presence of a defending army, using guns propped up over the walls of the fort and firing shots from different parts of the ramparts.

Some of the most elaborate displays of all are those involved in sexual reproduction, in particular those used by the male to attract a female. The bowerbirds of Australasia are an especially remarkable group. The birds themselves are on the whole not very conspicuous, but the males display by building complex and meticulously constructed buildings called 'bowers'. Bowers vary from species to species in shape and construction, but they often consist of a structure built out of twigs and leaves, which is then decorated with objects such as flowers, leaves, shells and feathers, according to species. The male satin bowerbird (Fig. 10.3), the most intensively studied species[6], builds a bower consisting of two rows of vertical twigs formed into an alleyway, the entrance to which is decorated with blue feathers, yellow leaves, snail shells and insect skins. Near camp sites the bowerbirds add various items of human debris such as clothes pegs, Foster's beer cans and toothbrushes (Fig. 10.4) to their decorations.

Males defend territories that include their bower, and when a female comes close to the bower she is courted, and if the male is successful mating takes place inside the bower. By filming the activities at a number of bowers over a mating season Gerald Borgia showed that different males have very different degrees of success: the most successful male mated 30 times, the least successful not at all. Mating success is directly related to bower quality. Successful males have more decorations and better constructed bowers than their less successful rivals. By shifting decorations from one bower to another it was possible to manipulate mating success experimentally and demonstrate a cause/effect relationship. How do the differences in bower quality come about? By placing individually marked feathers in a bower, it was discovered that males steal each other's decorations. The film records show that they also sometimes come and destroy each other's bowers. The upshot of this is that bower quality, the number of decorations and the quality of the construction, reflect a combination of a male's ability to filch from others and to keep rivals away. In other words, differences in overall bower quality are like a readout of the differences in male ability to defend and steal. In terms of our general points about animal language, the bower bird studies show both that complexity enhances the effectiveness of a signal and the elaborate signal is not arbitrary, but reflects differences in the quality of actors.

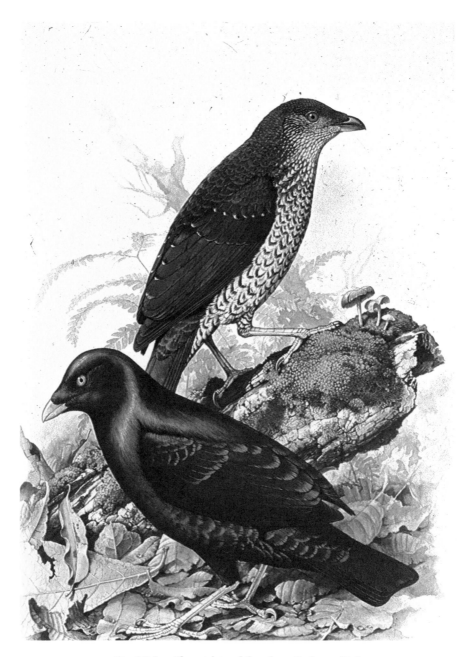

Fig. 10.3.   The male and female satin bowerbird.

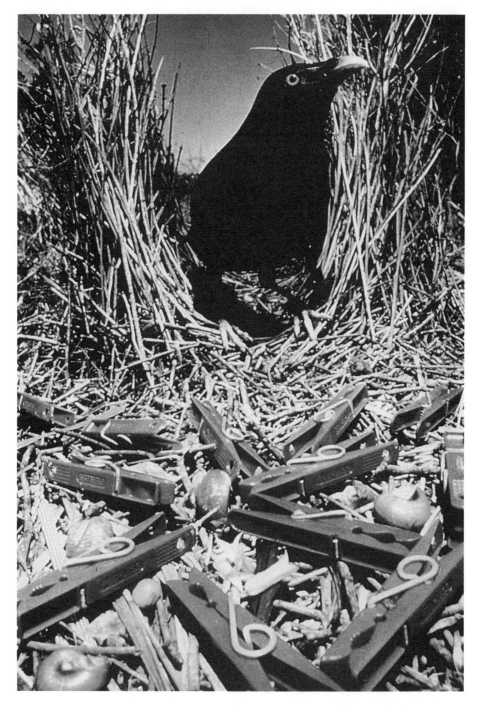

Fig. 10.4.   The male satin bowerbird builds a bower of vertical twigs and decorates it with blue objects. Here he has used clothes pegs. Females prefer to mate with males that have elaborately decorated bowers.

Language and awareness

One of the characteristics of human communication is that people are usually aware of what they are communicating about. They may have mental images of the objects; feelings they describe in words; they may use words to talk about events that have not actually happened or that may happen in the future. They may also, as I am doing, describe their awareness of what they are communicating. Is there evidence for even primordial states of awareness in animal language? Given the fact that our cognitive abilities in general are derived from those of our non-human ancestors, one ought to be able to recognise some of the characteristics of human language, albeit in primitive, undeveloped form, amongst animals. As Daniel Dennett has put it, we should be able to recognise *intentionality* in animal communication[7]. Yet the picture I have presented up to now is one in which animal language consists of automaton-like knee-jerk responses to stereotyped signals. It is of course very hard to find out about how aware animals are of their language, because by its nature the question is most easily accessible by introspection and by using human language to interrogate others. The best one can do is to seek instances which suggest a greater degree of flexibility in the use of language than one might have postulated on the basis of examples described so far[8].

An intriguing case of communication that *may* be an example indicating more than knee-jerk responses is that of an African bird, the greater honeyguide. The honeyguide is an extraordinary bird in several respects: it is a brood parasite (like the cuckoo it lays its eggs in the nests of other species), it can live on beeswax (it has micro-organisms in its gut to digest the wax) and it is heavily dependent on a commensal relationship with man to obtain its food.

The honeyguide's staple food is the wax, honey and larvae of wild bees' nests. Although the bird is adept at consuming the contents of a bees' nest, its feeding is often limited by its ability to gain access to nests. Nests are often located inside hollow trees and are always well defended by bees that are ready to sting an intruder. The honeyguide gets around this difficulty by literally calling on man to help. Man is a willing helper because for him, unlike the bird, the limiting step in harvesting honey from wild nests is finding the nests in the first place and not gaining access to the nest once found. Thus the relationship between bird and man is symbiotic: the bird provides its searching skills and man his brute force to get into the tree to open up the nest.

Honeyguides (the origin of their name should now be apparent!) have been studied in Northern Kenya by Hussein Isack[9]. Here the nomadic Boran people use honeyguides when they go out to collect honey. An interaction may be initiated either by the bird, by flying up to a man and making a persistent 'tirr tirr' call, or by a honey hunter going out into the woods and making a special whistle (called *Fuulido* in Boran language) with clasped fists, a modified snail shell or a palm nut. Other kinds of noise such as shouting or knocking on wood may also be used to attract the birds. Once a honeyguide has found a honey hunter it starts to lead him towards a bees' nest by flying in short flights and perching every few metres to give the guiding call. The bird sets off again when the follower catches up, and repeats the process until it reaches the nest. The bird signals the presence of the nest by changing to another call, and then it waits silently whilst the honey hunter looks for the nest. If the hunter, accidentally or deliberately, walks away from the nest, the bird will set off in front of the honey hunter and then fly in a loop back to the nest as if trying to lead him back. This may be repeated several times, until eventually the bird gives up and leads the honey hunter to another nest, a fact which is used by honey hunters to get the bird to guide them to more than one nest in a day. Some idea of the time saved for the honey hunter is given by the fact that the estimated average time to find a nest without a honeyguide is about nine hours, but with a honeyguide the time is reduced to three hours. This three hours includes the time taken to find a honeyguide and the time spent following the bird to the nest. The duration of the actual guiding is about 15 min and the average distance covered is betweeen 0.2 and 1.2 km.

It is tempting to conclude immediately that the honeyguide must be aware of what it is doing: it not only gives a special signal to lead a honey hunter in an apparently purposeful way to a site that is some distance way, but it also shows the flexibility to modify continually its behaviour as it goes along, for example by leading the man back to the nest if he strays in the wrong direction. However, one has to be careful in jumping to hasty conclusions, since even quite complex signalling interactions, which give the appearance of cognition, may be produced by automaton-like responses. Let me give one final example to illustrate this point.

Fireflies attract their sexual partners by flashing in the dark. Each species has its own particular morse code – a sequence of flashes of characteristic duration and intensity with characteristic intervals between flashes (Fig. 10.5). In one species that has been studied in detail, called *Photinus pyralis*, the male gives two short flashes separated by a six-second interval. The female responds with a flash two seconds after the male's second flash; the male flies towards the female and repeats his signal. The interaction goes on until the male arrives at the female or loses track of her position. It is hard work being an ardent male firefly. Jim Lloyd[10] estimates that the average male takes seven nights, five miles and 4000 flashes to get a single female (in contrast it takes an average female six minutes to get a male!). Not only is it

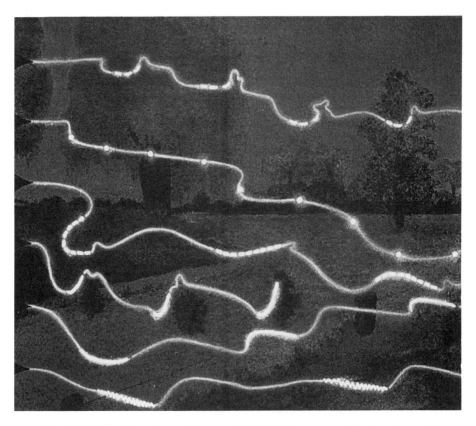

Fig. 10.5. The lines show schematically the flight paths and flash patterns of several species of firefly in Florida. Each species has its own flashing code, but some species prey on others by mimicking the flash code of females and luring males to their death.

hard work, but it is also dangerous work being a male *Photinus*. Females of another species of firefly, *Photuris*, are predators on male *Photinus* and they lure their victims to their death by mimicking the flash response of the female *Photinus*. This, however, is not the end of the story. Males of the predatory *Photuris* species also get in on the act. They sometimes mimic the male flash pattern of the prey species, so that when the female predator flashes to attract a putative victim, it sometimes turns out that the male on the other end of the line is one of her own species ready to mate! Here then is a complex set of signalling interactions involving deception and counterdeception with a similar appearance of 'purposiveness' as the honeyguides' interaction with man. Yet no one would seriously ascribe the attribute of awareness to fireflies.

So is there any basis on which to distinguish the honeyguide case from the firefly case? I think an essential difference is that the firefly interactions *rely* on the fact that the actors and reactors behave in a fixed automaton-like way, whilst the honeyguide – honey hunter interaction relies on flexibility, continual adjustment of behaviour by both partners, for its success. Whether this is sufficient evidence for conclusions about awareness is beyond the scope of this chapter.

Summary

Animals communicate by means of stereotyped behaviours or structure called signals. Signals generally convey simple messages about immediate events associated with the signaller and they are not arbitrary in the sense that they are derived from evolutionarily ancestral behaviours that allowed reactors to predict the behaviour of actors. The elaboration and complexity of animal signals can be understood in terms of an evolutionary race between manipulative actors and sales-resistance reactors. Given the fact of evolutionary continuity, animal language must show in embryonic form some of the characteristics of human communication. The difficulty in inferring the existence of one such property, awareness about the communication system, is illustrated by the seemingly purposeful use of signals by the honeyguide.

11

Are the signs of language arbitrary?

MARGARET DEUCHAR

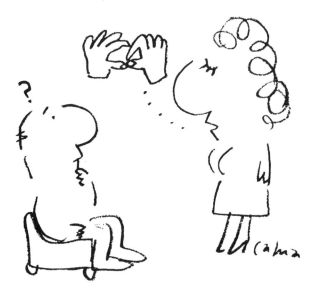

Introduction

Linguists of the twentieth century take it for granted that language is basically arbitrary, that is, there is an arbitrary relationship between the words of language and what they represent. In this chapter[1] I want to use an unusual form of language, the sign language of the deaf, to look again at our ideas about arbitrariness. I shall suggest that 20th century linguists are wrong in putting so much emphasis on this characteristic, and that in doing so they have ignored the important role of the users of a language.

Twentieth century structural linguistics

Although there have been debates since the time of the Greeks about the relation between words and their meanings, 20th century linguists often assume that the question was settled once and for all by the famous linguist Ferdinand de Saussure, who gave a course in general linguistics at the University of Geneva between 1906 and 1911. His course was published as a book after his death by two of his students², and the influence of the ideas contained in it has been so great that he is considered to be the founder of modern linguistics.

Modern linguistics is often described as structural (or even 'structuralist') because of the way in which language is viewed as a structure or system. Saussure contributed to this view in his description of language as a system of signs. By 'sign' Saussure meant a unit of language roughly equivalent to a word, but consisting of two related facets, a concept and a sound-image. The sound-image and the concept were referred to more technically by the terms 'signifier' and 'signified'. Saussure illustrated his view of a sign as in Fig. 11.1.

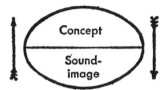

Fig. 11.1.   Saussure's view of the sign. Reprinted by permission from *Course in General Linguistics* by Ferdinand de Saussure, Fontana/Collins 1959.

His famous principle of arbitrariness applies to the relationship between the concept and the sound-image of the sign, which he claimed to be arbitrary. Thus there is no direct relationship, he argued, between a word such as 'tree' and the idea of a tree which it represents. The sequence of sounds in the word 'tree' could equally well be replaced by another sequence, such as 'arbor' (the Latin word), or even, one might add, 'X'. Possible ways of representing the idea of 'tree' are shown in Fig. 11.2.

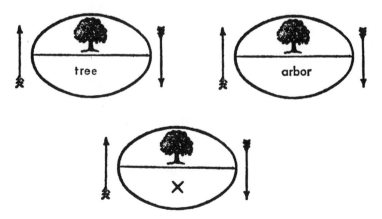

Fig. 11.2.   Ways of representing the idea of 'tree'. Adapted from *Course in General Linguistics* by Ferdinand de Saussure, Fontana/Collins 1959.

One can of course immediately think of words which appear to be an exception to Saussure's arbitrariness principle, which do seem to bear some relationship to what is represented. For example, English words such as 'crash'. 'boom', 'swish', could be said to sound like the sounds they represent, and bird names such as 'cuckoo' and 'peewit' are usually taken to represent the sound characteristically made by these birds. Saussure, however, dismisses onomatopoeic words of this kind as being limited in number, chosen somewhat arbitrarily, and being only conventional imitations of sounds. Later we shall see that if he had focussed on the conventional aspect of these words, he would not have had to dismiss them.

Saussure's principle of the arbitrary nature of the sign has had tremendous influence on 20th century linguistics. The American structural linguist Charles Hockett used arbitrariness in an influential article published in 1960[3] as one of the thirteen design features which he considered could be used to distinguish human languages from animal communication systems. Hockett's understanding of the meaning of 'arbitrary' is in line with Saussure's, though he defines it negatively[4] as meaning the absence of iconicity. This is made clear in the following quotation:

> A symbol means what it does iconically to the extent that it resembles its meaning in physical contours, or to the extent that the whole repertory of symbols in the system show a geometrical similarity to the whole repertory of meanings. To the extent that a symbol or system is not iconic, it is arbitrary.

This quotation shows how the notion 'arbitrary' has come to mean non-iconic rather than having a more positive meaning. If we assume, with both Saussure and Hockett, that arbitrariness is fundamental to language, then we are led to the conclusion that what is iconic is not language.

So what about iconic aspects of language such as onomatopoeia? We have seen that Saussure dismissed these as marginal to language, but what would Saussure have done if confronted with a visual system of language with an apparently higher degree of iconicity than spoken language? Unfortunately he is not here to tell us, but his work has certainly led linguists to assume that iconicity in a language system must raise doubts about whether or not the system can be considered a real language.

Sign languages of the deaf

One of the advances made in linguistics of the second half of the 20th century is that sign languages of the deaf have been studied in detail and recognized as languages in their own right, albeit in a visual medium. It has been known that manual communication systems of the deaf existed ever since they developed in institutions for the deaf established in the 18th and 19th centuries[5], but these were not studied seriously by linguists until this century. Pioneering work was done in the 1960s on American Sign Language (ASL)[6], and was followed by work in the 1970s and 1980s in various European countries including Britain, and in a few countries outside Europe[7].

One of the problems encountered by the first linguists to work on sign language was how to reconcile the apparently iconic aspects of sign languages with the conviction that these were indeed true languages. Taking British Sign Language (BSL) as an example, the signs illustrated in Fig. 11.3 might be said to be iconic to some extent.

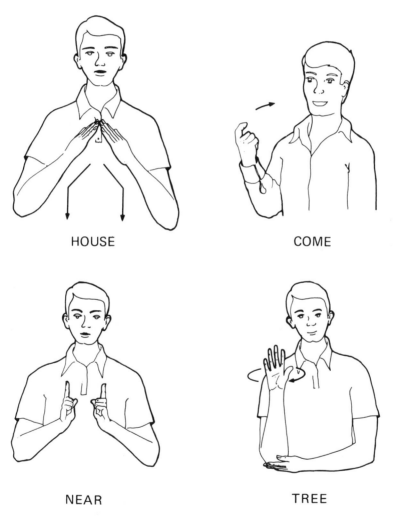

HOUSE   COME

NEAR   TREE

Fig. 11.3.   Iconic signs from British Sign Language. (Based on illustrations in Deuchar 1984, see note 5.)

In all four of the signs illustrated we can see a structural resemblance between the sign itself and what it is supposed to represent. So what did linguists investigating sign language do about this apparent departure from the arbitrariness principle so dear to Saussure's heart? Well, their basic argument was that the iconicity of sign language was less significant than it appeared, rather like Saussure's argument about the insignificance of ono-matopoeia. This argument took various forms, some of which are listed in Table 1.

I shall explain the gist of these arguments one by one.

Table 1. *Arguments against the significance of iconicity in sign language*

1. Not all signs are iconic
2. Iconicity diminishes over time
3. Iconicity has little psychological significance
4. Iconicity is not an all-or-nothing concept
5. The forms of iconic signs are not pre-determined

1 Not all signs are iconic

It is difficult to assess the proportion of signs in a given sign language vocabulary which are iconic, because one's results depend on the type and size of the sample taken. However, research[8] suggests that at least 40% of a vocabulary of basic signs in various sign languages show some degree of iconicity. One might expect more iconicity in a basic vocabulary than in the vocabulary as a whole because of the higher proportion of signs for concrete objects that you would expect in a basic vocabulary. My own research on a sample of 664 signs in ASL revealed that 34% could be said to be iconic, so we could guess that not more than one-third of the sign vocabulary of a particular sign language would be iconic. To make this discussion more concrete, examples of non-iconic signs from BSL are given in Fig. 11.4.

In Hockett's terms these signs would be described as arbitrary precisely because they lack iconicity. Saussure would also describe them as arbitrary because of the lack of a direct relationship between the form of each sign and what it represents. A Saussurean who knew something about Japanese or American Sign Language could also point out that the form of the sign meaning 'good' in BSL actually means 'male' in Japanese sign language, while the form of the sign meaning 'true' in BSL means 'stop' in American Sign Language. We would expect signs of the type illustrated in Fig. 11.4 to make up at least two-thirds of a sign language vocabulary, which means that iconic signs are actually in the minority.

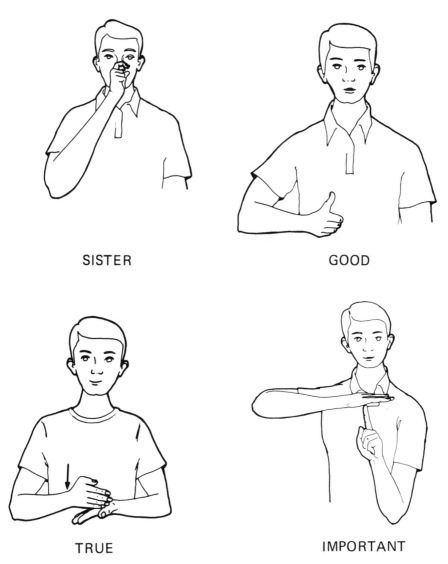

SISTER

GOOD

TRUE

IMPORTANT

Fig. 11.4.   Non-iconic signs from British Sign Language. (Based on illustrations
in Deuchar 1984, see note 5.)

2 Iconicity diminishes over time

This argument has been put most forcefully by the linguist Nancy Frishberg, working on American Sign Language[9]. By comparing older versions of American signs with their modern equivalents, she discovered a general trend for the modern signs to be less iconic than the earlier ones. So, for example, the American sign for TOMATO in 1918 was a combination of that for RED and that for SLICE, each of these two signs being to some extent

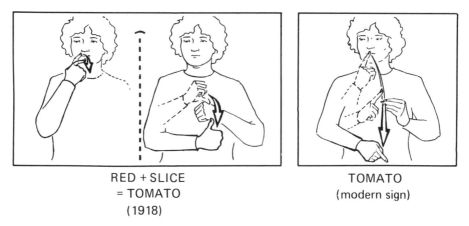

RED + SLICE
= TOMATO
(1918)

TOMATO
(modern sign)

Fig. 11.5. Ancient and modern TOMATO in American Sign Language. Reprinted from *The Signs of Language* by E.S. Klima & U. Bellugi, Harvard University Press 1979, by kind permission of the authors and publishers.

iconic. The modern sign, however, had fused the two parts to such an extent
that it now virtually lacked any trace of iconicity. The older and the more
modern signs are shown in Fig. 11.5.

Frishberg's discovery is supported by other research on spontaneous sign
systems which develop among children: these appear to show a greater
degree of iconicity in the early stages than later, when they have become
more established[10].

3 Iconicity has little psychological significance

This argument can be paraphrased as saying that iconicity does not play an
important role in the psychological aspects of sign language use. These
psychological aspects would include the processes of learning sign language,
and of recognition and memory for signs.

One interesting fact about the learning of sign language by young babies
whose parents sign to them is that the first sign is learned at an earlier average
age than the first word[11]. It has been suggested[12] that this is because the
greater iconicity of signs makes them easier to learn. There is some evidence
that this may be true for those learning sign language as a second language
beyond infancy[12, 13]. However, there is no evidence that I know of to show
that iconicity helps infants learning sign language as a first language[14]. In
fact Bates[15], who has studied the emergence of symbols in infancy, suggests
that the early learning of names for objects is by association rather than by
perception of similarity. Her work leads to the conclusion that an understanding of the nature of the relationship between a name and what it represents

requires an analytical approach which is not found in the earliest stages. We can conclude from this that iconic signs will not be understood to be iconic by infants in the early stages of language acquisition.

A study by Klima & Bellugi on deaf signers' ability to remember a list of signs shown to them on video-tape[16] revealed that when the signers failed to remember signs which were apparently iconic, the mistakes they made suggested that these signs were not stored in memory in an iconic form. Thus mistakes in remembering BIRD, for example, shown in Fig. 11.6, did not give rise to wrong signs which were similar in form and meaning, and also iconic, but instead to signs which were quite similar in form but very different in meaning. One sign remembered instead of BIRD in fact meant 'newspaper', which has a very different meaning. However, as you can see in Fig. 11.6, the sign for 'newspaper' is similar in both handshape and movement to that for 'bird', but it is made on a different part of the body.

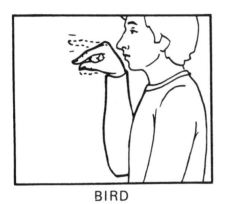 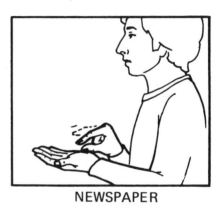

BIRD   NEWSPAPER

Fig. 11.6. BIRD and NEWSPAPER in American Sign Language. Reprinted from *The Signs of Language* by E.S. Klima & U. Bellugi, Harvard University Press 1979, by kind permission of the authors and publisher.

Klima & Bellugi conclude that signs are stored in memory as abstract combinations of movement, handshape and place, rather than in terms of meaning, or an iconic relationship between form and meaning.

4 Iconicity is not an all-or-nothing concept

We saw earlier that the notion 'arbitrary' has come to mean non-iconic as if iconicity was a binary concept such that signs clearly have it or they don't. However, there are various types and degrees of iconicity.

The relationship between an iconic sign and what it represents can be of many different types. For example, we can make a distinction between what we might call full and partial icons. The form of an iconic sign may represent all of the form of what it refers to, or it may represent only part of this form. For example, the BSL sign TREE as illustrated in Fig. 11.3 could be said to be a full icon, in that the shape of an entire tree is represented by the arm and hand, whereas the sign HOUSE is a partial icon in that the hands outline only the roof rather than the entire building. It could be argued that signs incorporating full icons are more iconic than those with only partial icons. The entire outline of a tree, for example, is represented roughly in the sign TREE, whereas only the roof appears in the sign HOUSE. One might argue that a partially iconic sign like HOUSE in fact shows a greater degree of arbitrariness in that it is arbitrary that the roof, rather than say the walls, have been selected for depiction. Thus the form of the icon itself can be arbitrary to some extent. We shall take up this point further under section 5 below.

Another way of working out how iconic particular signs are is by testing their 'guessability' among people who do not know sign language. Klima & Bellugi[16] showed a videotape of 90 ASL signs to people who had no previous knowledge of sign language. It turned out that people were extremely poor at guessing what these signs might mean, although once they were told the meaning they could often make a reasonable guess at the particular relation between a form and its meaning. To take an example, the sign TREE, which was on the video-tape and is similar to the BSL sign illustrated in Fig. 11.3, was not guessed correctly by anyone, although once people knew its meaning they were fairly easily able to agree that the form represented the trunk and branches of a tree. Klima & Bellugi's results provided support for a distinction between what they called 'transparent' and 'translucent' signs. Transparent signs could be understood from their form alone, while in the case of translucent signs, nonsigners could at least agree on the basis for the relation between form and meaning. Their results showed that only about 10% of the 90 signs on their video-tape could be considered transparent, while over half were translucent. The fact that the translucent signs were not guessable suggests that these were more arbitrary than the transparent signs. This all goes to show that our view of the extent of iconicity in a sign language will depend on how it is measured.

5 *The forms of signs are not pre-determined*

Bellugi & Klima[17] were also responsible for pointing out that even if we consider a sign to be iconic, that does not mean that its particular form is predetermined. We saw in the case of the sign HOUSE illustrated in Fig. 11.3 that it was somewhat arbitrary that its roof had been selected for representation rather than any other part of the house. The sign TREE, on the other hand, included a full representation of TREE, but not even the form of full icons is pre-determined. Bellugi & Klima's example of the signs for 'tree' in three sign languages, reproduced in Fig. 11.7, can be used to illustrate this point.

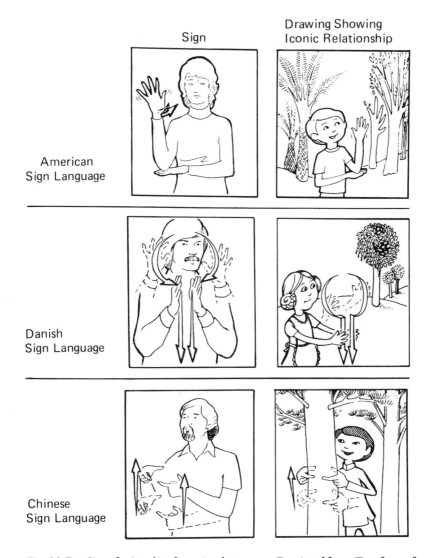

Fig. 11.7. Signs for 'tree' in three sign languages. Reprinted from 'Two faces of sign: iconic and abstract' by U. Bellugi & E.S. Klima in *Annals of the New York Academy of Sciences*, 280, 1976, by kind permission of the authors and the New York Academy of Sciences.

The signs in Fig. 11.7 could all be considered iconic, and yet they are not identical. The American and Danish signs both include full icons, and yet represent different shapes by different means. In ASL it is the arm itself which represents the tree, while in Danish Sign Language, the tree outline is drawn by the hands. The Chinese sign is only a partial icon in that only part of the tree, its trunk, is represented, and only one aspect of that, a cross-section.

These examples show that signs can be iconic without their forms being pre-determined. We can see that the *selection* of a particular form rather than another is arbitrary. Each form, however, has become a conventional sign to mean 'tree' in one of the sign languages, though the particular convention chosen varies from language to language. A similar point can also be made in relation to onomatopoeia in spoken language. Eco[18] points out that the sound made by humans to illustrate a cock crowing is different in different languages: 'cock-a-doodle-doo' in English, 'cocquerico' in French, and 'chicchiricchi' in Italian. As we saw earlier, Saussure pointed out that words of this kind were actually conventional, though he did not use this fact, as I shall, to conclude that conventionality in language is more important than arbitrariness.

We have now looked at five arguments relating to iconicity in sign language. We have seen that iconicity is not as significant as it might at first sight appear, and that it is a complex notion which does not entirely exclude arbitrariness. Signs may in fact have a varying mix of arbitrary and iconic aspects, but what all have in common is the *conventional nature of the relationship between form and meaning*.

Conventionality

What do I mean by saying that the relationship between form and meaning is conventional? By using this term I wish to draw attention to two important characteristics of language: one is the regular, rule-governed nature of language, and the other is the fact that these rules are shared.

The first of these two characteristics is fairly uncontroversial among linguists, most of whom would agree that language is rule-governed. If we confine our attention to the vocabulary, as we have been doing so far, it is clear that words or signs do not radically change their meaning each time they are used. So if I use the sign TREE to refer to a tree today, you would be justifiably surprised if I appeared to be using it to refer to a house tomorrow. Of course I might idiosyncratically use the sign TREE on all occasions to refer to a house, but you would still be able to detect a regular relation in my system between form and meaning, even if it differed from yours. Thus if we look at a particular language system we will expect to find regularity.

The second claim I want to make about language is that, in the typical case, these regularities are shared between language users. They are conventional in that they are based on tacit agreement between users. We have already recognized the existence of idiosyncratic form-meaning relations: these are not typical, however, for although they may be conceivable they are unlikely to survive as viable means of communication.

This second claim about language, that it is conventional in the sense of being based on agreement, is in fact far more controversial than the claim about regularity. It is a question which has been debated since the time of the Greeks, and which continues to be debated today[19]. I cannot enter into the debate here, but can at least point out that scholars who would accept that language depends on agreement are likely to be as much interested in language use, and the nature of the relationship between language users, as in the nature of the language system itself. Structural linguists like Saussure, on the other hand, tend to focus on the properties of the system itself independently of its users. From this perspective the question of whether language is based on agreement scarcely arises.

So Saussure's focus on arbitrariness at the expense of conventionality can perhaps be explained by his concern with the system as such rather than with its users. Why should he have picked on arbitrariness as basic to language, rather than some other notion, however? Andersen[20] provides an intriguing explanation in a recent paper. He suggests that scholars writing in the 17th century who described language as 'arbitrary' in fact meant something not all that different from what is meant by 'conventional' today. This is because the Greek word for convention (*nomos*) became translated in the European languages as 'arbitrary' or equivalent, which until after the 17th century meant 'voluntarily imposed'. After that, however, Andersen says that 'arbitrary' (and French *arbitraire*) changed in meaning to something like 'wilful, capricious, fortuitous', which is the meaning it would have had for Saussure. Thus in pursuing the debates of previous scholars Saussure may have been misled into a focus on arbitrariness rather on conventionality.

Conclusion

To sum up, I have argued that arbitrariness should not be a defining characteristic of language. What is important is a regular relationship between form and meaning, but this need not be arbitrary. Typically the relationship is conventional, though we can only recognize this if we are prepared to take the users of language into account.

12

Moving pictures

JONATHAN MILLER

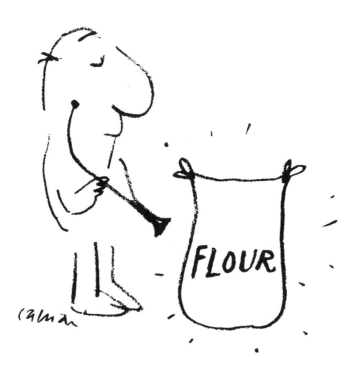

In his paper Horace Barlow says that this conference is devoted to images as they appear before the eye and the fate of images in the visual system which lies *behind* the retina (see p.5). In this chapter I would like to throw a bridge across these two domains by considering the way in which moving pictures are experienced and understood, since I believe that we can learn something about the behaviour of the visual system by considering the artificial images which we display to ourselves on the movie screen.

Movement in painting

For anyone who is interested in the mechanism of vision the structural peculiarities of the cinema are just as interesting as the stories which are told through this medium. You have only to remember how difficult it was to represent the world in action before the invention of cinematography. Because no matter how successful an artist might be in representing the *momentary* appearance of things, capturing, for example the sheen of silk, the lustre of pearls, the gleam of polished metal, not to mention perspective, the format of a picture is unavoidably frozen at an instant so that the spectator is bound to infer the previous and subsequent actions from tell-tale clues which the artist introduces. When Gotthold Lessing wrote his essay on the *Laöcoon*[1] in 1766 he pointed out that the representation of active reality was inescapably partitioned between literature and painting. 'Painting', he said, 'can only use a single moment of an action in its co-existing compositions and must therefore choose the one which is most suggestive from which the preceding and succeeding actions are most easily comprehensible.' Conversely literature, consisting as it does of words and sentences that follow one another, is better suited to conveying the consecutive change in the appearance of things and is relatively inefficient at representing 'the co-existing composition of momentary appearances'. This constraint did not, of course, rule out the possibility of representing actions and narratives in pictures. On the contrary, the very fact that 'still life' was distinguished as a representational genre proves that most Western artists worked within the limitations of their medium to represent a world in action. In fact, until painters like Chardin won grudging respect for their representation of stationary objects, it was widely assumed that it was the proper function of the visual arts to illustrate the dramatic events of history, myth and scripture. But Lessing's point still holds, because although the skilful painter could partly overcome the limitations of his motionless medium by showing postures from which the preceding and succeeding actions could be inferred, the picture was mobilised by the imagination of the spectator.

The spectator's ability to mobilize the otherwise still picture was partly dependent upon his or her familiarity with the relevant text – the Iliad, say, the Metamorphoses, or the Acts of the Apostles. But although these implicit texts provide a driving force without which narrative pictures would have lost much of their point, it would be wrong to assume that these images were a complete standstill as far as the illiterate spectator was concerned, because the artist could nevertheless arrange his figures to suggest movement which the static medium prevented him from representing directly. The most conspicuous example of this is the position of limbs at the extremity of strenuous movement. That is to say, in postures from which it is possible to predict a forthcoming event, or conversely postures from which it is possible to retrodict a movement which has just been completed – an arm upraised to

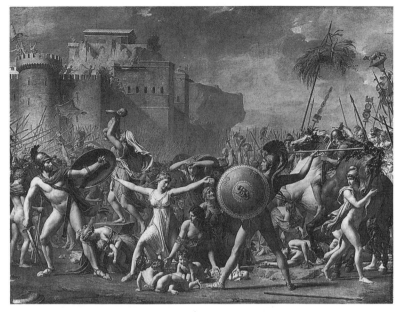

Fig. 12.1. *Intervention of the Sabine women* by David. Reproduced by kind
permission of the Louvre Museum, Paris.

deliver a blow or to hurl a spear, legs extended in a recently completed stride.
Frozen though they are, such artful arrangements are legible clues from
which the spectator can then supply the missing movement. Now although it
would be a misnomer to call this experience an *illusion* of movement, it is
nevertheless an *impression* of action. Such postures are emblems of action as
opposed to representations of them, and in some cases these emblems became
canonical representations of action even when they contradicted visual
reality. For instance, until Muybridge's photographs showed otherwise (see
Fig. 12.3a), the conventional representation of the galloping horse showed
the animal with legs extended fore and aft in the so-called rocking horse
position (see Fig. 12.3b). Although this is completely inaccurate, the representation of the limbs in this position suggested a forthcoming movement in
the opposite direction and the spectator supplied the rapid reciprocation of
the gallop without, of course, enjoying anything which might be called the
illusion of movement.

Movement in single images

A closer approximation to the *illusion* of movement came with the invention
of photography, and paradoxically it was the result of an imperfection in the
technique and might have been overlooked altogether if high-speed film had

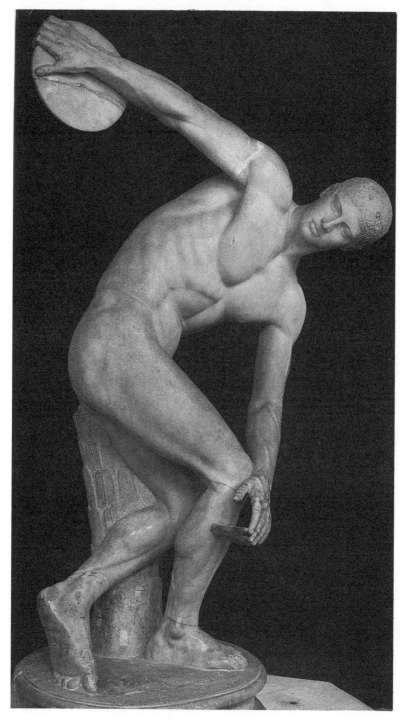

Fig. 12.2.   *The discus thrower* by Myron. Reproduced by kind permission of the
Museo Nazionale delle Terme, Rome.

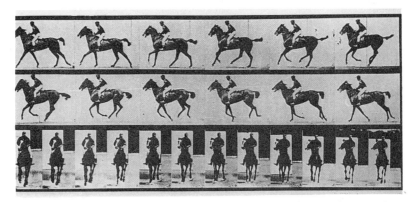

Fig. 12.3a.   *Annie G. in Canter* by Muybridge. From *Animal Locomotion*, 1887.

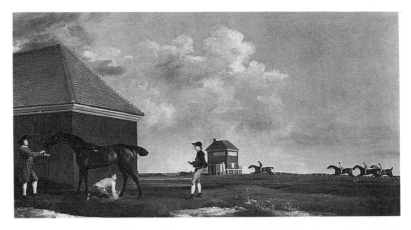

Fig. 12.3b.   *Gimcrack* by Stubbs, 1765. Reproduced by kind permission of the
Stewards of the Jockey Club.

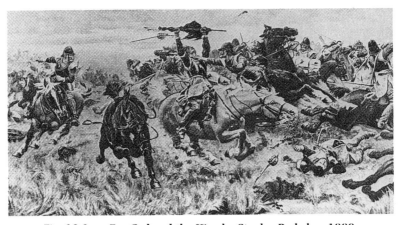

Fig. 12.3c.   *For God and the King* by Stanley Berkeley, 1889.

evolved without any of the intervening stages. This story has been admirably told by Aaron Scharf in his great work on *Art and Photography*[2]. He starts his enquiry with a question so obvious that it's surprising it never occurred to anyone before. Why is it that the mid-day photographs of Paris in the 1840s are so deserted? (See Fig. 12.4a.) Boulevards which ought to have been teeming with people are enigmatically empty. But as the years go by the streets appear to fill, not with people but with smudgy phantoms – smears in which one could eventually distinguish human outlines. What is happening? The answer is, of course, that the sensitivity of photographic emulsions is improving all the time and as the speed increases the rapidly moving population whose transit was unregistered by the long exposure of the early plates starts to leave incomplete traces on the film. For painters who are interested in representing the exciting activity of the teeming streets these blurry images offered an admirable pictorial cue for representing movement, certainly a novel advance on the postural emblems which had prevailed until then (see Fig. 12.4b). Here, it seemed, there was a much more convincing way of showing movement without having to show limbs frozen at the beginning and end of the excursion.

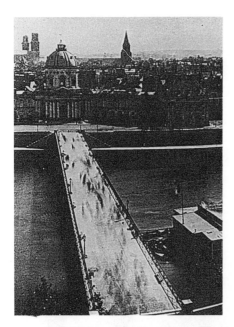 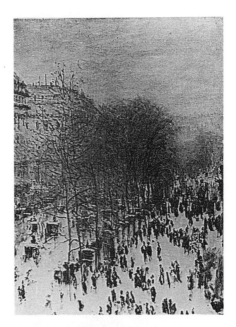

Fig. 12.4a. *The Pont des Arts* by Adolphe Braun, 1867. (Detail from a panoramic photograph of Paris.) Collection Société Française de Photographie, Paris.

Fig. 12.4b. *Boulevard des Capucines* by Monet, 1873. By permission of Mrs Marshall Field, Sen, New York.

The paradox is that these smeared images, which were the result of imperfections of the photographic craft, were more convincing representations of movement than the high-speed snaps which had evolved a few years later. We can see this as soon as we look at Muybridge's photographs of men and animals in motion. By 1870 photographic emulsions were fast enough to immobilize all but the most rapid actions without any trace of a blur. But by yielding a faithful record of each succeeding incident Muybridge's pictures failed to convey any sense of velocity. In other words one could tell exactly how the four limbs of a horse were disposed at any particular stage of the gallop or canter, but there was no impression of the speed of gait. This predicament is, to my mind at least, a pictorial counterpart of the situation which would later prevail in physics when it was discovered that one could record the velocity of a subatomic particle only at the expense of sacrificing precise knowledge of its position.

The birth of movies

It was only when photography had improved to the point where it could totally immobilize the image that it was possible to exploit these pictures to create the first genuine illusion of movement. Although the earlier smeared

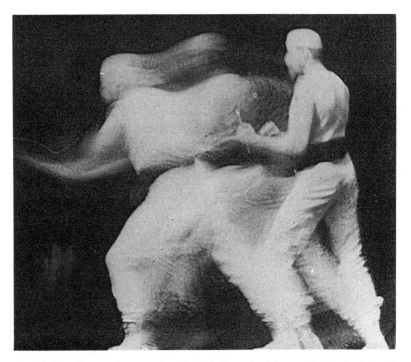

Fig. 12.5. *Chronophotograph of English Boxer* by Marey, 1880s. Archives de Cinémathique Française, Paris.

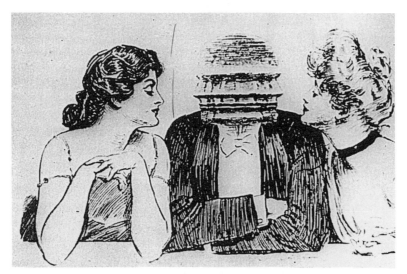

Fig. 12.6. *The Gentleman's Dilemma* by Gibson, 1900.

images gave a convincing *still* impression of movement, they would never have yielded the illusion which could now be created by the rapidly successive display of motionless frames. The point is that with the development of emulsions and shutter speeds fast enough to immobilize all the consecutive stages of an ongoing action it was possible for the first time to exploit a discovery which had previously yielded nothing better than an entertaining toy. I am referring, of course, to the zooetrope and other devices which virtually overcame the representational problem which Lessing had identified 80 years earlier. In these devices action was segmented into a consecutive series of still pictures and, by showing these one after another in rapid succession, it was possible to translate a segmented series into a continuously moving sequence. It was no longer necessary to partition the representation of action between still pictures and dynamic literature. The still frames took care of the 'co-existing compositions' whilst their successive display took care of their consecutiveness. Pictures, in other words, became self-animating and text became, or would soon become, superfluous. Strictly speaking, of course, the pictures were not self-animating at all. They were mobilized by the spectator's brain according to a psychophysical principle which psychologists had begun to elucidate by the end of the 19th century. Although movies are the most familiar expression of this principle, it does not need pictures to evoke it. In 1875 the Austrian physiologist, Sigmund Exner, elicited a comparable response by alternately switching between two lights placed side by side. As one light went out and the other one went on, the subject reported a lateral movement as if light A had actually moved to the position of light B. With the discovery of this principle there appeared a representational device which bore the same relationship to time as the discovery of geometrical perspective did to space.

In both cases we have a genuine illusion, which depends on something which Gombrich has described as 'the spectator's share'. But while a great deal of attention has been given to the cognitive work involved in perceiving *still* pictures, much less attention has been given to the spectator's share in the perception of movies. In fact, there is an implied assumption that it is just because they are moving, and therefore, more natural, that movies are much less of a perceptual problem. That is to say, by mobilizing the format it is assumed that cinematography has removed one obstacle against perceiving such pictures as representations of visual reality. And there is, of course, a sense in which this is perfectly true, because there are pictures whose representational significance remains ambiguous until they are made to move. The best known of these is one which figures in almost every textbook of experimental psychology. An arrangement of black and white flecks in which it is partly possible to recognize a dalmatian hound against a variegated background of light and shade, is effortlessly recognizable as soon as it begins to move (see Fig. 12.7). An even more dramatic example of movement

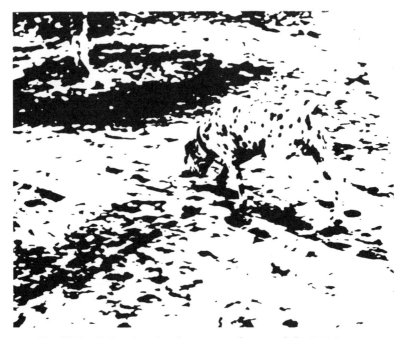

Fig. 12.7. Dalmatian dog dottogram, photograph by R.C. James.

as an aid to representational significance was reported by the Swedish psychologist, Gunnar Johansson. In a paper published in 1973 Johansson reported that an arrangement of lights placed on each of the main joints of a man's body were immediately recognizable as a human being as long as they were on the move, although the same format of lights was unidentifiable when static (see also p.98). Movement, in other words, adds an extra dimension of information from which pictorial significance can be derived.

The problem is that although movement is a source of information which can help us to pictorialize an otherwise non-pictorial array, there is no way in which movement itself can be pictorially represented. It can only be supplied in the form of an illusion, and this illusion, as I have already pointed out, depends on the successive display of pictures which are not moving. Illusion though it is, the sense of movement which results from such a display is quite inescapable and, unlike pictorial perception which has to be '*read*' before it can be appreciated, the impression of movement which is derived from the successive display of static frames cannot be eluded. In other words, it's not in any sense a pictorial convention with which the spectator has to be familiar before it becomes effective. In that sense it is quite unlike the cartoonist's device for representing movement. When a cartoonist wishes to give the impression of rapid action he will include 'whoosh lines' which describe the trajectory of an otherwise static limb. Although this gives an impression of dynamic acivity, it does so only because we have learnt to read or interpret the pictorial convention and a naive spectator might see it as a series of threads or pennants attached to the upraised limb. In the case of film there is no convention to be learned, no system of signs with which one must be familiar. To see such a picture is to see it move and that is all there is to it.

The problem of cuts and continuity

As cinematography developed, and when film-makers recognized it as a medium for telling stories, another level of pictorial discontinuity was introduced – a discontinuity which was altogether different from the segmentation upon which the illusion of movement depended. I am referring, of course, to the transition from shot to shot as opposed to the succession from frame to frame. In order to reconcile this type of discontinuity with the need to convey a continuous narrative, it is impossible to rely on psychophysics. With the introduction of editing or montage, involving a succession of shots taken from different angles, the interruption threatens the continuity of action, in spite of being its perceptual basis. As long as any particular shot goes on, the illusion of continuity is inescapable. The factors which contribute to the illusion arise from the 'bottom up' and the spectator cannot exempt himself from the perceptual effect, whereas the illusion of continuity which the spectator gets from shot to shot is all too escapable and without a substantial contribution made from the 'top down' – that is to say from a semantic level, the illusion of continuity can be lost altogether (Horace Barlow emphasizes the importance of these linking features on p.21, and Richard Gregory discusses perceptual processing in Chapter 20.).

I can illustrate the distinction by referring to an experience which everyone must have had, without necessarily paying much attention to it at the time. I originally became aware of it when I saw drive-in movies for the first time, but you can get the same effect by looking at TV programmes through a distant window. It goes like this. If you watch a film or a TV programme from so far away that you can neither hear the sound nor recognize the faces you will almost certainly be struck by a staccato interruptedness, something of which you are not aware if the same display is seen from close up. And between any two interruptions the images, unrecognizable though they are at such a distance, glide smoothly across the screen as the people and/or objects change their position. In fact, the illusion of movement survives even when it's impossible to tell *what's* moving. One can only conclude that whatever it is that guarantees the illusion of continuity from frame to frame is of a different order to the one which ensures the experience of continuity from shot to shot. As I have already said, the continuity which seems to fall apart at a distance is restored as the images get closer and one then needs to take a deliberate effort to see the *dis*continuities. When viewing a film from the correct distance, one becomes engrossed in the story and the continuity of its meaning overwhelms the discontinuity of its presentation. In other words, what we lose when we view a film at a distance is the *meaning* of what is going on and the appreciation of this aspect is, for obvious reasons, a 'top down' consideration. It presupposes 'grasp' or understanding.

So let me recapitulate the distinction. The medium of the movie has at least two levels of discontinuity, one of which is both unperceived and unperceivable, whereas the other one is optionally unperceived and if the psychological conditions are not favourable it is all too perceivable. As long as the movie is projected at the correct speed the experience of movement is unavoidable since it is guaranteed by a psychophysical process to which the spectator has no conscious access. The continuity that obtains from shot to shot – from wide shot to close-up, from one speaker's face to another and so on – is achieved by the viewer overlooking the interruption by his supplying more or less conscious knowledge or understanding of the fact that the situation is identifiable from one shot to the next and that what is shown is nothing more than various aspects of the same scene. The first level of discontinuity – frame to frame – has been the subject of considerable experimental investigation, if only because of the traditional interest in the psychophysics of apparent movement. But the level of pictorial integration – from shot to shot – has attracted much less interest, although the rapidly developing study of discourse promises the possibility of new understanding in this area. An important source of information is the intuitive folklore which is shared by movie editors, but up till now no one has bothered to make this practical wisdom explicit. There is, of course, a large literature dealing with stylistic issues in which film-makers and critics express their aesthetic preferences with regard to rhythm, tempo and tension – i.e. how to use film to tell a story in the most convincing or appealing way – but little has been written about the cognitive principles involved. The point is that below the *stylistic* level, that is to say the level at which film-makers and critics *argue* with one another, there is an area of unspoken agreement – various rules of thumb which all editors observe in the effort to maintain coherence and cohesion from shot to shot. Unfortunately, these practical principles have never been drawn up into anything resembling an explicit constitution and although movie editors recognize intuitively which cuts are possible and which ones are not, they usually find it difficult to put this wisdom into words.

Admittedly, editors and directors will often say that the rules are there to be broken, but this presupposes an editorial etiquette by contrast with which the viewer can recognize the violations as a deliberate effect. But for all normal story-telling the editor observes the unspoken rules, recognizing that unless he does so the viewer will get an uneasy sense of gratuitous discontinuity. The problem is that the more successful an editor is, that is to say the more practised he becomes, the harder it is to recognize how much craft has gone into the achievement. By the same token, the harder it is to recognize how much the viewer has to supply.

What glues the shots together?

As far as the spectator's share is concerned, I have already mentioned one condition which has to be satisfied before subjective continuity from shot to shot can be achieved. The spectator must be near enough to the screen to be able to mobilize his cognitive capacities – near enough, for example, to be able to recognize that the face he sees in a wide shot is the same one that follows it in close-up, or in the case of a switch from one person's face to another he must be near enough to hear the conversation so that he can tell that what one face is saying 'follows' what the previous face was saying.

Even if the spectator is viewing the screen under optimal conditions, the illusion of continuity may be lost if for some reason or other his cognitive abilities are impaired. In other words, if the spectator is unable to supply the understanding which glues the separate shots together, the film will fall apart at the joints and the sequence will look as discontinuous as it does to a normal subject who is viewing the film from afar. I once saw a vivid example of this in a patient who had sustained a left hemiplegia following a head injury. I saw the patient some months after her recovery, at a moment when there appeared to be no residual after-effects. She complained, however, that she was no longer able to understand films. The illusion of movement was intact, but she was completely bewildered by the sequence of cuts. She was unable to make sense of the succession from wide shot to close-up and was even more puzzled by the alternation from one speaking face to the other. As far as I could tell from questioning her, she was unable to reconstruct the three-dimensional space in which the successive images occurred. Now although it is unwise to theorize on the basis of a single case study, I would like to suggest that the injury had affected her capacity to build a three-dimensional mental model into which the successive images might otherwise have been slotted to create a representation of their spatial co-existence. Try to image what the cognitive problem is. Think of a conversational sequence in which two talking heads alternate with one another on the screen as the discussion passes from one speaker to the other. As far as the naive viewer is concerned, each face is looking in the same direction, i.e. out of the screen, so that in order to recognize that these two heads are facing one another as opposed to both looking in the same direction – that is to say that their succession on the *screen* is consistent with their simultaneous opposite presence on the *scene* – each of the two images has to be mentally rotated around its vertical axis and then placed at a speaking distance from the other. One can only assume that the intact brain creates a notional space, rather like one of those Perspex cubes on the faces of which one can stick family snapshots, except that in this case the two faces look inwards at one another from opposite walls of the transparent cube.

We know from the traditions of movie editing that the film-maker does everything he can to facilitate this model making by presenting the viewer with a so-called establishing shot, i.e. one which is wide enough to include both faces in the same frame. Presumably the memory of this arrangement helps to make sense of the successive close-ups of the separate faces which now follow. And more often than not, the editor will occasionally revert to the establishing shot as if to remind the spectator of the spatial set-up. The patient that I am referring to was presumably unable to take advantage of this establishing convention and was therefore bewildered by the succession of faces, all of which appeared to be looking the same way. In normal subjects the linguistic coherence of the conversation is enough to counteract the apparent discontinuity from one close-up to the next, so that even in the absence of an establishing shot the normal subject will recognize this sequence as a representation of two people simultaneously facing one another – which is why film sequences fall apart at the cuts when they are viewed from afar, especially when they are out of earshot. Robbed of their linguistic adhesive the images no longer hang together and the staccato rhythm which I mentioned earlier returns.

Although the linguistic coherence is often a necessary condition for maintaining the illusion of continuity from shot to shot, it is by no means a sufficient one, and the top down contribution which is based on semantic considerations can be converted by certain mechanical failures in editing. For example, failures to align the gaze may be very destructive. If 2 faces are to be seen addressing one another the eyeline of the first face must be accurately adjusted to the eyeline of the second. In other words, in order to convince the audience that the two faces are addressing one another it is important to guarantee that the eyeline of one engages or encounters the eyeline of the other. This means that if one head is looking screen left, the gaze of the second face must be directed screen right. When the two strips are supplied from two cameras which have been shooting the conversation simultaneously, this takes care of it because that is the direction in which each of the participants will be looking at each of the cameras respectively. But if, for some reason, one of the participants happens to be shot on one day and is merely cued 'off camera', the eyeline of the second actor may be a few degrees 'off'.

When the editor comes to splice the two pieces of footage the gazes will glide past one another and the viewer will then be disturbed by the uneasy feeling that A is not, in fact, addressing B but someone else for whose invisible presence the mental model of the conversational space has made no allowance. The accuracy with which the viewer can detect such failures and the fact that he can register discrepancies of gaze between successive images suggests that the brain might have feature detectors which are capable of comparing the direction of one conjugate gaze with another, even when the two images are exhibited consecutively. Perhaps the study by Dave Perrett and his colleagues is relevant to this issue (see Chapter 6).

Another paper which aroused my interest in this context was the one given by Anthony Movshon (see Chapter 8), whose identification of cells sensitive to movement both in the LGN and in area MT encourages me to ask whether there might be populations of cells sensitive to different velocities. My reason for asking this question is that movie editors often find that when they cut from a shot showing action from one angle to another shot which shows the ensuing phase of the action, the editing sometimes fails. And when it does the explanation usually turns out to be that the velocity of the arm movement, say, on the incoming shot is inconsistent with the velocity which you would expect it to have from the speed with which the arm was moving in the previous shot. Discrepancies of this sort are rarely, if ever, seen on TV, because the action is shared between two cameras shooting simultaneously – so that the action goes from one to the other in real time. But in film, where the action has to be repeated for the benefit of the second camera, unless great care is taken to replicate the velocity and trajectory, the two pieces of footage won't 'cut' and the spectator senses a discrepancy as the action passes from one shot to the next.

What can we learn?

These and other issues are part of the practical folklore of shooting and editing films, but because they do not impinge upon the stylistic considerations it's difficult to find any reference to them in the official literature of film. An apprentice editor learns it all in the cutting room and although there are manuals devoted to the subject, the questions that I have raised are scarcely mentioned. And yet it's on this 'craft' level that the management and mismanagement of moving images reveal so much about the functions of the working brain. The know-how of the cutting room depends upon cognitive principles, and could lead to scientific understanding of the way our minds construct a connected story from disconnected shots.

PART 4

Making images

CHRISTOPHER LONGUET-HIGGINS

The four chapters in this section illustrate the variety of interpretations that can be put upon the words 'image' and 'understanding'.

Michael Land's chapter draws our attention to the fact that in order to see, an animal does not have to be able to cast real images on to a sheet of light-sensitive cells or to use a lens for the purpose; and that the visual systems of some insects can detect not only the colour and the brightness but also the polarization of the incoming light. He also gives us a witty reminder of the biological uses of sight – for avoiding predators and distinguishing (though not infallibly) between a morsel of food and a potential mate.

At the opposite pole of the symposium is John Willats's essay on pictures – images of a supremely artificial kind. On the bold but hazardous assumption that pictures are the outcome of attempts to depict the real world, Willats invites us to distinguish between 'drawing systems' and 'denotation systems' – the latter being used to represent features of the world and the former to represent the spatial relations between them. To Willats, drawing a picture is to be compared with describing a scene rather than commenting on the visual process itself, as others have suggested. But perhaps the opposition should be thought of as applying not to alternative theories of draughtsmanship but to different kinds of picture.

John Lansdown and Andrew Witkin are children of the computer age, and some of the most striking examples of computer wizardry are to be found in the realm of computer graphics. Are computer-generated images just manifestations of The Higher Kitsch, or have they some deeper message for us? Lansdown's message is that the world of science fiction is closer than we thought; that we may soon be unable to distinguish computer-generated appearance from harsh reality. Possibly; but the artificial intelligentsia often find the real world to be a good deal more unruly than they had expected.

Witkin's pictures are no less impressive than Lansdown's, but his reflections take him in a quite different direction. In computer graphics, he argues, we build a three-dimensional model of something and use it for constructing a picture; in vision we start with the equivalent of a picture (J.J. Gibson's 'optic array') and derive from it a model of the outside world. If computer graphics depends on the principles of physical optics, does it not have something to teach us about vision, which has been described as 'inverse optics'? Assuming the answer to be yes, Witkin demonstrates the utility of mechanical as well as geometrical principles in the construction and manipulation of computer-generated pictures and movies, and suggests that an intuitive grasp of mechanical principles may be no less essential to an understanding of the visual images that the world and other people are continually presenting to us.

13

Vision in other animals

MICHAEL LAND

Introduction

A question that many people ask is: 'What does the world look like to an insect (or a fish, or a spider)?' Though seemingly straightforward, it is a difficult, and ultimately unanswerable question. We may know a great deal about an animal's eyes and even its behaviour, but in no case do we have a clear idea of the way the visual information is made available in the animal's brain. At one extreme, a robot with a perfectly good 'eye' may have no internal representation of the world other than that required to execute a series of set procedures, and at the other extreme our own internal image is so real and vivid that we routinely confuse it with the world itself. To what extent is another animal's visual world available for conscious scrutiny, as ours is? We have no way of finding out at present, partly no doubt because of our ignorance of the objective basis for our own internal image.

If we cannot give an answer to the most interesting question – it would, after all, be fun to know how the world looks to a bee – we can nevertheless answer two other slightly simpler ones. First, it is possible to assess the nature and quality of the optical image in most eyes, that is, the accuracy with which the eye's optical system separates out light coming from different parts of the visual field. We can also give the range of wavelengths to which the receptors are sensitive. For example, insect eyes provide images whose resolution is 10 to 100 times less acute than our own, and they usually have receptors sensitive to ultraviolet, as well as wavelengths visible to us. Should we wish to, we can use this kind of information to reconstruct the sort of internal image an animal would have *if it had a brain with a human-like visual consciousness*; that is, the way the world would appear to us if the optical and physiological structure of our eyes were the same as those of the animal in question. This is not of course the answer to the question we started with, but it is one that publishers and TV producers seem more than happy to accept in its place.

The second kind of question that can be answered concerns the uses that an animal makes of the information its eyes provide. Answering it usually involves much difficult experimental work, since one cannot ask animals direct questions. Karl von Frisch's long series of studies of bee behaviour is perhaps the most famous of all analyses of this kind[1]. By careful training he managed to show that bees had colour vision; that they could see and make use of landmarks when navigating between food and the hive; that they could detect the pattern of polarisation in sky light, and use it as a compass when the sun was not visible; and that they had considerable powers of shape discrimination, although exactly how great these are is still a matter of dispute. Studies like these leave us in no doubt that the visual world of insects is rich and complex, but, tantalisingly, they do not tell us whether bees have pictures in their heads as we do. Admittedly, the use of landmarks implies that bees do have a long-range and long-term representation of the world around them, but then one could argue that a cruise missile also has such a representation. I would not like to believe that the latter's computer consciously watches the world roll by beneath it, as it checks off the pattern of contours!

In this short essay I cannot provide a proper review of either the optical performance of animal eyes, or of visual behaviour. Instead I have decided to describe vision in a small selection of animals – a mollusc, an insect and a spider – chosen because they are as different from ourselves as I could manage. There are no vertebrates on the list because the basic pattern of the eye is remarkably uniform across the sub-phylum from fish to primate, and our own eye serves as a good model for the rest. I chose the scallop for its unique optics: an eye with a concave mirror instead of a lens. The water boatman (*Notonecta*) is an insect with a compound eye, but it is the unusual nature of its visual environment – the surface film of ponds and rivers – that singles it out as particularly interesting. Finally, I discuss vision in jumping spiders, the small zebra-striped hunters that live on walls. This is partly because their vision is the best of any terrestrial invertebrate, and partly because both the eyes and the behaviour resemble those of a vertebrate hunter. It is interesting to see how similar visual systems can become, where their evolutionary origins are so different.

Scallops and mirrors

A typical eye of a 'lower' invertebrate – a flatworm, say – is a small cup of black pigment partially surrounding a cluster of a few receptor cells[2]. The pigment shades the cells from light coming from all directions except one. The organ is thus a minute pinhole camera, but the pinhole is relatively so wide, and the number of receptors so small, that the resolution of the image such an eye can supply is very poor. There are three ways such an eye might be improved (Fig. 13.1). The first is to make the cup bigger, the hole relatively smaller, and the receptors more numerous, so that the eye becomes a 'proper' pinhole camera. This has been tried once, in *Nautilus*, the ancient molluscan relative of the octopus and squid and of the extinct ammonites. The eye is quite large (1 cm) and has a small pupil about 0.4 mm in diameter[3], which is simply a hole open to the sea. The weakness of this design, and undoubtedly the reason why it has not been more widely adopted, is that the image is very dim because the pupil must be small if the resolution is to be any good at all. The second type of improvement on the flatworm eye is to widen the pupil and put a lens in it. This overcomes the problem of the dim image, and at the same time provides better resolution than a pinhole can. In all essentials, this is the kind of eye that we have, and it has evolved many times: in the vertebrates, at least twice in the molluscs (octopus and snails), in some carnivorous worms, in certain jellyfish, in one water flea (*Labidocera*), and in insect larvae and spiders. There are basically two variations; in air, the curved cornea usually has enough optical power to form an image on its own, whereas in water the cornea is not effective and a powerful spherical lens is used instead[2]. There is a

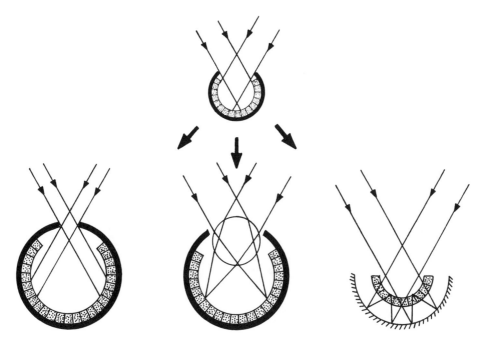

Fig. 13.1.   The simplest kind of pigment cup eye and three ways of improving its image: the pinhole eye of *Nautilus* (left), the lens eye of a fish (middle) and the mirror eye of a scallop (right).

third, and very much less common, way of providing a bright image – the use of a concave mirror – and we will consider that now.

The inedible part of a scallop, the frilly mantle attached to the edge of the shells, contains about 100 surprisingly eye-like eyes (Fig. 13.2). They enable the animal to shut its shell when the movement of a potential predator is detected, as SCUBA divers can attest. The eyes had been described many times, but because each has a lens of sorts most of the early anatomists thought that they were conventional lens eyes – like those of fish – and that was the situation when I first began to study them in 1963. One feature, however, puzzled me; there appeared to be no gap at all between the lens and the retina (Fig. 13.3), and unless the lens were implausibly refractile, it couldn't possibly have a focal length short enough to form an image on the retina. Shortly afterwards I noticed an even stranger phenomenon, which was that on looking into the eye through a microscope one sees an inverted image of oneself, apparently in the middle of the eye (Fig. 13.4). For a while this didn't strike me as peculiar; after all, there is an inverted image in the human eye. The difference is that when we look into our own eyes with an ophthalmoscope the view we have of the retina and images upon it appears to be located a long way behind the eye, not in the eye itself. The reason for this is that we are not looking at the retina directly, but through the eye's own optical system, and the effect is similar to the use of a magnifying glass. In a relaxed eye the retinal image appears to be at infinity. Nevertheless, in the scallop the image was definitely *in* the eye, not at infinity, and this means that it was not being seen through the same lens that produced it. The solution to this paradox, and to the absence of a focussing space between lens and retina turned out to be the same. The image is not produced by the lens, but by the

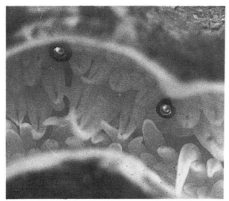

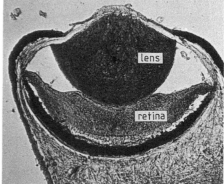

Fig. 13.2. Two eyes of the scallop *Pecten maximus*. Each is about 1 mm in diameter.

Fig. 13.3. Section through a scallop eye. Notice the dark 'lens', the thick retina, and the hemispherical rear surface.

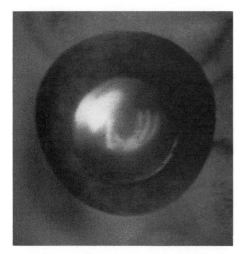

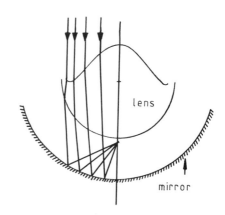

Fig. 13.4. Self portrait – well, hand anyway – photographed in the eye of a scallop.

Fig. 13.5. Image formation in *Pecten*. The image is formed by the mirror, as in a Newtonian telescope. The lens has little effect. From ref. 4.

reflecting layer that lines the back of the eye. As Fig. 13.3 shows, this is almost hemispherical, and, if we ignore the lens (which is actually made of rather low refractive index jelly), the mirror alone will form an inverted image in the distal region of the retina just beneath the lens. This gives us the optical diagram in Fig. 13.5, which is essentially the same as for a Newtonian reflecting astronomical telescope[4].

In the 1930s, with primitive recording apparatus and no knowledge of the eye's optics, H.K. Hartline showed that single nerve fibres from these eyes gave responses either to light going on or light going off, and that the 'off' responses came from the distal retina, where we now know that the image lies[5]. With this information, we can account for the animal's ability to see movement. If a dark object moves, then its leading edge will darken the cells that receive its image, and for a light object the trailing edge will do the same. In fact overall dimming works very well as a stimulus too, causing the scallop to shut. There is some evidence that scallops can also see the overall pattern of light and dark in the environment, probably using the 'on'-responding receptors in the proximal region of retina where there is no focussed image. However, the function of the scallop's unusual optical system is undoubtedly to provide an image for movement detection. Many other clams have individual receptors that respond to the dimming of light, but these are situated in the tissue of the body, not in specialised eyes. These animals respond when the whole animal is darkened, but unlike scallops they do not shut when an object merely moves without casting a shadow. The advantage of an image-forming eye is clear: it enables the scallop to respond to the presence of predators before they are, literally, on top of it.

It is most unlikely that scallops make any other use of the pictorial information in their images; I do not think they count the legs of starfish or anything like that. The point is that a good image is required for a simple task like predator detection, and the fact that an image exists in an eye does *not* mean that a usable internal representation of the environment exists too. The scallop is, I suspect, quite like the robot of the first paragraph.

Mirror eyes of the scallop type are very uncommon, probably because they are not a good design. The image contrast is poor because light has to go through the receptor layer unfocussed, before it returns focussed. There is, however, one other kind of mirror eye, and I will mention it briefly because, like the scallop eye, the discovery of the way it works is very recent. From the mid-1950s to the mid-1970s the eyes of the long-bodied decapod crustacea (shrimps, prawns, crayfish and lobsters) did not, apparently, work. The problem was that the structures in these compound eyes that were thought to be lenses actually turned out to be simple square blocks of jelly, without any usable optical properties. Eyes that don't work are embarrassing, and a solution had to be found. It came in 1975, when Klaus Vogt found that these square blocks in crayfish eyes have a mirror coating[6]. When one sketches out the paths of rays into the eye, reflecting the rays off the walls of the blocks, it rapidly becomes clear that such an array of mirrors will form an image on a hemisphere halfway out from the centre of the eye (Figs. 13.6, 13.7). The whole arrangement is a sort of inside-out scallop eye (compare Fig. 13.5). Shrimps can now see again, and are no doubt relieved.

Seeing in and out of water: the water boatman *Notonecta*

The main point of this section is to explore some of the oddities of vision in the vicinity of water surfaces, but as our subject is an insect I must say a little first about the way compound eyes form images. The shrimp eye just discussed is unusual in that all the facets in the optical array superimpose their contributions in a common image. This type of eye is known as a 'superposition' eye, in contrast to the more common 'apposition' compound eye, where each optical element forms a separate image (Fig. 13.8). In apposition eyes, each lens/rhabdom combination (a rhabdom is a photoreceptive structure formed from the membranes of eight or nine receptor cells) forms a separate functional element known as an ommatidium. In early studies of compound eyes there was some confusion about whether or not the insect sees the small inverted image in each ommatidium – Leeuwenhoek saw these images as

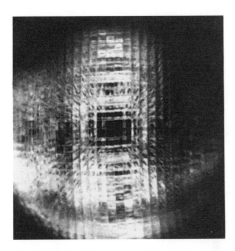

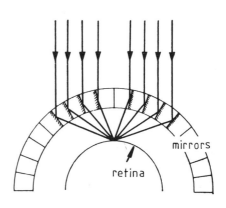

Fig. 13.6. The eye of the shrimp *Palaemonetes*. It seems obvious that it is made of mirrors, but this was not known until 1975.

Fig. 13.7. Optics of the shrimp eye. Rays are reflected to a focus on the retina by radially arranged mirrors.

early as 1695[7] – rather than the overall image across the eye surface, which is erect (Fig. 13.8). In most cases it seems that the inverted images are not seen, because the rhabdom is a single fused rod which simply measures the average intensity across its tip. However, in flies, and also in bugs like the water boatman, the situation is a little more complicated. The receptive structures that make up the rhabdom are not fused together, and so each can act as a separate receptor that does resolve a part of the inverted image behind each lens. However, this probably makes no difference to the overall picture because, in flies at least, the bundle of nerves from the receptors of each ommatidium has a twist in it. This has the effect of re-erecting each of the tiny inverted images, and fitting it into the overall erect image, so that the geometry of Fig. 13.9 is reinstated[8].

Notonecta catches insects that become trapped in the surface film of ponds and streams. It hangs from the surface with its head pointing obliquely down, and with four feet and the abdomen tip in contact with the surface. Usually, it first detects the surface ripples from the prey with its feet, and then homes in visually[9]. The view of the water surface from just underneath is very strange, because of the effects of refraction and total internal reflection (Figs. 13.10, 13.11). Up to an angle of 48.8° from the vertical, the aerial world above the surface can be seen in 'Snell's window' with a total width of 97.6°. At greater angles than this the surface acts as a mirror, and structures visible are either reflections of objects on the bottom, or they are the undersides of objects in the surface film. This leads to the very curious situation that the upper and lower

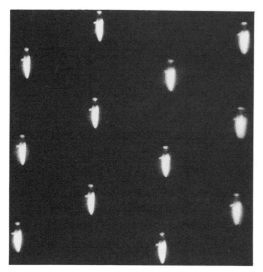

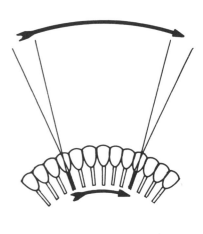

Fig. 13.8. In 1695 Leeuwenhoek wrote: 'What I observed by looking into the microscope were the inverted images of the burning flame: not one image, but some hundred images' [7]. This is my attempt to repeat his observation, using the cleaned cornea of a robber-fly (*Asilidae*).

Fig. 13.9. Optics of an apposition insect eye. The overall image is erect, and the small inverted images are typically not resolved by the receptors.

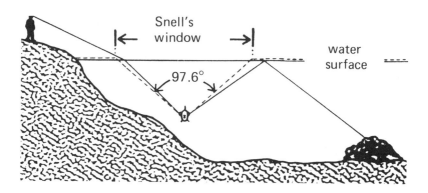

Fig. 13.10. The world of an aquatic animal. The aerial world occupies a circular region, 'Snell's window', above the animal. Below this objects on the bottom are seen by total internal reflection at the surface. After Walls[18].

parts of something floating on the surface are seen in different places, as the photograph in Fig. 13.11 shows.

The peculiar optical geometry of the water surface is reflected in the construction of the *Notonecta* eye, which is organised in such a way that special high-resolution regions are devoted to both the aerial and the aquatic

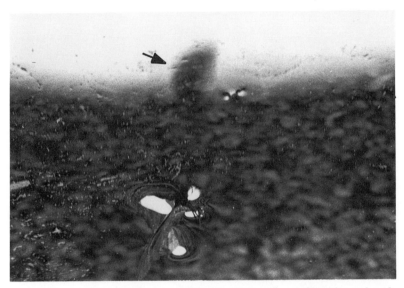

Fig. 13.11. A struggling insect, seen from just below the surface. The underside of the insect appears in the lower part of the picture, but the part in air is seen well above it (arrowed) inside Snell's window. To work out the orientation, imagine the fish in Fig. 13.10 looking at the S of SURFACE.

views of the surface film. Rudolf Schwind[10] discovered that the part of the eye that looks just above the surface has about twice the resolution of the rest of the eye, and that there is another region of enhanced resolution that looks in the horizontal direction when the animal is in its predatory posture (Fig. 13.12). These two regions will view the upper and lower parts of a stranded insect, respectively. Interestingly, there is also a surface-feeding fish (*Aplocheilus lineatus*) that has a similarly adapted eye, in that there are two horizontal 'areae' – regions where the density of both receptors and nerve cells in the retina is unusually high – which correspond to the regions just above and below the surface[11].

Notonecta lives a double life. If the pond dries up the adults will take to the air, in search of other stretches of water. The animals are now no longer upside down, in addition to being in a different medium, so that the way the world maps onto the eye is quite different. This presumably raises problems for the brain which we know little about. However, the eye itself has an ingenious adaptation to its new task: it has a built-in pond detector. Another optical property of water surfaces is that they polarise light, in such a way that the plane of vibration of the light waves is parallel to the surface. (This is why polaroid sunglasses are able to suppress reflections by only allowing

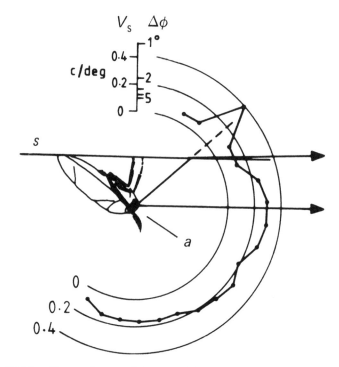

Fig. 13.12. The resolution of the eye of the water boatman *Notonecta*, as it hangs inverted from the water surface. The scale shows the angle between adjacent ommatidia ($\Delta\phi$), and the 'sampling frequency' of the retina $v_s = 1(2\Delta\phi)$. There are two directions of enhanced resolution, one corresponding to the region in air just above the surface, and the other to the region just below it. In Fig. 13.11 these would image the upper and lower parts of the insect. *a* is the body axis and *s* is the water surface. Based on Schwind[10].

through light polarised in the opposite plane, at right angles to the surface.) The receptors in the ventral region of the *Notonecta* eye have their light-sensitive molecules arranged so that some cells are maximally sensitive to light polarised parallel to the plane of the surface, and others to the plane at right angles as indicated in Fig. 13.13[12]. This means that when the eye views a non-polarising surface like earth, both sets of cells will respond equally. However, if they view a water surface, one set will be stimulated and the other not. A difference in activity between the two sets will then indicate the presence of water. Schwind was able to show that this was what happened[13]. He found that *Notonecta* would dive into water surfaces (the 'plunge reaction'), which is sensible enough. However, he also found that a simulated water surface – a sheet of illuminated polaroid – was just as effective, although presumably a little harder on the animal's head!

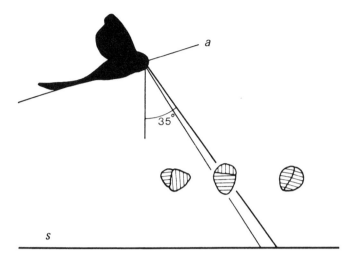

Fig. 13.13. *Notonecta* flying. In the region beneath the animal, the receptor molecules are arranged in two directions at right angles, but outside this region they are all parallel. The former arrangement allows the detection of polarised light from water sufaces. *a* and *s* as Fig. 13.12. Modified from Schwind[12].

A remarkable parallel: vision in jumping spiders

Very few animals, outside the mammals, look back at you when you look at them. Most ignore you, or, like birds, eye you obliquely in a way that seems to disguise their interest. Amongst invertebrates, praying mantids will fix you with a sinister but centred gaze, and so will jumping spiders (*Salticidae*), the subject of this section. These small (5 – 10 mm) common spiders are thoroughly untypical of their Order. They do not build webs, but stalk their prey – usually small insects – very much as a cat stalks a mouse. When they first see a movement they turn to face its source; they then approach it forwards, fast at first and then more slowly as the distance decreases. Finally, when 2 or 3 cm away, the spider crouches, waits, and completes the capture with an explosive jump. Sometimes they encounter other jumping spiders rather than flies, and then the behaviour is quite different. At most times of the year, once they have seen each other they turn away and avoid further contact. However, in the mating season, the males perform an elaborate and characteristic dance in front of the female. The front legs are raised, and the spider dances sideways in a series of arcs that slowly converge on the female (Fig. 13.16); the performance best resembles a highland fling[14].

Coordinating this highly visual behaviour are four pairs of eyes, although one pair is more or less vestigial in jumping spiders. The structure of the remaining six eyes is quite like the human eye. Each has a single chamber, with one lens forming an image on a retina at the back. However, they lack a mobile iris, a focussing mechanism, and eyelids. They are of two kinds (Figs. 13.14, 13.15). The four side eyes have between them a panoramic field of view, and they are fixed in the head. Their chief, and possibly only function is to detect movement, and to initiate turns that bring the other pair of eyes – the frontally situated principal eyes – to bear on whatever caused the movement. The resolution of the side eyes is fairly coarse, 0.5 to 1.5°, but that is quite adequate for the detection of a fly or another spider at half a metre[15]. At this stage, the identity of the stimulus is irrelevant: a spider, fly or car on the street produce the same turn. The principal eyes differ in several ways. They are much larger (although the focal length is still only about 1 mm), the field of view is very much smaller (about 5° wide by 20° high – these are 'telephoto' eyes), the resolution is much higher (about 0.1°), the receptors have a different structure and, most remarkably, these eyes are moveable. Like our own eyes, each has six eye muscles, and these move the retina up and down, side to side, and also cause it to rotate around the visual axis. However, unlike

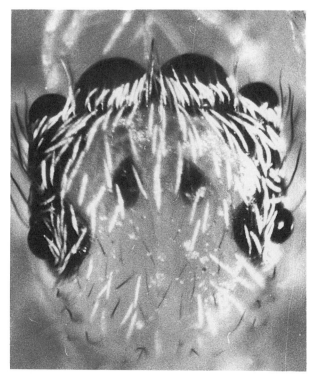

Fig. 13.14.   Head of a jumping spider (*Metaphiddipus*) from above, showing the eyes. Notice the ends of the eye-tubes of the AM eyes near the middle of the head. See Fig. 13.15.

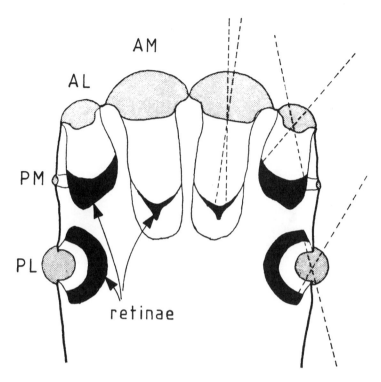

AM

AL

PM

PL

retinae

Fig. 13.15.   Diagram of a jumping spider's eyes. The fixed side eyes are the postero-laterals (PL), the antero-laterals (AL) and the vestigial postero-medians (PM). The antero-median (AM) or principal eyes are the largest pair. They have very narrow fields of view and are moveable. The horizontal extents of the fields of view are shown dotted on the right.

our eyes the lens remains fixed; it is only the retina that moves, not the globe as a whole.

It was the nature of the eye movements that excited me when I first studied these animals. During the few seconds that the spider takes to decide whether the object it has just seen is to be eaten, mated or ignored, the retinae go through a complicated but quite stereotyped scanning procedure[15, 16]. The muscles first centre the retinae on the target, then they make two kinds of oscillatory movements: to-and-fro sideways movements at about 1 per second, and much slower rotations (Fig. 13.19). The scanning is adjusted to the width of the target, but otherwise seems unaffected by its nature. In thinking about the function of this curious procedure, I was greatly helped by a study by Oskar Drees in the 1950s[17], in which he managed to work out the way the spider decides between flies and other spiders. It is on the basis of the legs, as Fig. 13.17 shows. The more legs at the right angles and in the right places, the less the spider is likely to pounce, and the sexier its behaviour. In contrast, almost any moving object of about the right size will be accepted as 'prey'

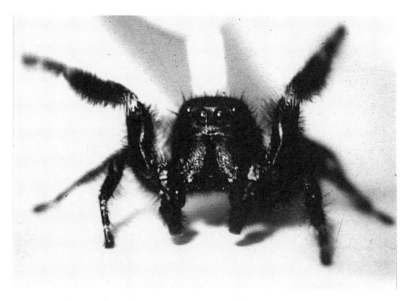

Fig. 13.16.   A male jumping spider (*Phiddipus*) in a courtship pose.

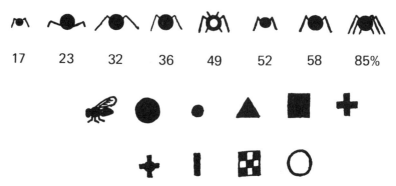

Fig. 13.17.   Drawing used by Drees[17] to evoke courtship behaviour (top row)
and prey capture (bottom rows) in jumping spiders. The numbers are the
percentages of courtship responses, so sexiness increases from left to right. It
seems that jumping spiders will attack most things, but will only mate with
objects that have legs in the right places.

(ball-bearings moved by a magnet work well). It seems, then, that the
function of the eye-movements is to search for contours in the target that
might be legs. If we assume that the retinae contain rows of receptors that link
up to 'line detectors', then the scanning pattern is understandable; the
rotational movements would provide the detectors with a range of orientations, and the lateral movements can be thought of as hunting for matches
between the detectors and the contours (Fig. 13.19).

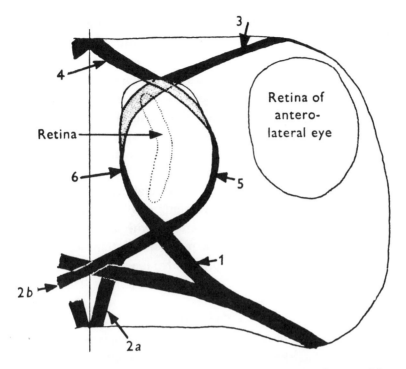

Fig. 13.18. The six muscles that move the retina of a principal eye. Each has a single nerve fibre, and between them they can move the retina up and down, side to side, and can also twist it through up to 50° around the eye's axis. The boomerang-shaped retina occupies about 5° by 20° in space. See Fig. 13.15 and reference[15].

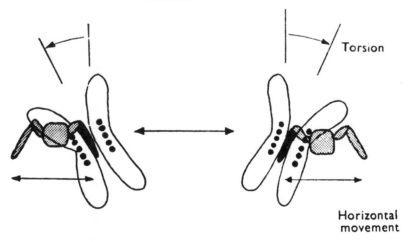

Fig. 13.19. Eye movements made by a jumping spider while examining a spider-like object (stippled). The two boomerang-shaped principal retinae move from side to side and also rotate (torsion), keeping parallel to each other. It is suggested that this procedure makes it possible for rows of receptors (black dots) to find the 'legs' in the retinal image. From[15].

We have seen that in the structure of the eyes themselves, the ways that they move, and in the form of the catching behaviour, there is an impressive resemblance between these spiders and mammalian predators, even though there are no evolutionary links of any kind. There are, however, interesting differences. In some ways the six-eye design for a visual system is much more economical than our two-eye design. Peripheral vision, where fairly low resolution is needed, can be put into the small side eyes, and the principal eyes which contain the equivalent of our 'fovea' can be made long and narrow. Where space is at a premium such an arrangement is less wasteful. Secondly, there is no equivalent in mammals to the special purpose scanning movements seen here; vertebrate eye movements are never linked to a single function such as mate detection. In an animal with a small nervous system (10^5 rather than 10^{11} cells) general purpose solutions to problems are perhaps too expensive, and special procedures for solving specific problems are more economical.

Conclusions

The camera-like design of the human eye is by no means the only way to produce an image, as the example of the scallop showed. The terrestrial environment we inhabit is not the only environment, and eyes like those of the water boatman are adapted in subtle ways to exploit the optical properties of other quite different habitats. Sometimes, convergence of habitat and lifestyle does lead to at least a superficial similarity in the way that animals from different groups organise their visual behaviour; cats and jumping spiders provide one example, and fish and squids another. The varying success of different evolutionary inventions is perhaps nowhere more clear than in the range of eyes and visual systems that the animal kingdom presents to us[18].

14

Linking perception and graphics: modeling with dynamic constraints

ANDREW WITKIN, MICHAEL KASS, DEMETRI TERZOPOULOS
AND ALAN BARR

Introduction

The goal of computer graphics is to build mathematical models of physical objects, then synthesize realistic pictures and movies of them. The goal of computer vision is to derive mathematical models describing the objects that appear in real pictures or movies. Both disciplines revolve around two key themes: the construction of three-dimensional models, and the relation between models and pictures. What's different is the direction: in graphics, we first build a model and then derive the picture. In vision, we're given the picture and need to derive a model for the objects that generated it.

In both graphics and vision, we find increasingly that the range and complexity of scenes we can deal with is limited by our ability to model the shapes and motions of physical objects. Current modeling techniques are simply inadequate to deal with the complexity, largely because they are so awkward to use. Many of the limitations of current modeling techniques stem from differences between the imaginary worlds they create and the real world of physical objects they purport to represent. Real objects are solid, with mass and inertia. They may deform or break under stress according to the materials of which they are composed. The way real objects move and deform is governed by their structure and by the forces applied to them. Physical attachments between parts, such as joints, transmit forces from part to part, linking their motions together in lawful and predictable ways. Ordinarily we take these properties completely for granted when we think about the way objects behave, and we rely on these properties when we shape real physical parts and assemble them together. In contrast, the 'computer world' in which we currently model objects is populated by massless geometric phantoms that move and deform only by direct modification of their position, orientation,

213

and shape parameters. Consequently, the entire stratum of real-world behavior due to simple mechanics is absent.

The lack of basic mechanics leads to models that don't *do* anything. Without the laws that govern and constrain the behavior of real objects, we cannot use our models to simulate, predict, or extrapolate to related situations. This is a serious limitation for both vision and graphics, becoming painfully evident when we attempt computer animation. To make geometric models behave realistically, we must move them by hand, guided by our own knowledge of physics. When we attempt to place a book on the table, it is liable to sink half-way in or float an inch above if we miscalculate. To make it appear that two parts are linked by a joint, we have to ensure manually that they stay joined. Truly complex articulated objects are eager to fall apart into a jumble of (probably interpenetrating) pieces. Getting them to move even plausibly is very difficult; truly realistic motion is the preserve of talented animators. By way of illustration, Fig. 14.1a shows a simplified model of a robot arm attached to a pedestal. We may be inclined to accept the image at face value – as a picture of a solid, articulated object connect by joints. When we attempt to move the arm to a new configuration it becomes clear that there is much less there than meets the eye. A small miscalculation in repositioning the parts leads to the ridiculous image shown in Fig. 14.1b: the joints have come apart, and the arm interpenetrates its base. The model is revealed for what it truly is – a collection of geometric forms floating in space. The model itself contains nothing to indicate that this configuration is wrong. It looks wrong to us because we expect the synthetic object to obey physical laws as would a real one.

Recognition of these difficulties led us to formulate a new approach to model building, in which we build and manipulate computer models much

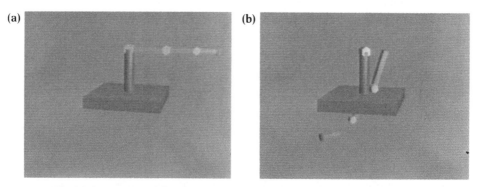

Fig. 14.1.   Some pitfalls of geometric models: (a) a simple robot arm; (b) interpenetration and disconnection of parts resulting from incorrect parameter settings.

the same way we build and manipulate real objects, by applying forces to them. We shape parts by applying forces to simulated materials, much as we might mold clay, bend metal wires or plates, stretch rubber sheets, etc. We assemble these parts into complex objects by imposing forces that hold the parts together in the manner of real joints and other attachments. This way, we can specify how the pieces are supposed to fit together without the need to compute their positions and orientations explicitly. Having constructed models in this way, we animate and manipulate them by applying additional forces corresponding to pushing, pulling, gravity, wind, etc.

This style of model building with *dynamic constraints* more nearly resembles the construction of scale models out of real materials than it does the unrealistic geometric manipulations of current modeling systems. However, since we are simulating materials and forces on the computer, we are freed from many of the hindrances we experience when we work with materials in the real world. We can easily design complex *shaping forces* and *assembling forces* that would be awkward to achieve in nature. We can even invent materials with no known physical counterparts to simplify the model-building process. Under the influence of these shaping and assembling forces, the parts of our models take shape and sail through space to their appointed positions and orientations. Once the model-building process is complete, we are left with a *working* model that responds realistically to imposed forces.

The possibility of *designing* forces and materials to aid model construction becomes particularly important in vision. It's in the nature of the visual interpretation process that the image provides many potential sources of evidence concerning the three-dimensional shapes and motions of the objects under view. Examples of this kind of evidence include the outline of an object, its shading and texture, and its apparent two-dimensional motion. In our paradigm of dynamic constraints, these and other sources of evidence are expressed as forces that act in concert on a simulated piece of three-dimensional material, molding it into a form consistent with the image data. The properties of the material itself – simple elasticity, as well as more elaborate symmetry- and rigidity-seeking properties – serve to combine the diverse constraints to create a specific, tangible model that represents a principled guess at the real object's form.

Within this framework, our research program – still in its early stages – is directed at designing specific shaping forces, assembly forces, and materials both for use by the human model-builder and by visual interpretation systems. In the remainder of this chapter, we present several examples that give the flavor of our work in progress.

Self-assembly

Our first example concerns the use of dynamic constraints to create and animate structures composed of rigid bodies connected by joints and other attachments. This example introduces the use of forces in model construction and illustrates some of the issues raised in designing such forces.

Many natural and man-made objects are well described as collections of rigid parts attached in various ways, for example by joints. In terms of its effect on the objects being connected, a joint can be described as a coupling force that pushes the connected objects back together if they begin to move apart or rotate in ways that the joint forbids. Alan Barr and Ronen Barzel[1] at Caltech have been developing simulated forces that model a variety of joints and attachments. Their approach to this problem offers a good illustration of the way a single force can be used both to assemble objects and to simulate them once assembled. To connect two real objects with a joint, we must first move the objects together, then fit and attach the joint. Barr and Barzel's simulated joints, however, are self-assembling. When the objects to be connected are far apart, the joint force pulls the objects smoothly through space until they coincide. Once they arrive, its behavior simulates that of a physical joint, holding the objects together, but leaving them free to pivot around the attachment. Thus, a single elegantly designed force serves both in the assembly process and in the simulation of the assembled object.

The technical issues involved in designing these forces are rather involved. A naive approach might be to model the force as a simple spring or rubberband that pulls together the points to be connected. However, this solution gives rise to undesirable oscillations and fails to maintain accurately positioned connections when the finished object is pushed or pulled. Barr and Barzel's solution uses critical damping to overcome these difficulties.

Using self-assembling joint forces, Barr and Barzel have so far been able to specify fairly complex objects just in terms of their connective topology – which part attaches to which. With the parts initially positioned at random, or layed out in rows, turning on the joint forces causes the parts to self-assemble, then to behave realistically as any external forces are applied to them. The final configuration is achieved without any of the parts' final positions and orientations having been specified explicitly. Figure 14.2 shows several stages in the self-assembly of a tower built of rigid rods. Figure 14.3 shows the construction of a 'bridge' of linked rods between two towers.

These examples illustrate the use of dynamic constraints to assemble complex objects composed of rigid parts. Although the positions and orienta-

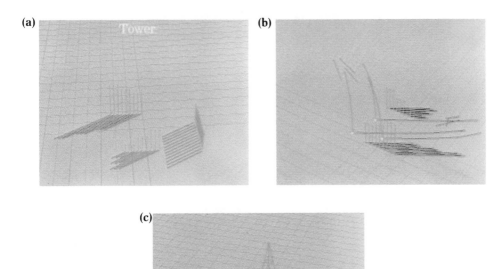

Fig. 14.2. Sequence illustrating a self-assembling tower. (a) Initial configuration: three members comprising base of tower are anchored to ground, remaining
parts are aligned in two rows awaiting assembly. Dark lines represent shadows.
(b) Tower at intermediate stages of assembly. Note how the tower structure
distorts in the direction of new parts, under influence of the symmetrically acting
assembly forces. (c) Fully-assembled tower. Additional forces can now be applied
to analyse how the tower will behave under various simulated conditions (e.g. a
high wind).

tions of the parts were determined automatically, the dimensions of the parts
– specifically, the lengths of the rods forming the tower and chain – had to be
specified manually in advance. Ideally, we would like the parts' dimensions,
as well as their positions and orientations, to be derived automatically from a
specification of constraints. For instance, knowing the desired height of the
tower, its width at the base, the symmetries it must possess, and so on, might
allow us to compute the dimensions of many or all of the constituent parts.

In fact, is is quite straightforward to extend the use of dynamic constraints
to the determination of parts' dimensions as well as their positions and
orientations in space[9]. In the rigid case, parts respond to constraint forces by
undergoing translations and rotations. Additionally, most of the geometric
shapes we use to build models come equipped with a small number of shape

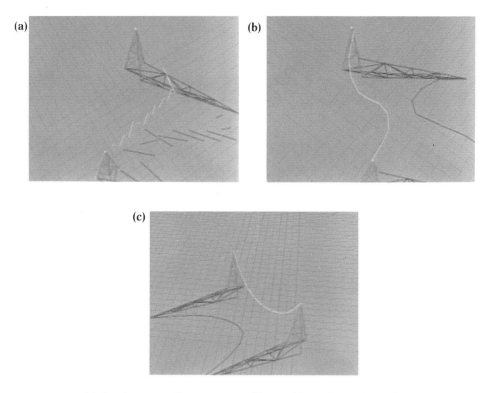

Fig. 14.3. Sequence illustrating a self-assembling chain. (a) Links coming together to form chain connecting towers; (b) completed chain continues to sway, working off the excess energy accumulated during assembly; (c) converging to a catenary at equilibrium.

parameters. For example, a sphere has a single shape parameter – its radius, while a cylinder has two parameters – length and radius. Just as we vary position and orientation in response to constraint forces, we can vary these shape parameters as well. This results in parts that may, if necessary, stretch or otherwise change their shapes to satisfy attachment constraints. An illustrative example is shown in Fig. 14.4: a pipe is to be fitted to other pipes at either end. The pipe is modeled so as to be able to stretch and bend as well as translate and rotate. The constraint forces cause the pipe to undergo just the stretching and bending required to make the pieces fit.

Snakes

In vision, we would like to build models by the use of similar shaping and assembling forces, but derive the forces automatically from images of the objects being modeled. As an initial experiment in visual modeling, we chose

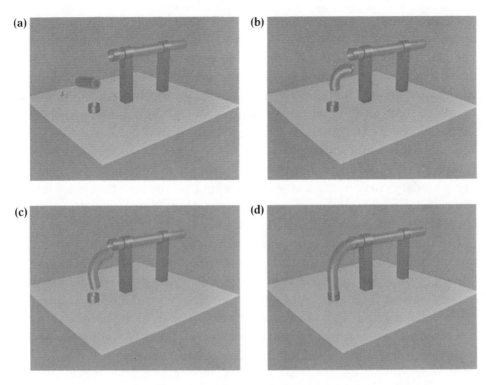

Fig. 14.4.   Dynamic constraints are used to adjust both the shape and position to
fit a pipe. (a) The initial condition; (b–c) the pipe in the process of bending,
stretching, translating, and rotating; and (d) the final condition with the attachment constraints satisfied.

a simple two-dimensional example. Our approach is to find the boundaries of
objects and other line-like features by immersing simulated pieces of springy,
stretchy wire (which we call 'snakes') in an image-derived force field that
attracts the wires to nearby features of interest[2]. The image forces provide a
type of *power assist* to a user, in pointing out the image features. If the user
moves the snake close enough to a particular image feature, then the image
forces take over and pull the snake in the rest of the way.

The effectiveness of the power assist depends on how well the image forces
capture the user's perception of the relevant image features. So far, we have
designed well-behaved forces for localizing lines and edges in complicated
imagery. As our understanding of image features improves, we will be able to
design increasingly powerful forces capable of homing in on more complex
features from longer distances away.

The line and edge forces we use are conservative, so they can be represented by potential energy functions. Under their influence, the snake seeks the

nearest local minimum in potential energy. If the image force is properly designed, then the intended image feature will lie at a local energy minimum. The trick is to get the snake close enough to the intended image feature so that the nearest energy minimum will be the correct one. To accomplish this, we let the user apply forces directly to the snake – dragging it around with simulated rope, pushing on it with repulsive forces, or tying it down with springs. When the snake gets close enough to the desired line or edge, it rolls down into the proper energy well.

Figure 14.5 shows a simulated wire positioned over the boundary of a pear. The boundary curve in the image exerts a force on the wire that holds it in place. The user is able to overcome this force and pull the wire away from the boundary, but it snaps back when released.

This interactive approach becomes particularly interesting when applied to a motion sequence – the successive frames of a movie. As the features of interest move, their corresponding energy wells also move. If the frame-to-frame displacement is small enough, snakes initially positioned on a feature are dragged along by the moving energy well. The result is that the snake tracks the feature's motion through the sequence. Figure 14.6 shows the use of snakes to track lip motion automatically during speech.

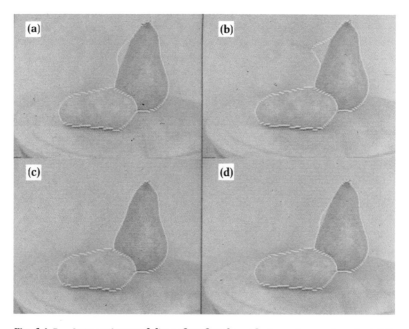

Fig. 14.5.   Interactive modeling of surface boundaries using snakes. In (a) the user has pulled the snake off the pear's boundary. In (b–d) the snake snaps back to the edge.

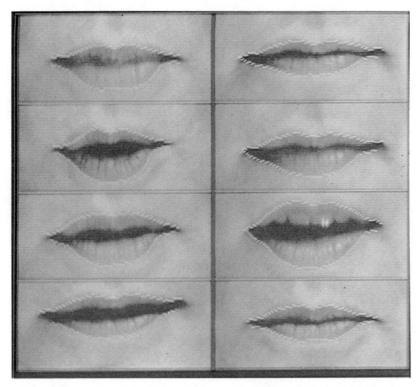

Fig. 14.6. A snake tracking a moving contour through a time-sequence of image frames. This capability is useful for a variety of movie-data reduction tasks (e.g. computing the changing volume of heart chambers in a cineradiogram).

Sheets

Our next experiment with the use of non-rigid materials concerns the simulation of thin sheets in three-dimensional space. To begin, we developed a general sheet model that can be used to simulate the behavior of a variety of materials, including paper, cloth, rubber sheets, and springy metal plates[5, 6]. The specific material we simulate is determined by the choice of several parameters of the model, governing the resistance to stretch, resistance to bending, and mass-density of the material.

These simulated materials let us predict and visualize the behavior of real deformable objects and allow us to create images and movies of such things as a flag waving in the wind (Fig. 14.7) or a piece of cloth draping over other objects (Fig. 14.8). Although the behavior of such objects is sufficiently complex that considerable artistic skill is required to make a natural-appear-

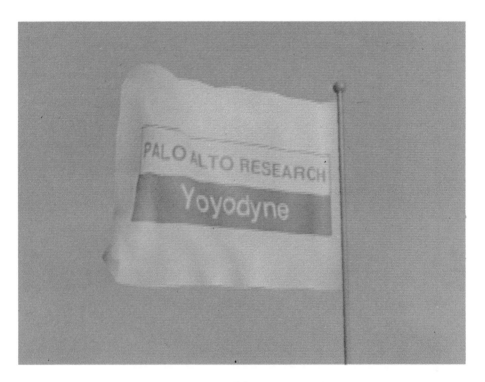

Fig. 14.7.   A simulated flag waving in the wind.

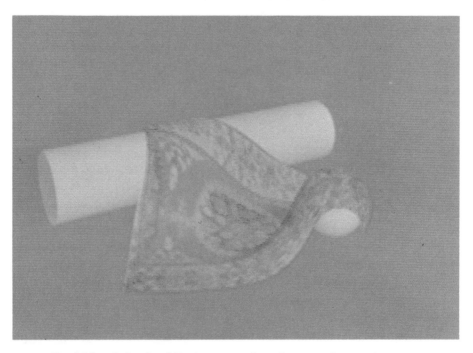

Fig. 14.8.   A simulated Persian carpet draped over a sphere and cylinder.

ing drawing of a draping piece of cloth, the simulated materials allow us to mimic the behavior and appearance of the real objects by applying the appropriate time-varying forces to them.

In graphics we wish to predict the deformation of a surface, given the applied forces. In vision, we wish to solve the inverse problem: given a moving image of a deforming sheet, or a static image of a sheet that has been deformed, we would like to compute the forces and material parameters that gave rise to the deformation. Having done so, we can predict the object's behavior in other situations. In general, this is a very difficult problem which remains unsolved. However, in restricted cases we have been able to get good solutions[3, 4, 10].

One such case is depicted in Fig. 14.10(a) which shows a piece of wood containing a knot. As the wood developed, the initially straight grain lines were deformed by the growth of the intruding knot. Given the final picture, we want to reconstruct this process, restoring the wood texture to its undeformed state and deleting the knot.

To do so, we start with a simulated elastic sheet overlayed on the picture. Imagine that the sheet is ruled with a series of horizontal lines, like notepad paper. Our first step is to immerse the sheet in a force field, inducing a deformation that causes the originally horizontal lines to line up with the curved grain lines in the image. By measuring the local direction of the grain at many locations in the image we produce a kind of flow field (Fig. 14.9) which is then used to apply rotational and translational forces to the sheet.

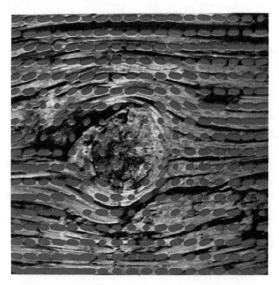

Fig. 14.9. A piece of wood with an automatically computed flow field superimposed. The red needles show the computed direction of the grain.

Having deformed the sheet, we then 'paint' the original picture on to the deformed sheet. When we remove the image forces the sheet is returned to its undeformed state, carrying the picture with it. A sequence beginning with the original picture and ending with the resulting 'straightened' image is shown in Fig. 14.10.

Axial shells

Our final example is an experiment in the design of specialized materials to simplify the task of model-building both for vision and graphics. Our premise is that global properties we want the shape of an object to have may be encoded into the properties of the material we use to form the object. Doing so reduces the amount of extra information that needs to be supplied to specify

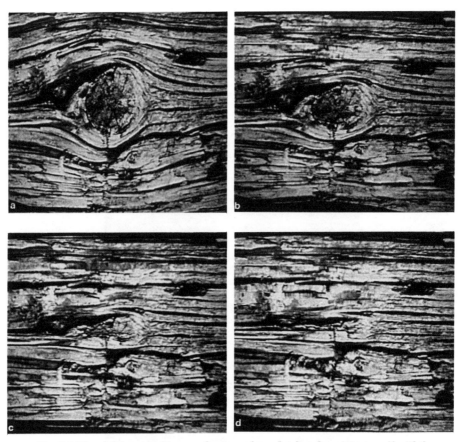

Fig. 14.10.   (a) A natural image of a piece of wood, taken from '*Textures*' by Phil Brodatz, Dover, 1966. An elastic sheet is used to model the forces responsible for bending the wood grain around the knot and to predict what would happen if the knot had been smaller (b–c) or absent altogether (d).

the shape, whether by a human model builder or by a vision system.

An interesting class of global properties are symmetries: many biological forms are approximately symmetric, as are many things we wish to build. To exploit this kind of regularity, we constructed a *symmetry-seeking* material for radial symmetries around an axis, based on the sheet model described above[3, 8]. First, we sew two opposite edges of a sheet together to form a tube, then cinch the ends of the tube to form a kind of sausage (all, of course, by the imposition of additional forces.) To create a symmetry-seeking object, we then run a wire down the middle of the tube, and impose two forces of interaction between the tube and the wire[7]. One force holds the wire in place within the tube. The

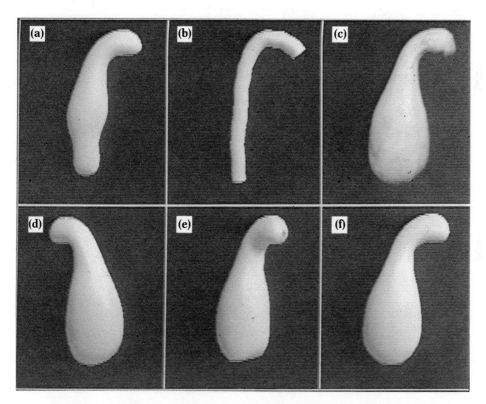

Fig. 14.11.   Interactive modeling of 3-D surfaces using axial shells. The squash (a) is modeled using an axial shell (b) that initially resembles a piece of macaroni. The shell was formed by rolling an elastic sheet into a tube. The tube was then bent interactively to conform roughly to the principal axis of the squash. The edges of this primitive tube are then attracted to the 2-D image boundaries of the squash. A pseudo force enforces symmetry in three dimensions, so that as the tube grows wider, it also grows in depth. Thus, the tube gradually inflates like an elastic balloon (c–d). The end result is a reasonable 3-D model of the squash, that can be displayed from a different viewpoint than the original image (e–f).

other influences the shape of the tube, making it tend toward symmetry around the wire. The resulting elastic body 'tries' to be radially symmetric around a flexible axis, although it can be coerced into non-symmetric forms by the application of sufficiently strong external forces.

Using these axial shells makes it easy to specify shapes that are approximately symmetric around an axis, or nearly so, because the material itself can do most of the work. For example, things we might form initially on a potter's wheel, then bend or pinch, can be economically specified by applying forces to just a few points.

Similarly, axial shells can be used to reconstruct roughly symmetric shapes from images, by imposing image-derived forces on the shell. By way of example, we show in Fig. 14.11 the 3-dimensional reconstruction of a crook-necked squash, derived from its outline in a static image. The reconstruction was made by extending the edge-attractor forces that we used for snakes (see above) into three dimensions, and applying these forces to axial shells.

Conclusions

Manipulating unconstrained models is an onerous task. The exact shape of each part has to be specified in detail. Every aspect of the way each part moves and interacts with other parts has to be completely described. If some part of the description is missing, then there is no automatic way to fill it in.

By contrast, constrained models allow for far simpler control. Pieces that are supposed to be attached stay attached without the need for further intervention. When you drop a suitably constrained model, it falls to the floor. You don't have explicitly to place it there. If one part collides with another, then ordinary physical constraints cause them to bounce. For models derived from vision, if part of the shape isn't visible, then symmetry and smoothness constraints can fill in a reasonable guess for the rest of the shape.

Whether the constraints come from physical forces, such as those involved in collisions, or non-physical sources, such as the symmetry force, their power lies in the way they allow a computer to turn partial descriptions of a model into the complete description it needs. The constraints fill in the missing information. They do this by incorporating dynamics into a model. Making a small change to some piece can cause other parts to move or deform so the constraints are satisfied. This dynamic behavior tremendously facilitates the model-building process, whether in graphics or vision.

15

Understanding the digital image

JOHN LANSDOWN

Introduction

Making drawn and painted images has always been part of our nature. There is evidence of picture-making going back to at least 15,000 BC but, as Sir Ernst Gombrich has pointed out, only for a few short periods in history has the goal of image-makers been to present, as it were, 'snapshot realism' – where one shows in a picture only that which could be seen from a single viewpoint as if photographed by an eyewitness with a snapshot camera. The main thrust of current research and development in making images by computer, so-called *computer graphics*, is towards such snapshot realism – often by computer scientists working on the mistaken belief that making 'realistic' images on the eyewitness principle is the preoccupation of artists[1].

It is hard to say what realism is – and I am not the one to try and make any useful statements about it – but it is clear that we judge the 'realism' of the scenes that surround us by using more information that can be acquired from a single viewpoint. Many of us do not regard photographs as a 'realistic' representation of the world at all and find more truth to our understanding of what something is when we see an artist's impression of it. But this essay is an introduction to the way in which computer graphics is being used to make images which try to emulate the realism obtainable in photographs and, except in the Conclusion, whenever the word 'realism' is used henceforth it is such photographic realism that is being implied.

Making computer drawings

There are basically two ways of creating images by computer. One is to sketch the desired pictures into the machine by using the computer analogues of paper, paint and pencil. Nowadays a large number of different systems exist which allow someone to sit at the equivalent of a drawing board and draw directly into the computer whilst watching the image being simultaneously displayed on a screen. Such devices are called *paint systems* and they give their users a range of tools and pallettes to help in such things as drawing straight lines, forming proper circles and ellipses, colouring-in areas without overlapping edges, easy editing of pictures, and so on. Once in the system, the images become two-dimensional digital representations which can be stored and then manipulated in ways which are not easy to achieve in conventional media. Paint systems, however, cannot be fully exploited unless their users have considerable prowess at drawing.

The other method of creating images by computer is very different. It might be called *modelled graphics* and, in this case, we do not give the computer a picture of the scene depicted but, rather, mathematical models of the objects that comprise the scene together with instructions on the laws of perspective, lighting, reflection, shadowing and so on. We then ask the computer to give us views of the scene which it derives from this knowledge and information. Whereas, in a paint system, the 'model' of what is to be depicted exists only in the draftsperson's head, in the modelled system it is the computer which holds the model and it creates its images from this. It is not necessary to have drawing skills in order to use a modelled system although, as I have pointed out elsewhere[2], visual literacy is an essential requirement. It is only modelled systems that will be dealt with in the rest of this essay.

Characteristics of the digital image

Perhaps the most important thing to realise about a digital image is that it is a sample. Just like a newspaper photograph, a digital image is built up not as a continuous surface but as an array of individual dots of different intensities and colours which, if you will, present a sample of the more properly continuous image. The dots in computer graphics are called 'pixels' – short for 'picture elements' – and the number of pixels a computer graphics system can display on a screen is a measure of the system's *resolution*. The resolution of many systems is no more than 512×512 pixels (comparable with a normal TV image). Sampling an image at such resolutions introduces some problems – not the least being that many of the lines drawn on the screen appear 'staircased' with jagged edges as illustrated in Fig. 15.1. This problem is a well-understood outcome of sampling theory known as *aliasing* and, to remove its effects, special anti-aliasing techniques have to be introduced. These techniques, which usually involve taking into account the contribution to the image of each individual pixel together with some of its surrounding pixels, greatly slow down the process of making the pictures.

It might be thought that screens of better resolution would be an answer to this problem. It can be shown that, for a 17-inch diagonal monitor viewed at a distance of 25 inches, a resolution of nearly 4000×4000 pixels is required

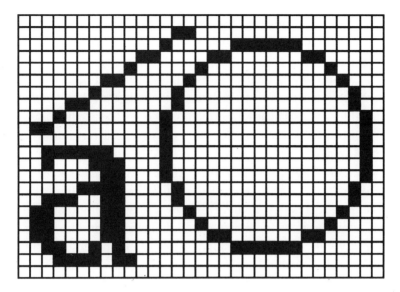

Fig. 15.1. Pixel-drawn line, circle and letter.

to meet the full requirements of the eye[3]. No one makes, or is planning to make, screens of such resolution. Even if they did, it would then be necessary to calculate the picture at a resolution of 4000×4000 (16 million) pixels and it is not clear that this would be faster than calculating at a resolution of 512×512 (262 thousand) pixels or 1000×1000 (1 million) pixels with anti-aliasing.

Ray tracing

For the time being in computer graphics the only method available for making realistic images is a somewhat 'brute force' technique known as *ray tracing*. The basic idea underlying ray tracing is to follow the paths of the many rays of light which illuminate a scene and to note the ways in which they are absorbed, reflected or refracted by the surfaces which they meet. Depending on their paths, some of these rays will finally meet the observer's eyepoint and, hence, contribute to the image. As most of the rays from the sources never reach the viewpoint, it would be computationally inefficient to trace from source to eye so, in the actual method, rays are traced from the eyepoint through each pixel out into the scene. (It is interesting to note that the Pythagoreans of the fourth century BC, also took the view that rays proceeded from the eye to the scene instead of vice versa.)

A ray projected from the eye into the space in which the objects lie will either intersect a surface or go out into the background. If there are transparent or shiny objects in the space, the ray that meets them will be refracted or reflected and then continue on to meet other objects or light sources which can be seen through or mirrored on the surfaces. A ray must be cast from the eye through each pixel point on the screen and checked against every object in the space to see whether it intersects it. If there are multiple objects, a given ray might intersect many of them and each intersection point must be calculated (Fig. 15.2). The intersection points have then to be sorted in order of distance from the eyepoint before it is possible to determine what colour should be displayed by a particular screen pixel. Sometimes scenes are ray traced on screens having a resolution of 1000×1000 pixels so as many as 1 million rays will be cast and some of these will intersect multiple surfaces or be reflected and refracted to spawn further rays. In addition, in order to display shadows, new rays have to be cast from light sources into the scene. It is not surprisng therefore that, even using the fastest computers available today, ray-traced pictures take a long time to produce.

Of course, many ingenious techniques have been devised to minimise computation and to speed up ray tracing – very few pictures are made using exactly the basic method just described[4]. However, even employing all the available short cuts, ray-traced pictures are expensive in terms of both money and computer resources. Images showing multiple objects having refractive and reflective surfaces can take two to three hours and longer to compute on very fast and costly machines.

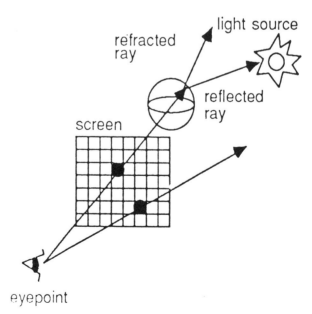

Fig. 15.2. **Ray-tracing method requires following path of all the light rays which meet the eye after being reflected or refracted by surfaces.**

Making ray-traced images

In broad terms there are six steps to be followed in making a ray-traced image. What has to be done is:

1. Create mathematical models of the objects to be depicted.
2. Place these in their required positions and orientations in space by means of the mathematical transformations of translation, rotation and scaling.
3. For each pixel, cast a ray from the eyepoint into the scene and calculate its intersection with any objects it meets in order to determine which surfaces are hidden and which visible. If the ray is refracted or reflected, continue the ray (and any of its progeny) until it strikes a light source, is absorbed by an object or goes off into the background.
4. Sort the intersections according to distance from the eyepoint. The closest intersection with a solid surface indicates the surface to be shown. This completes the testing for hidden surfaces – a process which, as has been shown in a seminal paper by Sutherland, Sproull & Schumacker[5], relies heavily on efficient sorting procedures.
5. Cast a ray from each visible surface to each light source to determine the areas which are in shadow.
6. For each pixel, compute the anti-aliased image and then display it.

It should be emphasised that the computer has no 'knowledge' about the scene other than that which it can compute from its model. Hence any ray sent out into the object space must be tested against *all* the objects to see whether it intersects them or not. An intelligent agent would know that a ray sent out, say, into the left-hand top corner of the scene would not meet a small object in the bottom right-hand corner but most ray-tracing programs are not intelligent and the only way they can learn which objects a ray hits is to test them all.

In attempting to make a realistic impression of a scene, then, we have to model both the objects in it and the behaviour of the light illuminating it.

Modelling objects

Two characteristics of an object influence the way it looks. These are its geometry and its surface finish (which, in turn, is influenced by its materials of construction). The geometry of certain objects is very easy to describe mathematically. The forms of cylinders, spheres, and similar regular solids, for example, can be specified by elementary mathematical formulae. Fortunately for computer graphics workers, many man-made objects are assembled from these simpler solids or *primitives* as they are known, and a whole new branch of applied mathematics called Constructive Solid

Geometry (CSG) has been built up to deal with this class of objects. Fig. 15.3 illustrates how a more complex shape can be made up from the addition and subtraction of primitives[6]. Two other solid forms are also easy to describe to a computer: those which have the same cross-sections throughout their lengths – such as extruded objects; and those which are formed by rotating a semi-cross-section 360° around an axis – such as objects which could be turned on a simple lathe (Fig. 15.4a, b). These two types are known as *swept forms*: those with the same-cross sections throughout their lengths are formed by *translational sweeping*, (a) and the others by *rotational sweeping* (b) Objects of freer form such as ship hulls and motor car bodies require rather more mathematics to describe but these forms too are now subject to well-understood geometrical treatment via an armoury of new surface specification techniques. The treatment of free form surfaces now goes under the name of *computational geometry*[7].

Objects which are not so easy to describe are natural forms such as trees, plants, mountains, and coastlines although here too great strides in descriptive methods are being made – particularly through the medium of the new mathematics of fractals invented by Benoit Mandelbrot[8].

Perhaps the most difficult object of all to describe to a computer is the human body. Indeed on all the evidence, we are still a very long way from being able to give a convincing rendering of any part of a person although there are some possibilities in sight[9]. (Don Pearson discusses computer-generated cartoon of human faces on pp.46–60.)

As far as computer graphics is concerned, the surface finish of an object has to be rendered by considering the way in which it reflects light. Matt surfaces appear matt because they reflect light in a diffuse way. Shiny surfaces appear shiny because they reflect much of the impinging light in a coherent way and,

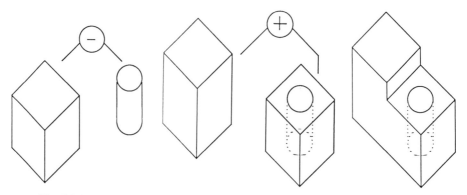

Fig. 15.3.   CSG method of building a complex object by adding and deducting simple primitives.

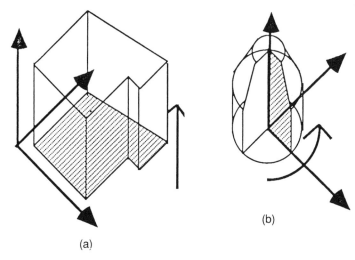

(a)

(b)

Fig. 15.4. (a) Translational sweeping. (b) Rotational sweeping.

if the surface is shiny enough, in a way that the light source itself can be seen.

For accuracy to the physics of the situation, a model of the illuminated surface must take into account energy equilibrium. That is to say, the energy reflected from the surface plus that passing through the surface must equal the illuminating energy. At any point on the surface of an object, the lightness of that point therefore depends on the roughness of the surface, its reflectivity and transmissivity, and the intensity of light reaching the point from all directions (including from other surfaces). A further complication is that reflectivity and transmissivity is wavelength-dependent: the colour of the light leaving the surface is not the same as that reaching it and different materials make the change in different ways (Fig. 15.5). Because of all this complexity, gross simplifications in modelling have to be adopted and much research goes into ways of making the simplifications rational without losing too much information[10].

Conclusion

Why is all this work on synthetic imagery being carried out? Primarily, of course, because of the intellectual challenge it affords. But it has its practical uses too. Designers frequently need to simulate the appearance of objects before making them; aeroplane pilots need flight training simulators which show convincing scenes; the entertainment industry wants to create realistic images of scenes for which it would be difficult to make full-sized or scaled physical models – indeed, it is probably from the entertainment industry that the maximum demand is arising.

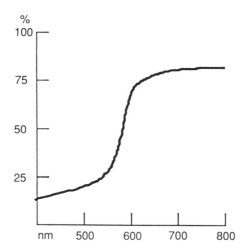

Fig. 15.5. **Percentage of light reflected from copper depends on wavelength of incident light.**

It is clear, though, that we are only just beginning to understand the ways of making synthetic images which match the *complexity* of reality. This is not the same as matching the *appearance* of it and I believe that we have a long way to go in both directions yet. To my mind it is more important to know how to deal with scenes of the same complexity as those captured by photographs than it is to model reality – even if that were, in the general case, possible. Above all, those who take a more broad view of the world than do many computer scientists should never cease to point out to them that the object of art is not to copy reality but to make sense of it. And making sense of a scene is something computers have scarcely begun to do.

16

The draughtsman's contract: how an artist creates an image

JOHN WILLATS

Introduction

What is the 'draughtsman's contract'? If it is the contract which the draughtsman makes to produce a picture which gives a truthful account of the world, how can this be done? How *do* artists create images?

'What is *The Draughtsman's Contract?*' is, on the other hand, an easier question to answer: it is the name of a film made by Peter Greenaway in 1981 for the British Film Institute. The film is set at the end of the 17th century and concerns an architectural draughtsman who is engaged, under rather unusual circumstances, to produce a set of drawings of a country house. The draughtsman, a Mr Neville, believes (at least so far as draughtsmanship is concerned) in fidelity; and to achieve this he makes use of a drawing machine (Fig. 16.1) which enables him to copy the appearance of the scene on to his paper. But to his dismay, various unexplained objects begin to intrude themselves into his pictures: a ladder appears, leaning against a window, and various items of clothing are discovered strewn about the landscape. When the owner of the house is murdered, the fidelity of Mr Neville's drawings (as well as his behaviour) is brought into question: are they to be accepted as truthful evidence?

Using a drawing machine would have been normal practice at the end of the 17th century, and in fact drawing machines had already been in common use by artists and draughtsmen for nearly 200 years. Albrecht Dürer[1] described several kinds of drawing machines, including one similar to that used in the film, and Leonardo da Vinci[2] showed a picture of a man using one in his *Notebooks*. During the 18th century drawing machines were improved by concentrating the light from the scene using a lens, and in the 19th century a way was found of capturing this light on film. The development of the drawing machine thus culminated in the invention of photography.

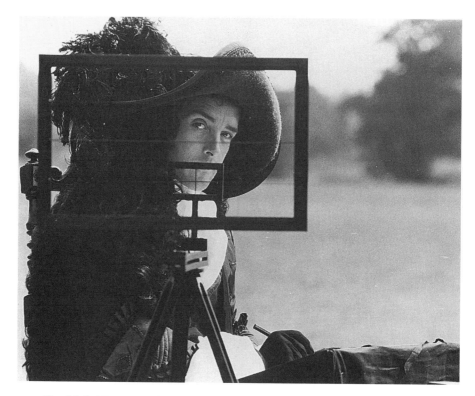

Fig. 16.1. Location photograph by Simon Archer for *The Draughtsman's Contract: Mr Neville (Anthony Higgins) drafting.* Courtesy of The British Film Institute.

The image captured by a drawing machine or camera is necessarily in perspective, and all through this period the optical basis of perspective was seen as a guarantee of its truth. In 1665 Robert Hooke[3], Curator of Experiments and sometime Secretary to the Royal Society, and himself the inventor of a drawing machine, argued that the exact recording of visual observations was the key to new and true knowledge:

> Shewing, that there is not so much requir'd towards it, any strength of *Imagination*, or exactness of *Method*, or depth of *Contemplation* (though the addition of these, where they can be had, musts needs produce a much more perfect composure) as a *sincere Hand*, and a *faithful Eye*, to examine, and to record, the things themselves as they appear.

Fifty years later Dr Brook Taylor in his famous book[4] on perspective commented:

> A Picture drawn in the utmost Degree of Perfection, and placed in a proper Position, ought so to appear to the Spectator, that he should not be able to distinguish what is there represented, from the real original

Objects actually placed where they are represented to be. In order to produce this effect, it is necessary that the Rays of Light ought to come from the several Parts of the Picture to the Spectator's Eye, with all the same Circumstances of Direction, Strength of Light and Shadow, and Colour, as they would so from the corresponding Parts of the real Objects seen in their proper Places.

In our own century the same sentiments find an echo in J.J. Gibson's[5] early definition of a 'faithful' picture – the definition which is likely to remain in most people's minds, in spite of all Gibson's subsequent efforts to correct it:

A delimited surface so processed that it yields a sheaf of light-rays to a given point which is the same as would be the sheaf of rays from the original scene to a given point.

If the optical basis of perspective is to be accepted as a guarantee of truth, as these authorities suggest, then our draughtsman Mr Neville would seem to be right: using a drawing machine or better still a camera is all that is necessary to make a truthful picture. If this were the case, then picture making, and analysing pictures, would indeed be trivial pursuits. But in fact photographs, or pictures which look realistic in a photographic way, only give one kind of truth: truth to appearances. Another kind of truth, equally important both to artists and to architects and engineers, is truth about the shapes of objects as they really are, independent of any particular viewpoint. This is the truth that Cézanne and later the Cubists were after: the kind of descriptions of objects that we arrive at in our minds after the visual system has processed and collated the immediate and transitory sensations available at the retina. David Marr[6], attempting to describe this end-point or goal of the visual process, called it the '3-D model' and described images of this kind as 'canonical'.

The attempt to depict this kind of 'canonical' image led artists after Cézanne, and especially those of our own century, to abandon perspective[7]:

Perspective is as accidental a thing as lighting. . . . Certainly reality shows us those objects mutilated in this way. But in reality, we can change position: a step to the right and a step to the left complete our vision. The knowledge we have of an object is, as I said before, a complex sum of perceptions. The plastic image does not move: it must be complete at first sight; therefore it must renounce perspective.

In practice, these different kinds of truths are expressed in pictures through different kinds of formal structures. The two main ones are the *drawings systems* which, like perspective, give an account of the spatial relationships between objects, and the *denotation systems* which say how the various marks on the picture surface are related to objects in the real world.

Drawing systems

Pictures can be based on any of a number of different drawing systems or combinations of systems. The following pictures, taken more or less at random from various periods and cultures, are simply intended to illustrate a few of the systems which are available.

Figure 16.2 shows a view of Venice drawn by Canaletto and illustrates what everyone knows about *perspective*: that the orthogonals, or lines representing edges in depth, converge to a vanishing point. Pictures of this kind give an optically true impression of the inclination of such edges and their projected lengths as they appear in the visual field.

Figure 16.3 is taken from a Chinese painting and is drawn in *oblique projection*. In this system the orthogonals are parallel instead of converging as they do in perspective. Pictures drawn in this system have the advantage over pictures in perspective in that they can be extended without distortion in any direction, whereas pictures in perspective can show only a limited field of view. Moreover, edges in depth, as well as edges in the other two (frontal) directions, can be shown as *true lengths*.

Figure 16.4 shows a detail from a 14th century Italian painting drawn in a

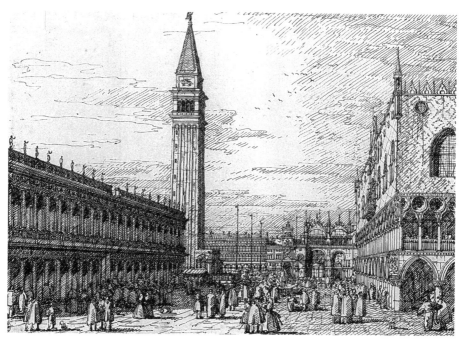

Fig. 16.2. *Perspective:* Canaletto, *Venice: The Libraria and Campanile from the Piazzetta*, mid 1730s. Ink over pencil, 27 × 37.5 cm. The Royal Library, Windsor Castle. Copyright reserved. Reproduced by gracious permission of Her Majesty The Queen.

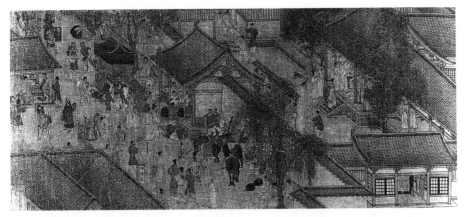

Fig. 16.3.   *Oblique projection: Lady Wen-chi's Return to China: Fourth Leaf*, ca. AD 1100, Northern Sung. Ink and colours on silk, 24.8 × 67.2 cm. Courtesy Museum of Fine Arts, Boston, Ross Collection.

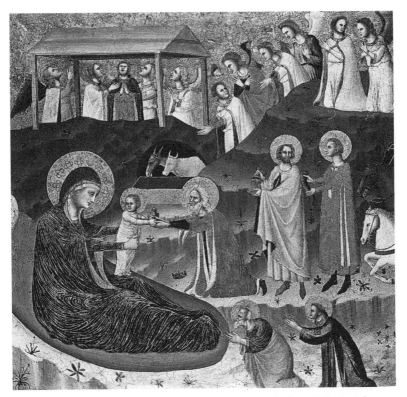

Fig. 16.4.   *Horizontal oblique projection*: Master of the Blessed Clare, *Adoration of the Magi*, mid-14th century, Riminese School. Oil on wood. Courtesy of Lowe Art Museum, University of Miami, Samuel H. Kress Collection.

system known as *horizontal oblique projection*. In this system the side and front faces of an object are joined together and shown as *true shapes*.

Horizontal oblique projection has a sister system called *vertical oblique projection* in which the top and front of an object are shown together. Two examples are shown here. In the first, a detail of a painting by David Hockney, the front of the house is shown as a true shape but the roof is somewhat foreshortened (Fig. 16.5). The second example (Fig. 16.6) is an architect's drawing and a strict version of vertical oblique projection; although in this context it would perhaps be better described as a variety of *axonometric*

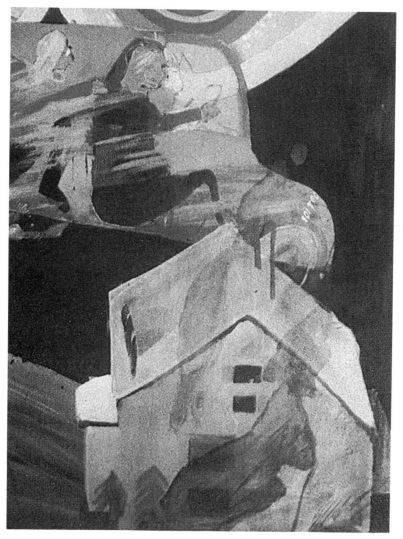

Fig. 16.5.   *Vertical oblique projection:* David Hockney, *Flight into Italy – Swiss Landscape*, 1962. (Detail.) Oil on canvas. Courtesy of the artist.

projection. (Rather confusingly, different disciplines have different names for the systems.) Normal axonometric projection with the plan of the building shown at an angle to the paper is in common use for architect's drawings, but a frontal view such as the one shown here is something of a rarity.

Pictures in *orthographic projection* (Figs. 16.7, 16.8) show only one face of an object, always as a *true shape*. Sometimes this true shape also corresponds to a possible view, as in the architect's drawing shown in Fig. 16.7, top. Figure 16.7, lower is a sectional plan of the same building and the idea of a

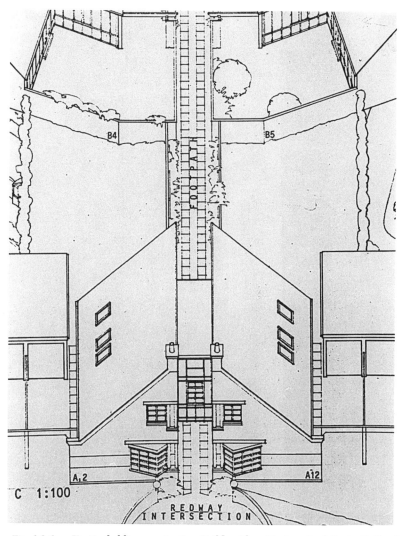

Fig. 16.6. *Vertical oblique projection:* Feilden Clegg Design, Architects, *Bolbeck Park, Milton Keynes, Commended Scheme,* 1984 (detail). Courtesy of the architects.

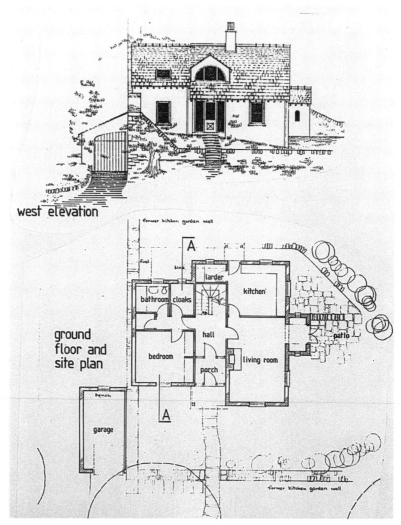

west elevation

ground
floor and
site plan

Fig. 16.7. *Orthographic projection.* Bob Mitchell, Architect, *Proprietor's Cottage, Hollens Hotel, Grassmere*, 1984. (Detail.) Courtesy of the architect.

view here is largely irrelevant, since the architect's intention is not to show an aerial view of the building with the roof taken off, but to show the shapes of the various rooms, and how they are connected. Similarly, the child's drawing of a house shown in Fig. 16.8 could be a sectional view through a snowdrift, but is more likely intended to show a house *surrounded* by snow: a *topological* rather than a projective relationship.

No picture on a two-dimensional surface can give the whole truth about the shape of a three-dimensional object. Instead, pictures in perspective are useful

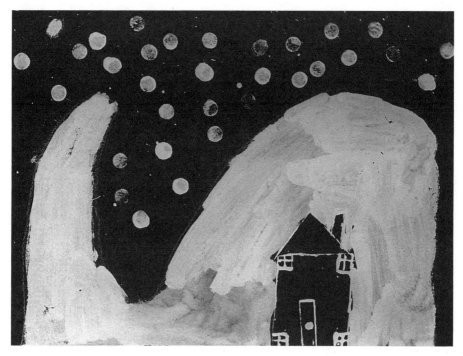

Fig. 16.8. *Orthographic projection.* Arfan Khan, aged 7.5, *House with a Huge Snowdrift.*

for showing the appearance of objects from a particular viewpoint, whereas pictures in some of the other systems show the true lengths of edges or the true shapes of surfaces. David Marr would say that pictures in perspective aim at giving a *viewer-centred* description of the world, while pictures in some of the other systems are intended to give *object-centred* descriptions.

Denotation systems

Each side in the long-standing dispute[8] about whether perspective is just one system among many or whether it is unique in giving a true account of the world has tended to take its arguments from the different drawing systems. But pictures can be described in another way: in terms of the different relationships between the marks on the surface and the features of the real world which these marks *denote*. Figure 16.7, like most architects' drawings, is based on a system in which *lines* stand for *edges*: edges such as the edges of windows and doors which have an objective existence independent of any particular viewpoint or lighting condition. Figure 16.9, a still taken from a videotape of *The Draughtsman's Contract*, is also a picture of a house, and here too we are inclined to say that the picture shows the edges of doors and

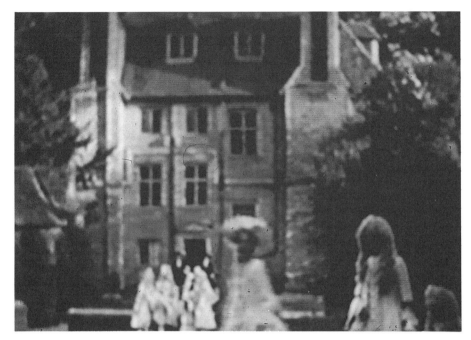

Fig. 16.9.   Still taken from a videotape of *The Draughtsman's Contract.* Courtesy of The British Film Institute.

windows. But an enlargement of part of the picture (Fig. 16.10) shows that these features are only represented indirectly. What the marks in pictures of this kind represent (at several stages removed in this case) is the pattern of light intensities which fell on the film as the house was photographed. Here, the marks (small *blobs* or patches of pigment) stand for or denote the *intercepts of small bundles of light rays* as they were received by the camera, or would have been received on the retina of a spectator at the same point. There is no representation of edges or similar features as such: the brain has to interpret the pattern of light intensities provided by the picture in order to extract features such as edges, just as it has to do when interpreting the array of light from a real scene as it falls on the retina. In pictures of this kind – photographs and Impressionist and Pointillist paintings – the artist or cameraman is passive so far as the representation of shape is concerned and all the work of interpretation has to be done by the person who views the picture. In architects' drawings (Fig. 16.7) and most children's drawings (Fig. 16.8) the draughtsman does the work of feature extraction and these features are directly represented in the picture.

Human beings are very good at extracting features such as edges from the varying intensity of light as it falls on the retina – so good that it is difficult at

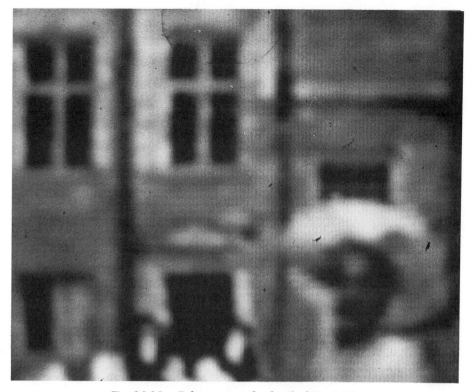

Fig. 16.10.   Enlargement of a detail of Fig. 16.9.

first to appreciate that the process of extracting edges must be a very complex one. Gibson would say that no such extraction is necessary, as such features are simply 'given' as invariants in the array of light. Just so; but what are these 'invariants' and how do human beings detect them? One thing we can say is that edges cannot be detected reliably just by looking for sharp changes in light intensity. Figure 16.11 shows a black and white photograph of a man under natural lighting conditions. Figure 16.12 shows what happens when lines are used to mark the places where sharp changes of light intensity occur. This process does pick out some genuine edges, but most of the lines mark the edges of shadows or highlights, and it is obvious that this does not result in an acceptable drawing. The same sort of effect can often be found in drawings by amateur artists and beginners in the life class.

Figure 16.13 is another line drawing of the head and shoulders of a man – this time *Igor Stravinsky* drawn by Picasso. In this drawing the lines denote: thin wire-like forms (such as hair), true edges (the edges of Stravinsky's glasses), 'soft' edges (the contours of the nose and cheek) and the boundaries of areas of differing local tones and colours (the pattern of spots on the tie).

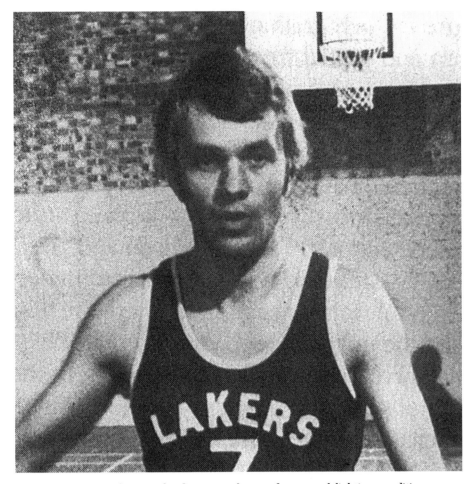

Fig. 16.11. Photograph of a man taken under normal lighting conditions.
Courtesy of BBC *Horizon*.

What lines are *not* used to stand for are the boundaries of shadows, areas of
tonal modelling, and highlights, although these would undoubtedly have
been present in Picasso's visual field. Much of the artistry of this drawing
comes from the exercise of informed choice. For some reason humans will
accept some denotation systems as the basis for convincing or 'realistic'
drawings, although the relationships between the marks and actual light
intensities from the scene are not at all direct. Others (like that used in
Fig. 16.12 where the lines stand for the positions of sharp changes in light
intensity) we will not accept, and it is part of an artist's training to learn
which is which.

I have given examples of two denotation systems: one in which the marks

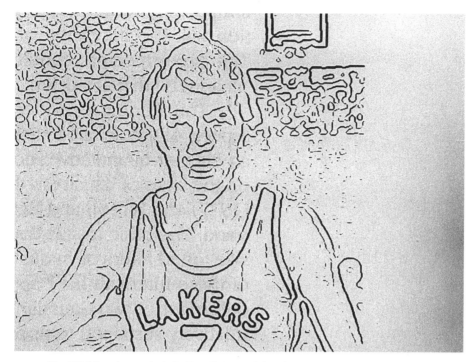

Fig. 16.12. An analysis by David Marr of the photograph shown in Fig. 16.11. The lines show the boundaries between areas of sharp tonal contrast. Courtesy of BBC *Horizon*.

stand for different colours and intensities in the optic array and another in which the marks stand for permanent features of the scene like true edges. Like the drawing systems, the denotation systems can also be grouped according to whether they form part of a transitory viewer-centred description or a more permanent object-centred description. Very often, related types of drawing systems and denotation systems are found together. In photographs the drawing system, perspective, is necessarily viewer-centred, and the marks, which stand for light intensities as they reach the eye or the camera, also form part of a viewer-centred description. In architects' drawings and children's drawings, on the other hand, the drawing systems form part of an object-centred description, and so do the marks.

This being so, it might seem superfluous to make a distinction between drawing systems and denotation systems. Why not just say that different pictures give more or less viewer-centred or object-centred accounts of the world? Such a scheme would be very economical. In addition, it is tempting to think of it as having far-reaching psychological implications. In Marr's account of the visual process the viewer-centred descriptions available at the

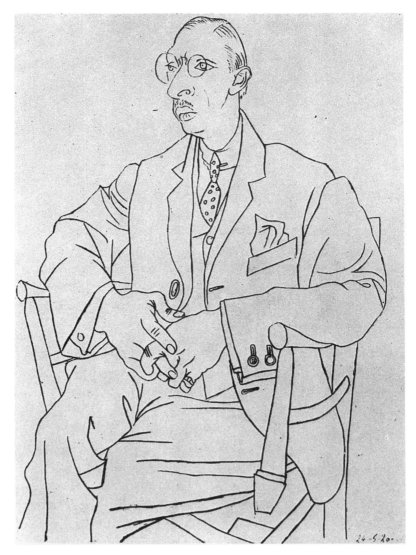

Fig. 16.13.   Picasso, *Igor Stravinsky*, 1920. (Detail.) Pencil. Private collection.
Copyright DACS.

retina are progressively changed, through a series of discrete stages, to give object-centred descriptions which are useful to humans in understanding the permanent shapes of objects (so that they can be recognized when seen from a new viewpoint or under new lighting conditions, for example). The design features of these stages – the co-ordinate systems on which they are based, the elements or 'primitives' of which they are composed – seem very similar to those found in the different drawing and denotation systems which form the basis of a picture: a point made by Marr himself.

Might this not be the key to a new kind of 'natural' theory of pictures, similar to Gibson's but taking account of other kinds of pictures as well as those in perspective? Photographs and Impressionist and Pointillist pictures would then correspond to the information available at the retina in the optic array (Gibson's[5] 'faithful' pictures) while other pictures (line drawings, for instance, like Picasso's drawing of Stravinsky) might correspond to the information available at other stages of the visual process – the $2\frac{1}{2}$-D sketch, perhaps, in Marr's scheme. This would provide a simple and economical theory of pictures: different kinds of pictures simply correspond to different stages in the visual process.

Too simple, unfortunately. Although related drawing and denotation systems often do go together they do not always do so. The Canaletto (Fig. 16.2) is an example: the drawing system is viewer-centred but the marks (lines) stand for edges which form part of an object-centred description. Conversely, the 19th century architects at the École des Beaux Arts often combined the use of strict object-centred orthographic projection with the whole repertoire of viewer-centred 'rendering': cast shadow, tonal modelling, highlights and colour. Many similar examples can be found, and it is hard to see how these 'hybrid' pictures could correspond in any direct way to simple intermediate stages in the visual system, whether in Marr's scheme or any other.

Hybrid pictures

Hybrids may occur accidentally or be more or less contrived. Natural hybrids often occur when the pictures produced by a culture are undergoing a change: for example, when the Italian artists of the 14th and 15th centuries were struggling to master perpective. In this period we often find pictures made up of mixtures of old and new drawing systems. Similarly, hybrids can occur during transitional stages as children learn to draw. The drawing systems and denotation systems seem to get 'out of step' and a child may try to graft a new drawing system on to an old denotation system with incongruous results. Hybrids also occur when one culture influences another: Persian miniature paintings, for example, which contain drawing and denotation systems from both East and West, or the marvellous 'botanical' drawings produced by local Indian and Chinese artists for officers of the East India Company. Figures 16.14 and 16.15 illustrate the contrasting ways in which Eastern art could be influenced by the West. In the first example the traditional denotation system is retained but allied to a new drawing system. In the second example the drawing system is traditional but is married to a new denotation system.

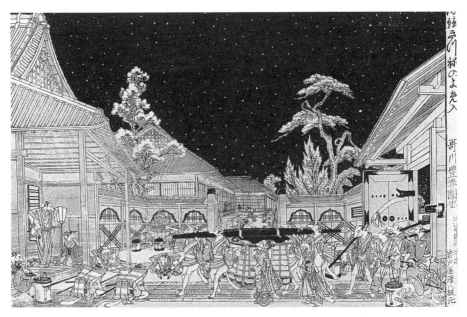

Fig. 16.14.   Utagawa Toyoharu, 1735–1814, *A Perspective Picture of the Foxes' Wedding Procession.* Woodcut, 23.3 × 33.7 cm. Nelson-Atkins Museum of Art, Kansas City, Missouri.

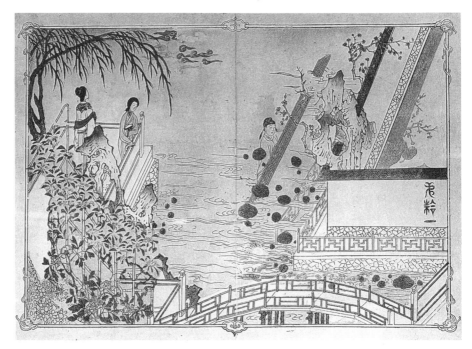

Fig. 16.15.   Min Qiji, *A Moonlight Scene from Xi Xian Ji, Dream of the Western Chamber,* 1640. Colour print. Courtesy of the Far Eastern Museum, Cologne (no. 702405).

Figure 16.14 is a Japanese woodcut which bears the inscription *A Perspective Picture of the Foxes' Wedding Procession*. The drawing system is straightforward linear perspective: commonplace in Western art but something of a novelty in Japanese pictures as the inclusion of the word 'perspective' in the title suggests. But the denotation system is completely traditional. The picture shows a night scene and the lamp on the left is alight. A Western artist would have seized on this as an excuse to show all sorts of lighting effects: cast shadow, tonal modelling and highlights. Instead, all the objects here, apart from the stars and the black sky, appear just as they would do in broad daylight; or rather an idealized daylight in which only the permanent, object-centred features of the scene are shown. In other words, the drawing system on which the picture is based – linear perspective – is well over to the viewer-centred end of the spectrum of drawing systems, but the marks in the picture depict features taken from an object-centred description.

Figure 16.15, a Chinese wood block colour print, also shows a night scene. Like the painting shown in Fig. 16.3, the drawing system used is oblique projection, probably the most commonly used system in Chinese pictures. What is quite extraordinary is that the artist has included a very realistic-looking shadow. The artist may have seen shadows in Western painting, or the idea of including a shadow may have been a personal discovery. In either case, the structure used in this picture is the reverse of that used in *The Foxes' Wedding Procession*: a drawing system towards the object-centred end of the spectrum is married to a denotation system towards the viewer-centred end.

In these hybrids the marriage of styles seems to have come about more or less by chance. In David Hockney's *The Second Marriage* (Fig. 16.16) the marriage has been arranged. The head of the woman was painted from a photograph (Fig. 16.17) and a number of other parts of the picture – the man's glasses, his face and his clothes and the bottle on the table – are painted in what Hockney elsewhere called 'an illusionistic style'. The strokes and blobs on the curtains and the sofa also seem to refer to the illusionistic effects of Impressionism and Pointillism, and the squarish marks on the floor recall both mosaics and the neo-impressionism of an early Matisse. But in fact all these marks form part of the *real* decoration of the surfaces:

> A curtain, after all, is exactly like a painting; you can take a painting off a stretcher, hang it up like a curtain, so a painted curtain could be very real All the philosophical things about flatness, if you go into it, are about reality, and if you cut out illusion then painting becomes completely 'real'.[9]

The inclusion of real wallpaper in the painting, an old trick taken over from the Cubists, carries the idea to its logical conclusion. So the picture contains

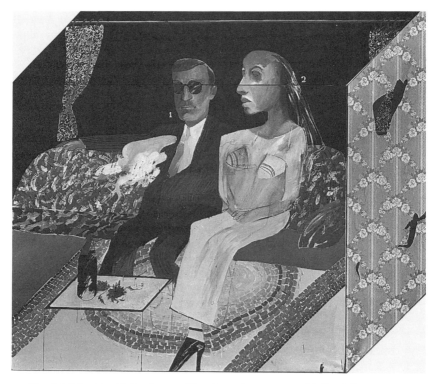

Fig. 16.16.   David Hockney, *The Second Marriage*, 1963. Oil on canvas,
183 × 183 cm. Courtesy of the artist.

examples taken from both extremes of the denotation systems: photography, capturing the transitory effects of light, and the inclusion of the real object itself.

The drawing systems used in the picture are equally complex. The bride's head is, inevitably, in perspective, since it is taken from a photograph. The picture as a whole is in oblique projection, by reason of its shape, and so is the table. But the bride's foot is shown perfectly flat and stands on the bottom of the picture, making this edge into the floor – just as children often make their houses and people stand on the bottom edge of the paper (Fig. 16.8).

In artificial hybrids like this – and hybrids are the rule rather than the exception in 20th century painting – the artist cannot simply be externalizing an internal image which could conceivably form some intermediate stage in the visual process. Still less is the artist 'copying' the array of light received on the retina, after the manner of Gibson's 'faithful' pictures. Rather, in pictures such as these, the elementary units of the perceptual system – the primitives, the coordinate systems – have been set free from the constraints of vision and reassembled as elements in a formal language.

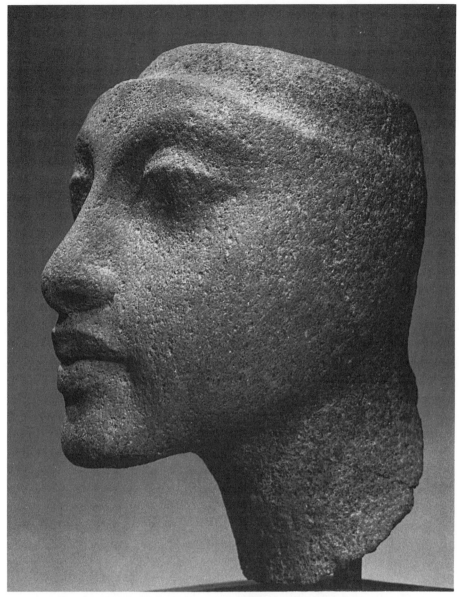

Fig. 16.17.   Photograph of *An Amarna Princess.* Plate 17 in *The Sculpture of Ancient Egypt* by C.N. Noblecourt, London: The Oldbourne Press, 1960. Courtesy of Macdonald Publishers.

Conclusions

Pictures can be described in terms of two kinds of formal systems: the drawing systems, which say where the marks in the picture go, and the denotation systems, which say what the marks in the picture stand for. Both systems can contribute to give either a viewer-centred or an object-centred description of the world. Drawing systems like perspective, for example, show the disposition of edges or other features as they appear in the visual field (viewer-centred) while some of the other drawing systems describe the direction of edges in real space, irrespective of any particular viewpoint (object-centred). Among the denotation systems some, such as impressionism, show the colour and intensity of light rays as they reach the eye (viewer-centred); others, such as those used by technical draughtsmen, use lines to stand for objective features such as edges and corners (object-centred).

Few pictures give purely viewer-centred or purely object-centred accounts of the world. Most pictures fall somewhere in between, and among them are those I have called 'hybrids': pictures in which, for example, the positions of the marks are determined by a viewer-centred drawing system such as perspective, while the marks themselves describe real objective features. Conversely, there are other hybrids in which the drawing system describes the location of features according to some objective frame of reference while the marks describe such transitory effects as highlights and shadows.

What can we deduce from the existence of these hybrids? Firstly that at least some pictures are not wholly 'natural', either in the crude sense of replicating the visual array as it impinges on the retina, or in the subtler sense of having been derived more or less directly from some internal representation which forms part of the visual system. Nor are these pictures wholly 'conventional' since either the drawing system or the denotation system will be taken fairly directly from the laws of optics. Pictures like this are in part artificial and in part taken from Nature.

Secondly, their existence suggests that there is no single ultimately truthful kind of picture: pictures say different things about the world, according to what systems they use. In the past, artists tried to give as true account as possible within the limitations of whatever drawing and denotation systems were available at the time. The results thus varied from one culture to another.

At first the different systems, like different species of roses, developed in isolation. Then, through the interactions of war and trade, systems used by one culture would be intermarried with those of another, just as hybrid roses came about when China or Damascus roses were brought to Europe. Nowadays painters and designers, like rose growers, can hybridize deliberately to produce whatever characteristics they wish. Choosing the right mix of systems to suit the job in hand is an important part of the draughtsman's contract.

PART 5

Images and thought

RICHARD HELD

We have distinguished between artists concerned with what is in front of the eye and vision scientists concerned with what is behind the eye. Now what is the relation between these approaches? I suggest the following without laying any claim as to its originality. By a complex inventive process the artist produces objects and events for the consumption of the viewer. Ernst Gombrich has masterfully described this process. Of course the viewer does not literally consume. I use the metaphor of consumption deliberately to emphasize a distinction between what can and cannot be incorporated into the experience of the perceiver. I do so to emphasize that not all conceivable objects and events are amenable to this process. In fact, I suspect that most are not. What, then, constrains acceptability of the artist's work, let alone the enjoyment and effect it may engender? To a considerable extent it must be the workings of the perceptual mechanism which, in the case of the visual arts, the vision scientist purports to understand.

The information processing equipment found in the eye and brain determines the constellation of visual stimuli originating from in front of the eye that can influence the visual system. As has been discussed by Michael Land (Chapter 13), the type of eye found in a particular species of animal determines the properties of light that excite the retina. So also do the more complex modes of processing in the brain determine its receptivity to objects and events in the world. In this sense there is reciprocity between what is in front of the eye and what lies behind it. An understanding of order in the visible world is to be found neither solely by analysis of properties of the world external to perception nor solely by understanding of the neuronal processing mechanism. The interaction of the two determines what can be seen. This interaction applies both in immediate perception and historically in the evolution of the receptive mechanisms. The visual system has evolved so as to be tuned to respond to life-sustaining features of the environment. But that function hardly limits its capabilities. The inventions of artists belie such a limitation.

Vision scientists study neuronal processes behind the eye in order to

understand the processing of visual information and provide an understanding of the light stimuli essential to such processes. They also utilize psychophysical methods to explore the capabilities of vision. How much light is
required just to detect a spot in the dark? What combinations of wavelength
yield similar colors? Psychophysicists rarely go beyond the study of simple
properties of the world as they impinge upon the visual system. Happily,
artists have no such inhibitions. They freely explore the extent of variations in
light, color, shape, and movement which are of interest to the educated visual
system. In this special sense they are performing a very sophisticated form of
psychophysics although they will not recognize their work as such. It is with
this logic, I suspect, that Jonathan Miller urged upon us the study of a
particular artifact, the film with its shifting perspectives made coherent by the
top-down processing capabilities of the brain.

Just as the visual system evolved in phylogeny to accommodate to the
different ecological niches occupied by various species, so the perceptive
abilities of the viewer adapt during a lifetime of viewing artifacts. Accord-
ingly, what appears to be chaos today may appear ordered tomorrow. The
tuning of vision to the properties of the artificial world is not passive but an
active process. The system is educable. The changing of styles bears out this
contention. But this form of learning also entails processes in the visual brain.
In summary, let me reiterate my belief that the relation between what is
outside and what is inside is reciprocal. Processes behind the eye and the
creation of artifacts in front of the eye co-determine each other. Study of the
interaction of the two should enrich our conceptions of both.

17

Understanding images in the brain

COLIN BLAKEMORE

The homunculus fallacy

If you have never read Ludwig Wittgenstein's great treatise *Philosophical Investigations*[1], I have just a single word of advice. Don't! Or, to be less facetious, do it with an open mind and a stiff drink. It is an extraordinary and puzzling book – a mixture of brilliant insight and frustrating conundrums.

Wittgenstein's enduring concern was for the nature of language and what it tells us about the minds of language-users. His arguments led him to one conclusion that seems trivial, maybe just plain wrong, but which has spawned worrying criticism of our use of everyday words to describe how the brain works. Wittgenstein wrote: 'Only of a living human being and what resembles (behaves like) a living human being can one say: it has sensations; it sees; is blind; hears; is conscious or unconscious' (Wittgenstein[1]).

Anthony Kenny[2], in his spirited defence of *The Legacy of Wittgenstein*, laments what he sees as the frequent rejection of this dictum by psychologists of perception, by neurophysiologists and by those who are interested in machine intelligence. He coined the term 'homunculus fallacy' to describe such false ascription of predicates that are valid only for *whole* human beings when talking about bits of animals or people (especially their brains), or about electronic circuits. What, exactly, is the problem, you might ask? After all, no-one would suggest that a one-legged man cannot *hear* (in the sense that we use that word to describe the auditory perceptions of an intact human being). And is it really a gross conceptual blunder to talk of a robot with an artificial eye as *seeing*? How complete must a human being be and how human-like must the behaviour of a machine be in order for the predicates of sensation and consciousness to be valid?

To clarify the issue we need an example, and the one that Anthony Kenny develops is the question of how the brain perceives the visual world (if you will, for the moment, forgive me for deliberately committing the homunculus fallacy!). Kenny thinks that present-day visual neurophysiologists and psychologists have still not escaped from a conceptual tangle first recognized by

257

René Descartes. In his description of the formation of the retinal image, in *La Dioptrique*[3] of 1637, and his subsequent suggestion that images of a sort are formed in the brain, Descartes both invented and acknowledged the major problem. 'The things we look at', he wrote, 'form quite perfect images in the back of our eyes.' Furthermore, such an image is 'not only produced in the back of the eye but also transmitted to the brain'.

Descartes did not, of course, know about nerve impulses or synaptic transmission and he followed ancient Aristotelian views about the importance of fluids or 'spirits' in the body. The clear cerebrospinal fluid, which fills the cavities or ventricles of the brain, had long been thought of as a pure and perfect distillation of blood and air. It was called *animal spirit* by the medieval philosophers, who believed it to be the source of the *anima* or soul. Descartes imagined that the myriad fibres in the optic nerves transmitted a coherent copy of the retinal image, in the form of a pattern of vibrations, on to the surface of the ventricles of the brain. Now, the traditional medieval Cell Doctrine had suggested that the ventricular system of the brain is divided into three cells, serving different aspects of mental function, from sensation (in the first cell) through thought and reason (middle cell) to memory or movement (last cell). Descartes' most famous addition to this scheme was his attribution of special status to the pineal gland, a tiny organ at the back of the ventricles (the true function of which is still obscure). He thought that the pineal gland secreted the animal spirit and acted as an interface between the soul and the mere physical machinery of the brain.

In *Les Passions de l'âme*[4], Descartes imagined that the two pictures of any particular shape in the outside world (one from each eye), formed on the lining of the ventricles, set up corresponding patterns of motion in the fluid, which 'radiate towards the little gland which is surrounded by these spirits. Thus the two images in the brain form only one image on the gland, which, acting directly on the soul, causes it to see the shape.' This single picture on the pineal gland not only fused the images of the two eyes into a single view of the world but even conveniently re-inverted it!

But then comes the problem of the homunculus fallacy. How can simply *having* an image in the brain constitute *seeing* that image? Descartes had earlier acknowledged this problem for the picture on the walls of the ventricles. 'The picture to some extent resembles the objects from which it originates... but we must not think that it is by means of this resemblance that the image makes us aware of the objects – as if we had another pair of eyes inside the brain to see it.' What was different about the image on the pineal gland was, presumably, its direct communion with the soul, which was, in effect, just such an internal pair of eyes – indeed an internal perceiver, thinker,

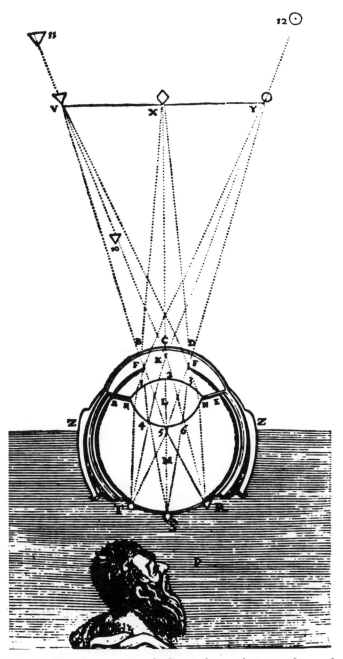

Fig. 17.1.   René Descartes was not the first to observe the inverted image formed on the retina of the eye, but Descartes' description in *La Dioptrique* of 1637 was the most complete at that time. This diagram shows the technique that Descartes used to reveal this image. He cut a window in the outer coat of the back of an ox eye and covered it with paper. He then saw the tiny inverted image formed on the paper screen.

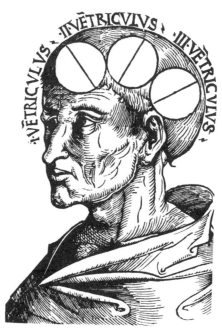

Fig. 17.2.   During the medieval period, under the influence of the Church, very
little experimental observation was carried out. Theories of brain function rested
largely on the writings of the Greeks and the dissections of Galen of Bergama
(129–199 AD). One dominant theme, which persisted until the 18th century,
was that mental processes take place in the fluid ('animal spirit') that fills the
chambers or ventricles of the brain. There are 3 such chambers, the first being
divided into a pair of lateral ventricles. According to the 'Cell Doctrine' of the Early
Christian Fathers, this first pair received messages from the sense organs; the
middle one was responsible for judgement, thought and reason; and the last was
the seat of memory and (sometimes) movement. This illustration of the Cell
Doctrine comes from the 1506 edition of *Philosophia pauperum* of Albertus
Magnus (1206–80), published as *Philosophia naturalis* by M. Furter, Basle. The
three ventricles are shown as simple circles, each divided in two.

chooser and knower. That, of course, is the essence of Cartesian Dualism. The
body, including the brain, is a machine; a delicate, complex, beautifully
interconnected machine – but merely a machine. In the *Traité de l'homme* of
1664 Descartes asks us to imagine that

> all the functions that I attribute to this machine such as . . . waking and
> sleeping; the reception of light, sounds, odours . . ., the impression of
> ideas, . . . the retention of those ideas in memory; . . . appetites and
> passions; and finally the movements of all the external members . . . occur
> naturally in this machine solely by the disposition of its organs, no less
> than the movements of a clock.

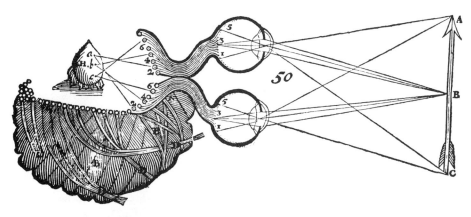

Fig. 17.3. In this famous diagram from the *Traité de l'homme* of 1664, Descartes got the anatomy very wrong but made a number of conceptual advances. He suggested that nerve fibres from each eye project into the brain in a coherent bundle, thus reproducing an array of activity (2,4,6) on the wall of the ventricles corresponding to the retinal image (1,3,5). He also proposed that combination of signals from the two eyes might occur to form a binocular image (a,b,c) on the pineal body (H), which Descartes saw as the site of communication between the spiritual soul and the machinery of the brain. In fact we now know that a binocular 'map' is indeed set up, not in the pineal, but in the primary visual cortex at the back of the cerebral hemispheres.

But, to Descartes, the essentially human features of existence and action – consciousness, perception, decision and will – were the domain of the soul, a mysterious, silent agent that watched the pictures in the brain and poked its invisible fingers into the clockwork from time to time to guide the mere machine.

If we resist the intellectual surrender of Dualism, is it possible to steer a course around the rocks of the homunculus fallacy on our way to a material explanation of behaviour and even of perception and consciousness?

Order and disorder in brains and machines

Computers can do very clever things without forming pictures in their chips. In the most general sense of the word *computer*, the brain is a computer – in the immortal words of Marvin Minsky, it is a 'meat machine'. Then could the brain not work perfectly well without having to depend on Cartesian inner images?

In June, 1986, a steering committee for a System Development Foundation Symposium on Computational Neuroscience composed a 'formulation of dialectics' in which two opposed positions were put forward in response to the question 'Is physical locality an essential part of neural computation?':

> Position 1 . . .: The anatomical structure of the brain has no more to do with its function than the shape of the cabinet of a Vax (a powerful computer), or the location of its pc boards. Brain function is determined by the logical and dynamic connection properties of its neurons. The actual physical structure, location, architecture, and geometry is irrelevant compared to its logical, connectionist aspects.
>
> Position 2: Significant recent work in brain research has been related to the discovery and elucidation of detailed forms of somatotopic mapping, laminar specialization in cortex, and columnar architectures representing sensory sub-modalities. These forms of functional architecture may represent a major mode of brain function: the formatting of sensory data in a manner which simplifies its further processing. One of the major differences in computational style of brain versus Vax may well be the indifference of the Vax to its geometry and the exquisite attention paid by the brain to its geometry[5].

Whether or not the physical, spatial arrangement of activity in the brain has *functional* significance is the issue that I want to address. Undoubtedly spatial order is a dominant feature of the brain, which is far from the random network that some theoreticians would have liked it to be. The handful of jelly that fills the human head is in fact a tightly packed conglomerate of separate clumps of nerve cells wrapped in huge bundles of axons (nerve fibres). The stem of the brain, the cerebellum, the cerebral hemispheres – they are all distinct structures with their own characteristic appearances in microscopic sections, all laid out and interconnected in a highly ordered fashion.

Even the cerebral cortex, the wrinkled mantle of grey matter that swaddles the cerebral hemispheres, is, in fact, a vast patchwork of distinct functional areas. In 1672, in Oxford, Thomas Willis first suggested, on the basis of anatomical evidence as well as the effects of brain damage, that mental functions take place in the cerebral cortex rather than in the fluid of the ventricles. But the first suggestion that specific functions are *localized* in different regions of the cerebral cortex came from the bogus science of phrenology, which claimed that various mental functions are performed in 'organs', distributed over the brain, whose development is reflected in the size of bumps on the skull. Franz Joseph Gall, the Austrian physician who founded phrenology at the start of the 19th century, was an expert and respected anatomist, who must at least take credit for drawing attention to the distinctive folds and creases in the cortex. Even the attempt to correlate individual differences in mental faculties with variations in the structure of the brain was remarkably original and far-sighted. Phrenology was scientific

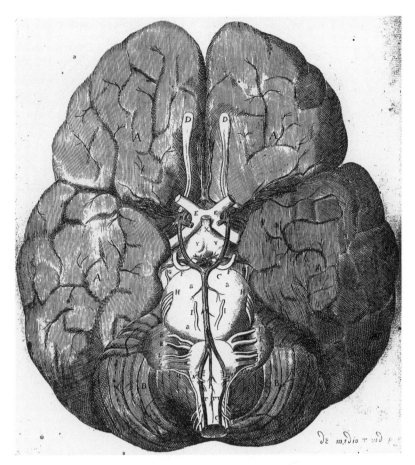

Fig. 17.4. This illustration, from the 1664 edition of *Cerebri Anatomie* of Thomas Willis (J. Martyn and J. Allestry, London), is perhaps the most famous 17th century diagram of the human brain. The original drawing was made by Christopher Wren, who worked for Willis in Oxford. The brain is shown from below, with the brainstem, surrounded by the cerebellum (B). Many of the cranial nerves, including the optic nerve (E) are seen emerging from the brainstem. The blood supply of the base of the brain is very clearly illustrated, as are the great cerebral hemispheres (A), with their many folds and grooves. Willis was the first to attribute mental functions to the cerebral hemispheres.

nonsense not because of a defect in its underlying logic but because of its dependence on anecdotal observations and inadequate samples.

Ironically, although the methods and conclusions of phrenology were soon discredited and ridiculed by the scientific community, the concept of functional localization subsequently became the bedrock of brain research. In the

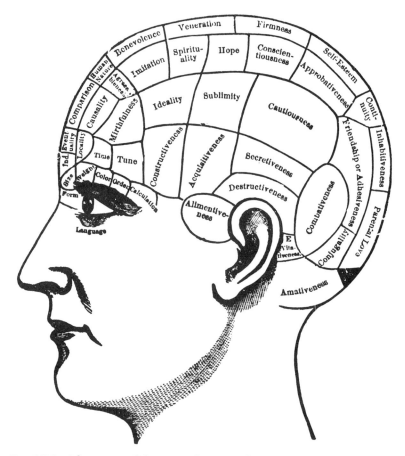

Fig. 17.5. This is one of the many diagrams illustrating the bogus theory of phrenology that were popular for more than a hundred years after the distinguished anatomist Franz Joseph Gall (1758–1828) first suggested that mental faculties were localized in distinct brain organs and that character could be diagnosed by feeling the bumps of the skull.

1860s, neurologists, especially John Hughlings Jackson in London and Pierre-Paul Broca in Paris, started to chart the surface of the cerebral hemispheres, using as their evidence the effects on behaviour, perception, language, movement and personality of localized damage to the brain. Broca described an area in the frontal lobes, usually on the left side, that now bears his name and which is essential for normal speech. Damage here (through stroke or injury) robs people of their ability to say more than a word or two, but not of their understanding of the spoken or written word.

In the context of images in the brain, Hughlings Jackson's findings were even more significant. He described the way in which epileptic seizures sometimes start with involuntary twitching in one particular group of muscles, often those of the thumb, the corner of the mouth or one of the toes, before spreading to other parts of the body. By relating the starting point of these 'Jacksonian fits' to small regions of degeneration and irritation, discovered *post mortem* in the brain, Jackson concluded that a strip of cortex, running down the middle of each cerebral hemisphere just behind Broca's area, is responsible for activation of the muscles on the opposite side of the body. What is more, the motor strip on each side is arranged *topographically*, the muscles of the toes and leg being controlled by the top of the strip, with the torso, arm, hand and face represented successively along the strip. This motor area of the cortex has now been explored in animals as well as humans, by a variety of experimental techniques, and they all confirm Hughlings Jackson's opinion that there is a kind of image of the body muscles in the brain.

Since Hughlings Jackson's time, the concept of functional sub-division and topographic representation has become a *sine qua non* of brain research. The task of charting the brain is far from complete but the successes of the past make one confident that each part of the brain (and especially the cerebral cortex) *is* likely to be organized in a spatially ordered fashion. Just as in the decoding of a cipher, the translation of Linear B or the reading of hieroglyphics, all that we need to recognize the order in the brain is a set of rules – rules that relate the activity of nerves to events in the outside world or in the animal's body.

The most fully explored spatial representations are those in the regions of cerebral cortex reserved for the three major senses – vision, hearing and bodily sensation (touch, pain, etc.). In Chapter 1, Horace Barlow has already described these sensory areas (see Fig. 1.2) and it is important to add that each primary sensory area is now known to be surrounded by a number of additional areas, each probably containing its own distinctive form of spatial arrangement of information-processing (but more of this later).

Faced with such overwhelming evidence for topographic patterns of activity in the brain it is hardly surprising that neurophysiologists and neuroanatomists have come to speak of the brain having *maps*, which are thought to play an essential part in the representation and interpretation of the world by the brain, just as the maps of an atlas do for the reader of them. The biologist J.Z. Young writes of the brain having a language of a pictographic kind: 'What goes on in the brain must provide a faithful representation of events outside, and the arrangement of the cells in it provides a detailed model of the world. It communicates meanings by topographical analogies'[6]. But is there a danger in the metaphorical use of such terms as 'language', 'grammar' and 'map' to describe the properties of the brain? Peter Hacker, the Oxford Wittgenstein scholar, sees it as an extreme example of the homunculus

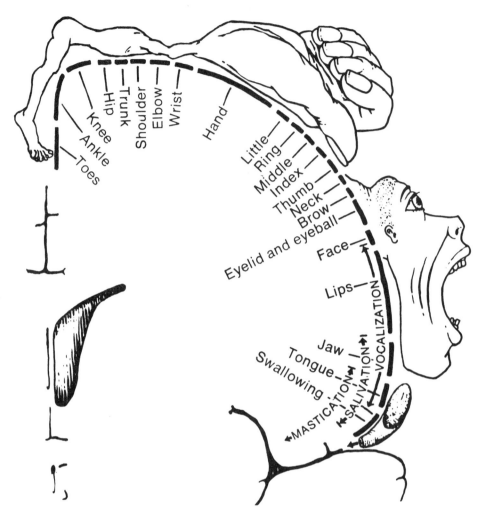

Fig. 17.6. Hughlings Jackson's idea that there is a motor map in the human cerebral hemispheres received strong support from the observations of the neurologists W. Penfield and T. Rasmussen in the 1940s. They described the effects of local electrical stimulation of the surface of the cortex in conscious human patients undergoing neurosurgical operations under local anaesthetic. Here is Penfield and Rasmussen's diagram of the motor 'homunculus'. Imagine that the brain has been cut in half, in a vertical plane lying approximately through the two ears, and we are looking from behind at a cross-section through the motor cortex on the right side of the brain. The labels show the various parts of the body that are caused to move by electrical stimulation at different points along the motor strip, from the tongue and face on the side of the hemisphere around to the toes on the part of the strip that lies buried in the cleft that runs along the middle of the hemispheres. The cartoon drawings indicate the relative areas of motor cortex devoted to different parts of the body. Notice the way in which the jaws and hands are vastly over-represented.

fallacy[7]. He finds it a 'startling, indeed amazing idea' that scientists should suggest that there are maps in the brain. He writes:

> there are no representing maps without conventions of representation. There are no conventions of representation without the *use*, by intelligent, symbol-employing creatures, of the representation. And to *use* a representation correctly one must *know* the conventions of representation, understand them, be able to explain them, recognize mistakes and correct or acknowledge them when they are printed out. Whether a certain array of lines is or is not a map is not an *intrinsic* feature of the lines ... but a *conventional* one (that is, the *actual* employment, by a person, of a convention of mapping)... the modern neurophysiologist ... comes perilously close to saying that when a person sees an object there is a map, a representation of the object, not on the pineal gland, but on the visual cortex. But now he must explain who or what sees or reads the map.

Frankly, I think that this concern is misplaced. I cannot believe that any neurophysiologist believes that there is a ghostly cartographer browsing through the cerebral atlas. Nor do I think that the employment of common language words (such as map, representation, code, information and even language) is a conceptual blunder of the kind that Peter Hacker imagines. Such metaphorical imagery is a mixture of empirical description, poetic licence and inadequate vocabulary. Yet an important question remains. If the existence of spatially ordered neural images is *useful* to the brain, what benefit does that order bestow? Indeed, is it possible that the presence of order (convenient though it may be to the neuroscientist) is no more than an epiphenomenon – perhaps an inevitable but useless consequence of the fact that nerve fibres, growing from the sense organs to their targets in the brain, tend to preserve the same spatial pattern as that of the receptors in the sense organ – rather like the individual glass fibres in a coherent fibre optic bundle?

Isomorphic maps

A tendency of nerve fibres to maintain spatial order as they grow would, of itself, generate *isomorphic* distributions in the brain – patterns topographically directly related to the array of receptor cells in the sense organ. Many cerebral maps are of this kind. Perhaps the map of the visual field on the primary visual cortex (described by Horace Barlow in Chapter 1) is simply a consequence of the fact that there is an orderly input of nerve fibres maintaining the neighbourly relations of the cells in the retina (though, as Barlow points out, the partial crossing-over of fibres from the two eyes as they enter the brain is a striking, and functionally appropriate, departure from strict isomorphism).

In the same terms, the somatic sensory area has on it a 'picture' of the opposite half of the body because sensory nerve fibres entering the spinal cord form an array corresponding to their origin on the body surface. Even the 'tonotopic' map in the primary auditory cortex (in which nerve cells are distributed in an orderly sequence according to the tone frequency to which they respond best) is isomorphic. The sound receptor cells are distributed along a membrane in the cochlea (the sense organ in the inner ear) and different frequencies of sound set up different patterns of vibration of this membrane, the point of maximum vibration (and thus maximum nerve activity) shifting along the membrane as the tone changes in pitch from high to low. So, as long as nerve fibres in the auditory pathway maintain the same general pattern as that of the array of receptor cells in the cochlea, a tonotopic map is inevitable.

It is well known that these cortical maps have spatial distortions, which appear as if they might be functionally important. For instance, the representation of the most acute, central *fovea* of the retina occupies a hugely disproportionate fraction of the visual cortex; and the most sensitive areas of the body surface – the fingers, toes and lips in humans, the snout in a pig – have expanded representations in the somatic sensory cortex. At first blush, it is tempting to think of these enlarged sub-maps as being like the large-scale inserts of major cities in a road atlas – a *functional* device to provide greater detail about things of most importance. In fact, though, even these apparently significant peculiarities of cortical maps might also be a simple consequence of patterned nerve growth. The fovea of the retina, the fingers, toes and so on all have a much denser innervation of sensory nerve fibres than the rest of the retina and skin. Hence, over-representation of those parts is an inevitable consequence of uniform topographic distribution of nerve fibres into the brain.

One of the most remarkable isomorphic maps is found in the somatic sensory area of the cortex of a mouse, or indeed any rodent that has large whiskers on its face, which it uses to explore its environment. The mouse has five rows of such whiskers and the sensory nerve that innervates them is much larger than the optic nerve from the eye. It is hard to imagine the perceptual world of a mouse but the sensations from its whiskers must surely play a major role in it. No surprise, then, to discover that a huge proportion of the somatic sensory area on the side of the cerebral hemispheres of a mouse (Fig. 17.7) is devoted to signals from the whiskers. But the isomorphism goes much further than the existence of a map of the body. Tom Woolsey and Hendrik Van der Loos[8] looked at microscopic sections of this whisker area, cut parallel to the flat surface of the cortex. The sections through the fourth cortical layer (where most of the incoming sensory nerve fibres terminate) have the remarkable appearance shown in Fig. 17.7 – a pattern of rings, each ring consisting of densely packed cortical nerve cell bodies surrounding a bunch of incoming fibres. They called these structures 'barrels' because their three-dimensional appearance is like rows of barrels. There are the same number of barrels as there are whiskers, and the barrels are distributed in a pattern just like that of the whiskers on the face. The obvious conclusion that each barrel of cells is a cortical 'organ' (a barrel organ?) corresponding to a single whisker has been amply confirmed by electrophysiologists, who have recorded activity from cortical cells in this area and have shown that the cells of each barrel respond when one particular whisker is touched.

Figure 17.8 is a further, elegant demonstration of this barrel/whisker isomorphism, performed by Margaret Kossut and Peter Hand at the University of Pennsylvania[9]. It is a computer-processed image of a cross-section (not a surface-parallel section) through the somatic sensory cortex of the left hemisphere of a rat (which also has barrels). The anaesthetized animal was given an injection of a radioactively-labelled analogue of glucose (2-deoxyglucose), which is taken up by any highly active nerve cells in the brain. After the injection, just one whisker on the opposite side of the face was vibrated gently, and the computer image (in which the colour scale indicates the level of radioactive labelling) shows one strongly labelled barrel in the middle of the cortex.

In a trivial sense, these brain maps do now have readers – the anatomists and physiologists who have discovered them. But the question remains: does the brain itself make use of its maps in a functional sense? Or are they all accidents of nerve growth? In the case of the whisker barrels there is good evidence that the map is not an inherent property of that bit of cortex but is imposed on it by the ingrowing sensory fibres. Van der Loos and Woolsey have shown that the cortical cells do not become assembled into barrels until about five days after birth in the mouse; if, before this age, one row of whiskers is plucked out, the corresponding row of barrels fails to form and the neighbouring barrels are larger than normal. This strongly suggests that the topographic order in the brain is determined by the pattern of incoming fibres.

If all maps in the brain were of this isomorphic form, it would be difficult to argue for their functional value. But if we were to find that the brain contained new forms of mapping, topologically related to some important aspect of the sensory stimulus, but not simply reflecting an anatomical pattern of ingrowing nerve fibres, that would surely indicate that maps have meaning.

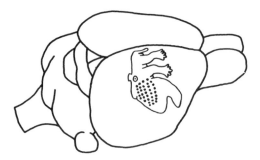

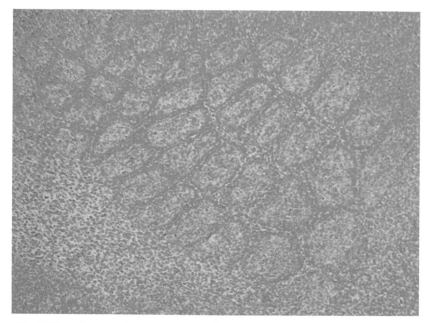

Fig. 17.7.   The somatic sensory area in the cortex of a mouse occupies a central strip down each side of the cerebral hemispheres. Each strip receives sensory information from the skin and other tissues of the opposite side of the body. The pattern of projection forms a crude, distorted map of the half-body, with the muzzle representation vastly magnified. The upper diagram shows the right side of the mouse brain, with the general arrangement of this body map. There is a huge area devoted to the whiskers.

Below is a photomicrograph (kindly supplied by Hendrik Van der Loos), taken at low magnification, of a single thin section through the cortex in the whisker area, cut parallel to the surface of the cortex. This particular section has glanced through the fourth layer, where the incoming sensory fibres arrive. It is stained to show the individual cortical nerve cells as small blue-green dots and they clearly form a distinct pattern of rings or 'barrels', with the same spatial arrangement as the array of whiskers on the muzzle.

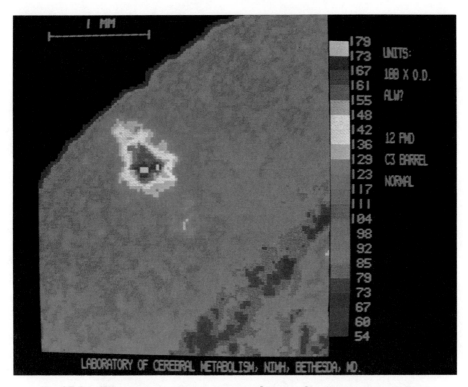

Fig. 17.8. Here we see a computer-processed image of a microscopic section cut in a vertical plane through the whisker area of the left hemisphere of a rat. The 1 mm scale bar indicates the size of this piece of cortex. The rat had received a small injection of a radioactive substance similar to glucose, which is taken up by active nerve cells. During the uptake period, one whisker on the right side of the face was gently stroked to stimulate its sensory nerve endings. The colour scale indicates the levels of radioactivity in the brain. The red spot in the middle layers of the cortex is presumably an individual 'barrel' of nerve cells activated by the stimulated whisker. (Computer image kindly supplied by Margaret Kossut and Peter Hand[9].)

Non-isomorphic maps

There are representations in the brain that are topographic in relation to the outside world, or to some aspect of the sensory stimulus, but which are not isomorphic, in the sense that they do not have the same spatial arrangement as the distribution of receptors. Horace Barlow, in Chapter 1 of this volume and elsewhere[10], has already discussed the principles behind (and advantages of) such forms of mapping. A few examples will make clear what I mean.

The first example – one already shown in Fig. 1.6 – is the way in which the orientations of the edges of shapes in the visual world are represented by a local system of sub-mapping within the visual cortex. Individual nerve cells in the primary visual cortex are selectively sensitive to the angles of lines and edges in the visual field: some cells respond best (produce the highest rate of impulses) when shown a vertical line, others a horizontal line and so on, for every possible angle of line. Moreover, these nerve cells are clustered together in 'columns' or 'slabs', so that if a microelectrode is put into the cortex perpendicular to the surface and recordings are taken from several cells in succession, then all of them, from the surface down to the bottom of the grey matter, respond best to roughly the same orientation. But if an electrode moves obliquely through the cortex, the preferred orientation shifts, usually in very small steps, from one cluster of column of cells to the next.

It seems, possible, then, that the primary visual cortex is 'decomposing' images into the orientations of their component contours and classifying shapes by the angles of their edges. For such a representation to be complete, in every part of the visual field, there are certain formal requirements for the form of mapping. Obviously, all orientations must be represented for each position on the visual field, otherwise the animal or human being would be blind to certain edges at certain points in space. This is achieved by superb efficiency of representation. First, there is sufficient sloppiness or scatter in the simple isomorphic map of the visual field to ensure that each point in space is represented over a *patch* of visual cortex about 2 mm in diameter. In turn, the orientation columns are laid down in such a way that a full sequence of all orientations is represented across about 0.75–1.00 mm. This means that there is a 'safety factor' of about 2 in the mapping[11]. Any particular edge in the visual field causes activity in at least two different columns of orientation-selective cells and the chance is very low that any particular orientation will be missed completely.

Now, orientation is a one-dimensional, cyclical variable – from vertical to oblique to horizontal to the other oblique, back to vertical and so on. On the other hand the visual field is two-dimensional. To represent both properties smoothly across a single two-dimensional surface (the cortex) poses a topo-logical problem. Figure 17.9 shows the way in which it seems to be solved in the primary visual cortex of the cat. We are looking down on the surface of a small patch of cortex explored by the neurophysiologist Klaus Albus[12]; each short line indicates the preferred orientation of the column of nerve cells lying beneath that point. (Some of these orientations were obtained empirically, by recording with a microelectrode at that point; the rest were filled in by inspired guesswork.) The pattern has a number of interesting features; first, the preferred orientation usually, but not always, shifts in small steps from one column to all its neighbours; second, each complete cycle of orientations occupies 1 mm or less across the cortex; third, there is an element of

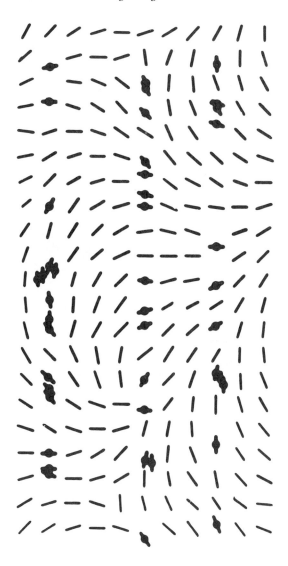

Fig. 17.9. This diagram, based on experiments by Klaus Albus[12], represents a small part (about 1mm × 0.5 mm) of the surface of the primary visual cortex of a cat. Each short line shows the angle at which an edge must appear in the appropriate part of the visual field to stimulate the tiny column of nerve cells lying below that point on the surface. The lines with dots in the middle are actual experimental results, showing the preferred orientation of the first nerve cell recorded with a microelectrode introduced into the cortex at that point. The other orientations were added on the basis of the experimental observation that, on average, the preferred orientation of adjacent columns of neurons changes by about 10° for a movement of 50 μm across the cortical surface. This piece of visual cortex receives information from a single patch of visual field. Thus each edge of any object appearing in this region would set up activity in a number of columns of cells 'tuned' to the appropriate angle.

randomness, manifest in occasional reversals in sequences of orientation and in sudden large jumps.

Compare this pattern with Figure 17.10, a graphic exercise by the artist Bridget Riley. She has apparently set herself the same task as that of the map of orientation in the visual cortex, namely representing steady progressive shifts of angle of lines on a two-dimensional surface. And she arrives at much the same solution.

My other example of a non-isomorphic map comes from the auditory system. We can use our ears not only to distinguish tones (and hence more complex sounds, including speech) but also to judge the *position* in space of a sound source – surely an important skill to an animal attacking or under attack. Now, the pitch of a sound, as I have already described, is reflected in the position of maximum vibration in the organ of hearing, and hence the *place* at which nerve cells are most active in the isomorphic tone map of the primary auditory cortex. But distinguishing the position of a sound source is a much more subtle affair. It depends on a comparison of differences in the intensity and time of arrival of the sound wave at the *two* ears (for the horizontal position) or of the relative intensities of different components of

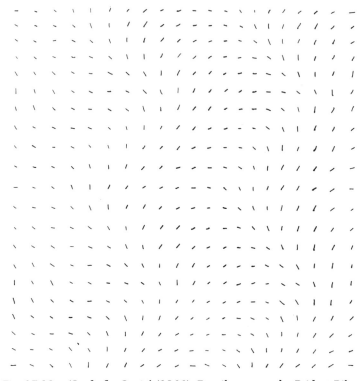

Fig. 17.10. 'Study for Static' (1966). Pencil on paper by Bridget Riley.

complex sounds reflected from the crevices of the outer ear (for vertical as well as horizontal position).

No simple isomorphism between sound receptors and nerve cells in the brain could create a map of auditory space, yet such maps do exist in the brains of birds and mammals. On the back of the midbrain of mammals (the top of the brainstem, underneath the cerebral hemispheres) there are two pairs of little bumps, the *superior* and *inferior colliculi*, both of which have input from the ears. The inferior colliculus has a beautiful isomorphic map of tone frequency (like that in the primary auditory cortex); each individual nerve cell responds preferentially to a particular pitch but is almost insensitive to the position of sound in space. The situation is just the opposite in the deeper layers of the superior colliculus. Here the nerve cells respond best to complex 'natural' sounds rather than pure tones, and most of them need the sound source to be placed at a particular *position* in space to give their best response. Moreover, the best position shifts progressively from cell to cell, forming a 2-dimensional map of auditory space across this brain structure[13].

It turns out that the superior colliculus is primarily a *visual* centre, involved in the control of movements of the eyes, head and body. The incoming visual fibres are distributed in an isomorphic map of the visual field, which is neatly in register with the non-isomorphic map of auditory space. And both of these sensory maps are aligned with a motor map, such that activation of one group of nerve cells in this structure (whether through the occurrence of a sound or a visual stimulus at a particular point in space) causes the eyes to move across to look in the direction of that stimulus. A perfect little neuronal machine, whose actions depend on those two, superimposed sensory maps, sharing the same motor output.

The construction of a non-isomorphic map of auditory space requires much more than the simple ordered growth of bundles of nerve fibres. In fact, Andrew King and his colleagues at Oxford[14] have evidence that the map of auditory space in the superior colliculus of the ferret is not purely innately determined, but is partly dependent on interplay between auditory and visual signals early in life, leading to the establishment of an auditory map aligned with the visual one. This kind of construction of a spatial representation that bears a relationship to the world but not to any simple feature of the sense organ seems to me strong evidence that maps, as such, are useful to the brain.

Why have maps?

The operations performed by a nerve cell are determined not only by its inherent electrical and chemical properties but also by the connections that it receives, just like any component in an electronic circuit. What value could

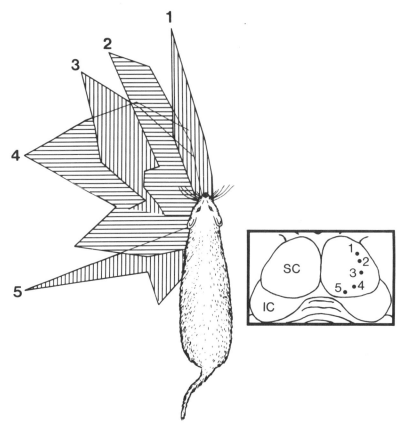

Fig. 17.11. In the deep layers of the superior colliculus (a visual centre in the brainstem) of mammals there are nerve cells that respond to sounds at particular positions in space, and they are distributed to form a map of auditory space aligned with the visual map formed by input from the eyes. Here we see a ferret viewed from above. The inset diagram represents the surface of the midbrain, consisting of the inferior colliculi (IC), which have purely auditory input, and the superior colliculi (SC). The numbered dots show the positions at which nerve cells were recorded in the deep layers. Each cell responded best to sound presented at the position on the opposite side of space, shown in the diagram on the left. Each curve (enclosing a striped area) represents the relative strength of response of the nerve cell for sounds presented at different positions around the animal's head.
(Based on results of A.J. King and M.E. Hutchings[13].)

there be in having these unitary nerve cells arranged in topographic order? Perhaps it has something to do with the fact that most of the connections in the brain are short, local fibres, such that cells are either excited or inhibited by their close neighbours. The nature of any computation accomplished by such local connections will obviously depend on the relationship between the properties of *neighbouring* nerve cells.

Consider the kind of processing that is known to go on in the primary visual cortex. Individual nerve cells, in a single column, respond to a line of a particular orientation. This very property of orientation selectivity seems to depend, at least in part, on short-range inhibitory connections from cells in neighbouring columns (which respond best to other orientations). Administration of a drug that blocks inhibition in the cortex makes cortical cells partly or completely lose their selectivity for the angle of a line[15]. Some cortical cells respond best to an edge of a particular angle that *moves* across a region of the visual field and they may achieve this property by receiving excitatory connections from a number of nearby cells in the same column, which all prefer lines of a particular angle, but each at a slightly different position in the field.

Of course, interconnected elements in the brain, just as in a computer, need not necessarily lie *close* to each other. One could imagine a brain in which all the cells are redistributed randomly, but maintaining all the same connections. Would it not work just as well? In at least one respect it would not. Nerve fibres conduct impulses at very slow speeds (between about 0.5 and 100 m/s), compared with the speed of transmission in electronic circuitry. So, the inevitable lengthening of nerve fibres introduced by scrambling a brain would severely slow down the operations of the brain and would introduce differences and errors of timing between the various inputs to each cell, which might seriously interfere with the process it performs.

Another advantage of topography is that it simplifies the problem of getting some *other* input into register with the sensory array. Imagine a visual area in the cortex that receives not only an input of fibres carrying the visual messages from the eyes forming a map of the visual field but also a much coarser array of 'activating' fibres that adjust the excitability of nerve cells so as to turn visual attention on or off selectively in different parts of the visual field. (Actually this is not wild speculation: almost certainly there are such activating inputs.) As long as there is a map, any other spatially distributed input to the area will have its influence topologically patterned in relation to the coordinates of the map. If there were a non-isomorphic map in which all red objects (whatever their position in the visual field) were represented in one sub-division of the map (or all birds, all mice, all human faces, etc.), then a set of 'activating' fibres distributed topographically across such a map could confine attention to one sub-division of experience. Whatever the mechanism of storing memories, that too might depend on a system of 'this-is-worth-remembering fibres' distributed across the maps of sensory experience.

Finally there is the overriding problem of economy in the specification of instructions for building the brain. The chromosomes of a human being, which have to be sufficient to specify the structure of the entire body, may contain as few as 50,000 functional genes. Some of the genetic instructions for building the brain may, however, be very simple, such as 'make all nerve cells inhibit their immediate neighbours on either side', or 'link together nearby cells that tend to fire off at the same time'. The theoretical modellers of brain function have shown that such simple rules for local interaction replicate certain properties of real nerve cells (such as selectivity for elongated lines at particular orientations) but only if the input to the network is topographically arranged.

Indeed it is a very attractive notion that the basic circuitry of each local 'module' of cortex might be identical, or at least very similar, in every cortical region. The very different functions of different cortical areas may depend mainly on the nature of the inputs received and their topographical distributions. If this is true, the intrinsic circuitry of the whole cerebral cortex may be specified by a surprisingly small number of genes.

Meaning from maps?

Horace Barlow[10] has already argued that the value of maps may be to bring together new associations of activity that can reveal interesting properties of the original image. The idea that the existence of a map in a brain structure allows local circuitry to discover useful relationships between the activity of neighbouring nerve cells may resolve a recent puzzling finding. The somatic sensory area of the cerebral cortex of a fruit bat, the flying fox, has a map of the body surface, like that in other mammals, but with one surprising difference. Figure 17.12 shows, on the left, the typical arrangement, in the somatic sensory cortex of the rat. Both hindlimbs and forelimbs are represented at the *front* of the strip of cortex, while the animal's back is represented behind. The map in the bat (shown on the right) has the representations of the head, hind limb and back disposed much as in other mammals, but the forelimb (wing) representation lies at the *back* of the strip. Mike Calford and his colleagues[16], who discovered this odd pattern, pointed out that the disposition of the parts of the body in the map mimicks the posture of this animal, which habitually hangs with its wings folded over its back. They inferred that the very existence of this topographic arangement may have meaning for the animal in terms of its body posture. But how could this be without a Cartesian inner eye to look at it? An alternative possibility is that the arrangement allows local interactions between signals from parts of the body surface that usually lie close to each other and are therefore likely to be touched simultaneously or sequentially. Imagine, for instance, a branch brushing against the bat as it hangs in a tree. It is likely to touch both the fur of the animal's back and its wing

A   B

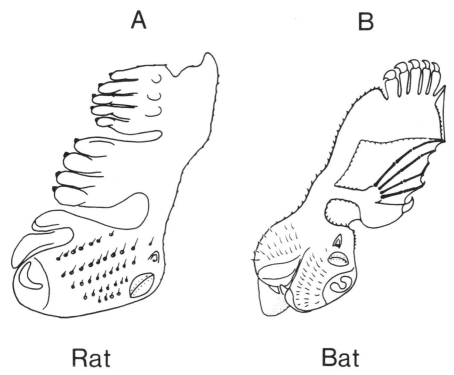

Rat   Bat

Fig. 17.12.   There are certain fundamental similarities in the nature of the map
of the body of the somatic sensory cortex in virtually all mammals so far studied.
The somatic cortex lies in the middle of the cerebral hemisphere, with the head
represented at the bottom of the strip (see Fig. 17.7). The diagram on the left
shows the typical arrangement of the body map on the left side of the hemispheres
of a rat. The representations of the forelimbs and the hindlimbs point *forwards*. In
the fruit bat, however, Mike Calford and his colleagues[16] found that there is a
small but significant variation on this general theme. As shown on the right, the
representation of the forelimb (the wing) points *backwards*, close to the representation of the animal's back. In other words, the map reflects the habitual posture
of the bat as it roosts, hanging with its wings folded over its back.

successively. Perhaps local interconnection between the closely spaced
regions of cortex representing these two regions of skin allows some nerve
cells to detect and respond selectively to such a stimulus.

Multiple sensory maps

I have already mentioned that each primary sensory area is surrounded by
additional areas, in which the same basic sensory information may be re-cast
on different spatial coordinates.

For instance, in the *auditory* region of the cortex of the moustached bat

(which uses echo-location to guide its flight and hunting), the primary area
has a simple (isomorphic) map of tone frequency, with a much enlarged
representation (an auditory 'fovea') for frequencies around the strongest
harmonic component of the bat's own echolocating cries. This area is flanked
by others in which important functional characteristics of the sound are
mapped out. One consists of nerve cells that respond only when the locating
cry is followed by a *delayed* echo, and they are arranged in a map in which the
required delay (in other words the required *distance* of a target) varies across
the cortex. Another area contains cells that respond preferentially to the first
harmonic of the emitted cry plus another pitch, slightly shifted from either the
second or the third harmonic. These cells would respond best as the bat
approaches a target which reflects an echo that has all its harmonic components Doppler-shifted to a slightly higher frequency (like the siren of a police
car as it approaches you). In this area there are two maps, each with one axis
corresponding to a small range of frequency around one of the higher
harmonics. This arrangement results in the *velocity* of approach being represented systematically along each sub-area[17].

The monkey's cerebral cortex is now known to be filled with a profusion of
sensory areas[18, 19]. Figure 17.13 gives a 1985 version of the cerebral atlas of
the rhesus monkey[19] (though new areas are being discovered all the time).
The many separate visual areas contain complete or partial representations
of the visual field but the assumption is that each of them is serving a special
purpose in the interpretation of the visual image. Semir Zeki at University
College London has evidence that one of them, the fourth visual area (V4), is
especially interested in the colour of visual stimuli[16], and another one (V5 or
'MT'), described by Tony Movshon in Chapter 8, is concerned with the
analysis of movement in the visual scene.

Interestingly, the number of such additional cortical areas appears to have
increased up the evolutionary scale. A monkey may have as many as twenty
extra visual areas, whereas a mouse probably has only two. Indeed, the
ballooning expansion of the cerebral hemispheres that has occurred during
mammalian evolution may have been achieved largely by the addition of
more and more *sensory* areas, each with its own map of a particular sensory
property or properties. The conventional wisdom of comparative psychology
is that the intelligence of animals (i.e. the richness and sophistication of their
behavioural repertoires) is correlated with the size of their cerebral hemispheres. Could it be that each additional *sensory* area gives a quantal incre-
ment of *understanding* of the world?

It is surely significant that *visual* areas occupy more than half of the entire
surface of the cerebral hemispheres of a monkey. For we now know that,

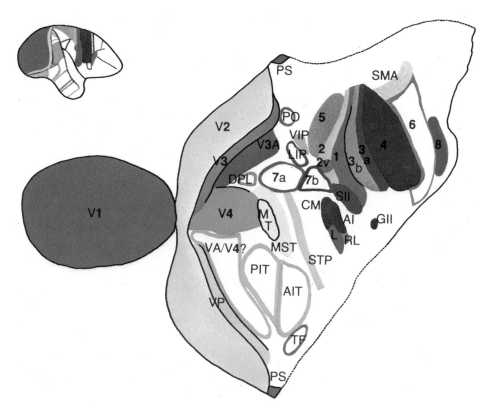

Fig. 17.13. One of the most exciting discoveries of the last few years is that there are many different sensory and motor areas in the cerebral cortex. In the monkey brain, illustrated here, a large number of visual areas fill up more than half of the entire surface of the cerebral hemispheres. The small diagram at the top left is a view of the right side of the cerebral hemispheres of a monkey, showing the major folds and creases, with colours representing the various areas visible on the surface. The rest of this diagram is an imaginary unfolded view of the entire cortical surface, revealing many other areas that are buried out of sight in the clefts of the cortex. Motor areas appear grey, somatic sensory areas blue and auditory areas green. All the other colours, shades of red and yellow, represent individual areas concerned with vision. Some of these are thought to be specialized for the analysis of particular aspects of the visual scene – motion in the area labelled MT, form and colour in V4[18]. (Kindly supplied by David Van Essen[19]).

although vision *feels* as if it is a simple and effortless process, it is extraordinarily complicated in computational terms. Writing computer programs to do things that we think of as being intellectually demanding, such as playing chess or doing advanced calculus, has proved relatively simple compared with the monstrous problem of making a machine that can *see*.

The ultimate enigma of perception

After all of this, how do we stand with Wittgenstein? There *are* topographically arranged sensory areas in the brain. Some of them have spatial coordinates that bear no simple relationship to the pattern of sensory receptors. In these terms, the brain does contain images of the outside world and it seems likely that these images are of functional value in the brain's task of analysing sensory signals. With deference to Wittgenstein, is it really misleading to call such things maps?

We are making slow but steady progress towards an account of how the structure and organization of the brain allow the owner of that brain to respond appropriately to the visual world. One day we might even be able to build a machine that simulates vision by having the same kind of structure as the brain. But will it *see*? Will it have conscious awareness of its visual world? According to Wittgenstein, it is appropriate to use the language of the mental only when talking of people or of other animals (or even, presumably, machines) whose behaviour is indistinguishable from that of human beings. As far as the privy world of conscious perception is concerned, this argument is flawless. Indeed one could go further: how can one be truly confident about the nature of the perceptual experiences of *any* creature but oneself?

The *nature* of perceptual experience is rightly a question for philosophy (see Chapter 22 by Nelson Goodman). There is every reason for philosophers to be interested in such classical conundrums as 'when I say that I see red and you say that you see red, are we having the same experience?'; and 'is "pain" a property of noxious stimuli or a creation of the conscious mind?' But the *mechanisms* by which a creature understands the world around it (i.e. responds appropriately to things and events) is surely a matter for empirical investigation. The brain is a machine that accomplishes behaviour. The challenge faced by brain research is to provide a plausible account, backed by experimental evidence, of the workings of this machine.

It should be no surprise to find that science – especially a branch of science that is rapidly throwing up new discoveries – runs out of words. Everyday language is an invention to deal with everyday events. It works well as a means of communication between people who share a common view of the world and of their own conscious experiences and motives. It is, in its simplest form, at the level of individual words, a convention of categorical descriptions. Therefore language, even everyday language, has grown and changed as new views about the world have developed and as the need for new categories has arisen. The thing I am sitting/kneeling on, as I write this, is neither a chair nor a stool. It is one of those new-fangled 'contraptions for sitting/kneeling on', which is supposed to be good for your back. I need a new word for it but I carry on calling it a chair, until a better noun comes along.

Science is constantly generating new categories and new notions, beyond previous experience. Sometimes it invents neologisms for them (Supernova, protoplasm, quark, molecule, entropy, isotope, gene); sometimes it sticks to everyday words, beating them into new meanings (Black Hole, mass, nucleus, power, cell, current, inertia). Is it really a greater conceptual confusion for brain researchers to call the distribution of activity in the visual cortex a 'map' than for me to call the thing that I am sitting/kneeling on a 'chair' (or to call the *black* birds that swim on the Swan River in Western Australia 'swans')?

One of the most profoundly enigmatic aspects of science is that it often has to use everyday language to formulate questions and concepts concerning a world beyond everyday experience. It is true that some areas of intellectual effort (such as mathematics, logic and music) have devised new systems of notation because everyday language has proved inadequate as a medium of communication of questions and ideas in these disciplines. But most areas of science stumble along, using ordinary language to 'bootstrap' themselves up to new concepts. Nowhere is the problem of language greater than in brain research, but the difficulty is not so much a deep conceptual confusion as an inadequacy of vocabulary and notation.

Ultimately, it should be the objective of brain research to provide an account of the function of the nervous system that even includes the mechanism of consciousness. But that is, I fear, a long way off (not least because the everyday language of consciousness gives little clue as to how to formulate questions about its mechanism). In the meantime, it would be a major achievement to give an empirical description of the mechanisms in the brain that allow animals and people to respond *as if they understand* the visual world.

18

Images of the functioning human brain

MARCUS RAICHLE

Introduction

Beginning with the pioneering work of the great British physiologist, Sir Charles Sherrington, and his collaborator, C.S. Roy[1], scientists have appreciated the fact that functional activity, for example, movements of all types, speaking, listening, and vision, cause striking changes in local brain blood flow[2]. The first clinical demonstration of this interesting and highly useful relationship between local neuronal activity and blood flow occurred in 1928. In that year the neurologist John Fulton working with the famed neurosurgeon, Harvey Cushing, at the Peter Bent Brigham Hospital in Boston, had occasion to study a patient with a large vascular malformation sitting at the back of the brain in the region of the viual cortex[3]. The patient came to the attention of Dr Cushing because of headaches and failing vision. In addition, the patient reported that he heard a loud blowing sound or *bruit* in his head which became more noticeable when he used his eyes. Surgery was performed with the intention of removing this malformation but, because of its size, it was left in place. Following the surgical procedure, the patient had a small bony defect beneath the scalp in the region of the malformation that permitted his physicians to listen to this *bruit*, which resulted from blood flowing through the vascular malformation to the part of the brain serving vision. Recordings of what they heard provided a most remarkable demonstration of changes in local blood flow to the brain associated with the visual activity. With his eyes closed, the *bruit* was quite soft and barely audible either to the physicians or the patient; however, when the patient was reading the intensity of the *bruit* increased noticeably as both reported by the patient and heard by his physicians. This remarkable case remained the only demonstration in a human subject of the close coupling between local blood flow and function until the advent of more sophisticated techniques using radioisotopes[2].

Creating an image of the brain in action

Scientific developments over the past 40 years have culminated in the development of imaging techniques that permit the safe visualization of local blood flow and metabolism (i.e. the local consumption of oxygen and glucose supporting neuronal work) in the living human brain. Because blood flow and metabolism are closely linked to the activity of nerve cells, it is possible to monitor highly localized changes in nerve cell activity within the human brain during various types of functional activity. In addition the effect of various disease states on neuronal activity can be determined and related to changes in human behavior. The most successful and accurate technique for this type of imaging involves the use of radioisotopes which have been produced in a cyclotron.

The radioisotopes

Cyclotron-produced radioisotopes used in medical imaging are unique in several respects. First, the most commonly used isotopes are carbon-11, oxygen-15, nitrogen-13 and fluorine-18. Three of these represent natural building blocks of biological molecules and, therefore, can be incorporated into a variety of radiopharmaceutical substances that will behave like the naturally occurring compounds once they have been administered to a human subject. Second, these isotopes have an extremely short physical half-life ranging from two min for oxygen-15 to 110 min for fluorine-18. As a result they impart relatively low radiation dose to a human subject and therefore can be administered quite safely. (One disadvantage of the short half-life is the necessity for a cyclotron to be on the spot for their production. As a result, this type of research has been restricted to major medical centers with sophisticated radiochemical laboratories that include an in-house cyclotron.) Third, these radioisotopes decay by the emission of a positively charged particle the size of an electron which is known, not surprisingly, as a positron, and from it comes the name positron emission tomography or PET as the general designation for this type of imaging of the living brain.

The scanner

The detection of compounds labeled with positron-emitting radioisotopes is based on the behavior of the positron as it leaves the nucleus of the isotope and wanders out into the tissue[2]. As it comes to rest several millimeters from its origin, the positron interacts with a negatively charged electron with the resulting annihilation of both particles. This annihilation event produces secondary radiation that is of sufficiently high energy that it escapes the tissue in the form of two annihilation photons traveling in opposite directions. The schemes used for imaging the brain take advantage of this fact by using radiation detectors in pairs on opposite sides of the head, which signal an event within the tissue only when they detect radioactivity simultaneously. Such an arrangement is known as a coincidence circuit. The events recorded with it allow one to establish the origin of the radioactive event along a line between the two detectors. Imaging devices using this principle (Fig. 18.1) are composed of hundreds of such detector pairs which allow many lines to be drawn through the tissue, and mathematical techniques to be applied to such data, which result in the creation of an image of the distribution of radioactivity within the tissue. Such an image is entirely equivalent to tissue autoradiography used in many laboratories throughout the world in which scientists remove the brain following the administration of a radioisotope to an animal, slice it up and lay it on X-ray film. The resulting

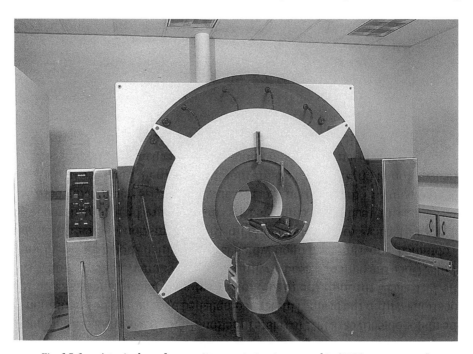

Fig. 18.1.   A typical, modern positron emission tomographic (PET) scanner used to obtain images of the distribution of radioactive substances in the brain of a human subject. The subject lies on the couch in the foreground with his head supported in the head-holder. The couch is positioned so that his head is just within the aperture in the center of the scanner. Surrounding this aperture are hundreds of small radiation detectors (hidden from view by the frame of the scanner) which send radioactive counting information to a large computer which uses this information to construct a three-dimensional image of the distribution of the radioactivity in the brain.

exposure provides an image of the distribution of radioactivity within the brain in the plane of the section. Positron emission tomography permits the identical image to be generated but substitutes computer-based reconstruction techniques for decapitation. Obviously, this is a highly desirable feature when studies in human subjects are contemplated. Using this general approach, a variety of measurements have been accomplished in human subjects[2].

Blood flow

I would like to focus on measurements of local blood flow using a technique initially developed by Seymour Kety and his associates for tissue autoradiographic measurements in laboratory animals[4]. In these early, pioneering studies, Dr Kety and his associates administered radiolabeled trifluoroiodomethane to animals and obtained striking images of blood flow in the brain. The present-day equivalent of this procedure is to administer ^{15}O-labeled water intravenously to a human subject and obtain an image of its distribution over the ensuing 40 seconds[5]. This image (Fig. 18.2) is a faithful representation of local blood flow within the human brain and can be converted into an actual quantitative image in units of blood flow (i.e., ml, min^{-1}, 100 g of tissue^{-1}) as long as one obtains a simultaneous record of the history of radioactive events in arterial blood. Such data are usually obtained from a peripheral artery at the time these studies are performed. This very simple measurement is, as you will see, most useful in studies of the function of the human brain. Before discussing such studies, it is important to understand one additional feature of this type of work.

Anatomical localization

In discussing some of the results obtained with PET, I will note with great precision the anatomical localization of these responses. It is, after all, one of the major objectives of PET to relate functional changes to specific anatomical locations within the brain. This is accomplished by relating the orientation of the PET slices through the tissue, to known anatomical landmarks on the skull[6]. Once the patient's head is within the PET scanner, a lateral skull X-ray is obtained, superimposed upon which is a grid which shows the orientation of the PET slices to be obtained. With this information one can then use stereotaxis (a technique employed for many years by neurosurgeons to localize points in the brain) in order to obtain a precise relationship between the location of physiological events monitored with PET and the underlying anatomy of the brain[6]. It is always important to keep in mind the importance of such a strategy. It is easy to be deceived by PET images that appear to depict

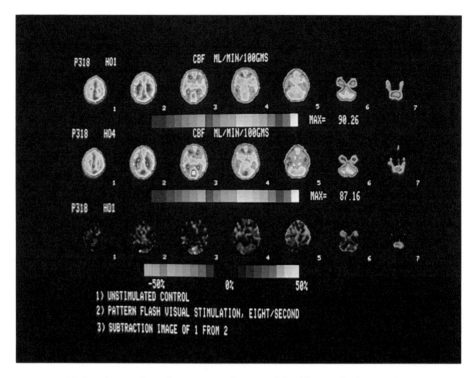

Fig. 18.2.   A typical set of PET images depicting blood flow in the human brain at rest with the eyes closed (top row) and during visual stimulation produced by viewing a simple pattern of flashing lights (middle row). The images are oriented with the subject's left to the reader's left and the subject's nose at 12 o'clock. The PET scanner used in this study obtained 7 simultaneous horizontal images of the brain beginning (left) with the uppermost part of the brain and extending down to include the base of the brain (right). In these images, color is used to depict the amount of blood flow to a particular region of the brain. The color scale for each set of images appears below the images along with the maximum value (in ml of blood flowing per 100 g of brain per min) for that scale. The scales consist of 20 divisions which divide up the maximum value (represented as white) into 20 equal increments. During visual stimulation (middle row) close inspection of image 3 will reveal increased blood flow to the visual cortex which is situated at approximately 6 o'clock. To make it easier for the viewer of these images to locate the exact center of increased blood flow the third row of images is created which represents the percent change in blood flow caused by visual stimulation. The color scale now represents percent difference between rows one and two and ranges from minus to plus 50%. Areas with no change appear black.

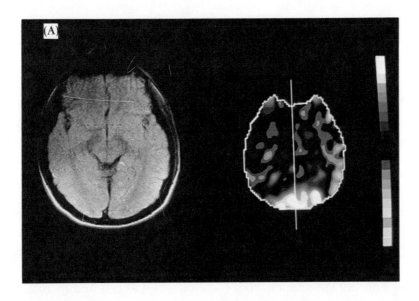

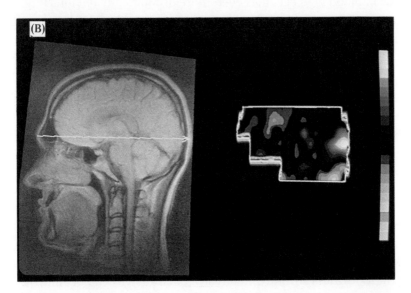

Fig. 18.3. An indication of the anatomical location of the responses depicted in Fig. 18.2 can be obtained by comparing these PET images with anatomical images obtained in the same individual using a clinical imaging technique known as nuclear magnetic resonance (NMR). In (A) a horizontal NMR and PET (percent change due to visual stimulation) image are shown. Both were obtained in the same individual and are anatomically made in the same plane. In (B) these same data are presented in a saggital plane (i.e. a slice down the middle of the brain) which shows even more clearly that the visually stimulated activity is occurring in visual cortex which resides at the back of the brain along the medial banks of the two cerebral hemispheres. The horizontal line through the NMR image in (B) gives the orientation of the two images in (A).

anatomy when, in fact, they are exhibiting physiology that may change from moment to moment or with disease states.

Responses of the normal brain

In our laboratory we have been able to monitor local blood flow in the visual cortex of the brain of normal subjects during precisely controlled visual stimulation. In this study the individual subject wears goggles that resemble simple swimming goggles but they contain light-emitting diodes instead of lenses. These diodes can be made to produce repetitive flashing lights which provoke a remarkable increase in local blood flow in the visual cortex. Comparing measurements of blood flow obtained at rest and during stimulation in the same subject reveals, without any special processing, local changes in the blood flow of a considerable degree (Fig. 18.2). Our ability to perceive these changes, however, is enhanced by subtracting the images obtained during stimulation from those obtained at rest and then the local increase in blood flow becomes even more dramatically obvious (Fig. 18.2). Because these data are electronic they can be manipulated on a computer and so 'viewed' from any direction. Under these circumstances, it is possible to compare these functional images with anatomical images obtained with other imaging techniques such as nuclear magnetic resonance (Fig. 18.3).

Local changes in blood flow as well as of metabolism in response to a variety of other kinds of stimulation have been demonstrated in our laboratory and others[2]. For example, it turns out that profound changes in the circulation of blood through the brain can be produced by a simple vibratory stimulation of any part of the body. We know from anatomical studies in a variety of species, as well as experience of patients suffering from strokes and other diseases that have discretely injured the human brain, that the representation of bodily sensation occurs in a very orderly manner on the surface of the brain. Each half of the body is represented in the opposite hemisphere of the brain. This map can be depicted as a homunculus with the feet at the top of the brain and the body stretched out with the face and the hands around towards the side (see Fig. 17.6). If one then stimulates a human body, beginning with the toes and proceeding to the hands and then the lips, one sees an orderly movement of activity in the PET scan from the very top of the brain to a position somewhat more laterally to, finally, a position considerably more laterally (Fig. 18.4), thus depicting the exact organization of incoming sensory information in the living brain of a normal human subject[7]. The ability to make such simple maps portends much more sophisticated studies of functions that, as I will discuss in a moment, are uniquely human.

As this work has progressed it has become apparent to us that it can be

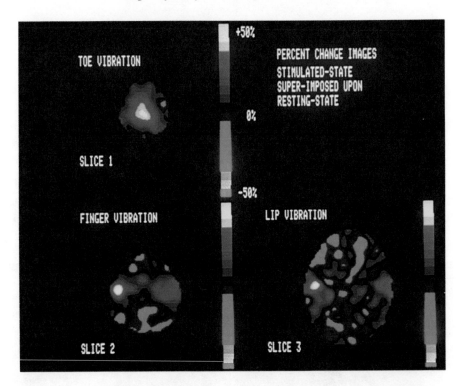

Fig. 18.4. Stimulation of body surfaces with a simple vibrator produces intense neuronal activity and, hence, changes in local blood flow in those regions of the brain receiving and processing such information. From PET images obtained during this type of stimulation it is possible to develop a map of these areas. Shown in these images are the responses (i.e. percent change from control) observed in the brain of a single individual stimulated on the toes (upper left), fingers of the right hand (lower left) and on the right side of the lips (lower right). Note that these responses appear opposite the side of the body stimulated in the case of the fingers and the lips and occur at different levels along the surface of the cerebral hemispheres.

accomplished with spatial precision that far exceeds our original expectations based upon the inherent resolution of the PET scanner. This may seem like getting something for nothing, but it has a logical explanation. Let me illustrate the phenomenon first and then give you the explanation. If one takes a visual stimulus consisting of a colored checkerboard in the form of an annulus and presents it first to the center of the visual field as a very small reversing checkerboard and then gradually increases the size of the annulus, having the subject always stare fixedly at its center, the visual cortex is stimulated with information initially coming from the center of the retina followed by information coming from its periphery (Fig. 18.5). Until this study was performed with PET we had only indirect evidence that the primary visual cortex of the human brain is organized in a very systematic manner with the center of the retina represented at the back of the brain and the periphery of the retina represented more towards the front of the brain[8]. Using these stimuli, we were able to map very precisely the progression of activity along the visual cortex in the human brain as it moved from the most posterior part of the visual cortex with stimulation of the center of the retina, more anteriorly with peripheral stimulation[8] (Fig. 18.5).

The movement of this response could be detected with an accuracy approaching 1 mm, yet the operational resolution of the PET scanning device employed for this work was 18 mm. In order to understand how we were able to accomplish this, it is important to understand what we mean by resolution.

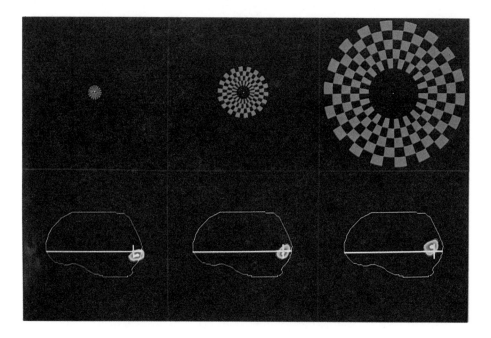

Fig. 18.5.   The ability to localize responses accurately in the human brain can be quite precise with PET. In the study depicted in these images[8] the retina was stimulated, first, at its center (left) and then at two positions in the periphery by having the subjects view the black-and-red checkerboards in which the colors reversed 16 times per s during the measurement of local blood flow. The images presented here represent the summed responses from seven individuals. The responses observed in blood flow represent the difference between the control and stimulated states in each individual. The outline of the brain is shown for orientation along with a horizontal and vertical line for reference. The movement of the area of activation from the back of the brain forward as the stimulus is moved from the center of the retina outwards is apparent. Localization of responses such as these can be accurate to within 1 mm[8].

If a PET scanner is presented a point source of activity it blurs that activity depending upon its resolution. The resulting image is a point spread function which is maximum at its center. Resolution is defined as the width of this blurred activity at half of its maximum value. If two points are separated by no more than the width of these distributions at half of their maximum value, it is impossible to detect them as two separate sources of activity. However, when presented sequentially it is quite possible to detect the center of such activity with great precision. This phenomenon has been well described in signal detection theory and is thought to underlie the phenomenon of hyperacuity in the human visual system (such as the detection of a vernier break in a line) where the anatomical structure of the retina would initially suggest a much poorer resolution than we are accustomed to in our everyday life. The ability to make such precise estimates of the location of a response in the human brain with PET portends very sophisticated studies of neuronal function using such imaging techniques. There is every reason to believe that as the resolution of PET scanners improves, our ability to localize areas of increased neuronal activity through changes in local blood flow or metabolism may approach 300 μm.

PET is unique in its ability to help us study the human brain and those functions that are uniquely human. In this regard, language is the most obvious candidate. The study of language might, at first, seem an easy task; for example, why not simply ask the subject to talk and measure local blood flow with the PET scanner? A moment's consideration will reveal, however, that such an activity is likely to activate many areas within the brain simultaneously. If the task involves reading one can envisage blood flow in the visual cortex increasing, as we have previously seen (Figs. 18.2 and 18.3), along with areas concerned with the lips and tongue (Fig. 18.4) and the processing of sounds that are produced. Thus to begin to understand how language is truly organized in the brain, it is important to develop a strategy for such studies. This has been undertaken in our laboratory by Steve Petersen, Peter Fox, Mark Mintun, Michael Posner and myself[9]. Using a variety of tasks we have developed activation paradigms that permit one sequentially to subtract various components of the language task and allow us to begin to understand the role of different areas of the brain in the complex task of language generation. For example, if a subject is to view and repeat words (in a study designed to unravel the processing of single words) that are shown on a television screen while in the PET scanner, the study would begin with an eyes-closed control. These data are subtracted from a second study performed in which the subject simply views, passively, the nouns to be repeated. The second task (i.e. passively viewing nouns on the monitor) becomes the control for the task in which the subject repeats the nouns. Finally, subjects are asked to generate an appropriate verb for each noun, subtracting, as the control task, the simple repeating of the nouns. By following such a sequential paradigm one can see activity in areas of the brain that are uniquely involved in the component processes of speaking a written word. Some of the areas of activity that are revealed, like the primary visual cortex (viewing the words) and the primary sensorimotor mouth area in both hemispheres (speaking the words), are not surprising. Other findings, admittedly preliminary, indicate that areas in frontal cortex, parietal cortex and lateral cerebellum, may contribute significantly to the interpretation and internal processing of language. Such studies are too preliminary to allow any general conclusions to be made but nevertheless indicate that tasks as sophisticated as cognition and language can be effectively studied in human subjects with PET.

Studies in disease

In addition to providing new insights into the function of the normal human brain, PET has contributed to an understanding of the diseased human brain. As expected, dramatic changes have been observed in important diseases such as stroke[10], epilepsy[11], and aging and dementia[12]. More surprising have been recent findings that disturbances in emotional function can be related to highly localized abnormalities in brain blood flow and metabolism. I would like to review one of these findings.

Anxiety must be considered the most common emotional disturbance afflicting mankind. Some patients suffer from a particularly disabling form of anxiety which has most recently been called panic disorder[13]. Patients with this devastating disorder experience spontaneous episodes of severe anxiety accompanied by a variety of symptoms that usually include shortness of breath, a lump in the throat, a choking sensation, lightheadedness, numbness, a pounding heart, and occasionally chest pain. Such attacks are usually brief but may be frequent. They are never provoked by a frightening stimulus. This is a surprisingly common condition affecting 2–3% of the general population worldwide.

An underlying biological basis for panic disorder has been suspected for quite some time. This is based primarily on the observation that attacks of panic can be precipitated by the intravenous infusion of the chemical sodium DL-lactate. This remarkable observation resulted from earlier work indicating that during exercise patients with panic disorder had a higher blood lactate than normal individuals. Although this was probably a spurious observation it prompted two enterprising psychiatrists at Washington

University in St Louis, Ferris Pitts and J.N. McClure, Jr, to reason that lactate might have something to do with the production of panic attacks[14]. To test their hypothesis Pitts and McClure infused sodium DL-lactate into subjects with a history of this disease and found, to their amazement, that symptoms were produced which absolutely duplicated the attacks of anxiety. Normal individuals did not respond to this challenge.

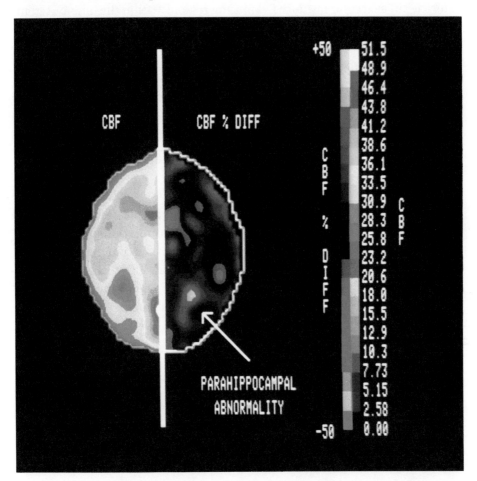

Fig. 18.6. Positron emission tomographic image of local blood flow in the brain of a resting, awake subject with panic disorder, a severe form of anxiety[13]. The left half of the image is a quantitative representation of blood flow corresponding to the left side of the calibrated color scale. The right half of the image represents the difference between the right and left hemispheres expressed as a percent of the left hemisphere blood flow in the right half of the calibrated color scale. Note the striking asymmetry in the posterior aspect of the image. With a complex anatomical localization technique[6] this regional asymmetry was established as residing in the region of the parahippocampal gyrus[15]. Other asymmetries appearing in the image varied randomly among subjects.

Prompted by these observations, we have studied a group of patients with panic disorder before and during the administration of sodium DL-lactate[15] (exactly in the manner of Pitts and McClure). Using our technique for anatomical localization, we decided to explore regions of the brain that were thought to be related to the expression of emotion. These regions lie within what is known as the limbic system, an area of the brain that surrounds its ventricles in a circular fashion. Examining regions within the limbic system, we made the observation that in patients with panic disorder who were sensitive to sodium lactate, there was an abnormality in the parahippocampal region. This abnormality consisted of an increase in blood flow and metabolism in the right hemisphere in the parahippocampal gyrus (Fig. 18.6). It must be recalled that such changes in blood flow and metabolism reflect complex alterations in underlying neuronal activity. At this time we do not know the exact nature of these abnormalities. They await further research in both human subjects and experimental animals.

Conclusions

The material I have presented gives only a brief glimpse of the possibilities that exist for brain imaging with positron emission tomography in human subjects. I have not even touched on the fascinating area of neuropharmacology in which it has been possible to view, using PET techniques in the living brain, the activity of neurotransmitters and their receptors[16]. Coupling such measurements with the functional studies that I have described will give an increasingly detailed view of the human brain. Ultimately, such information should be of considerable use in the understanding of human disease and the alleviation of suffering.

19

Thinking with a computer

DANIEL DENNETT

Imagining and conceiving

According to Descartes, conceiving is one thing and imagining is quite another. What we cannot imagine we may well conceive. His famous example was the chiliagon, a regular 1000-sided figure, which is indistinguishable *in imagination* from a regular 999-sided figure. Both look (see Fig. 19.1) just like circles to the naked eye – and to the naked mind's eye, as Descartes suggested. But conception, he insisted, was a distinct faculty, purified of dependence on the fallible bodily senses and hence more powerful. The image of a chiliagon may be easily confused with the image of a 999-sided figure, but the concept of a chiliagon is as distinct from the concept of a 999-sided figure as any two clear and distinct concepts can be.

This idea that pure conception is a superior faculty of the mind, capable of

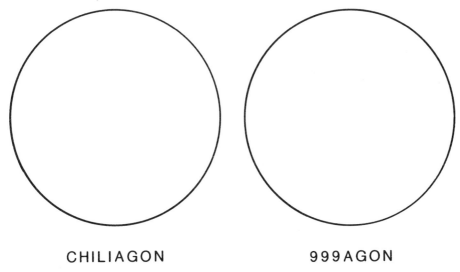

CHILIAGON   999AGON

Fig. 19.1. Since vision cannot distinguish these two figures without the aid of their labels, neither can imagination.

297

taking us far beyond the limits of sensation, has confused and intimidated generations of hapless imaginers, would-be conceivers, who have wondered what it must be like to conceive of the unimaginable: seven-dimensional cubes, the curvature of space, grades of infinity, or – more concretely – the operation of the network composed of trillions of synapses in their own heads. At the risk of unmasking myself as one of the handicapped, I declare my suspicion that Descartes' highly touted act of pure conception is a myth, unattained by Descartes himself and by the deepest, most adroit thinkers ever since. There is no such thing. I can ask you to imagine a hexagon, or a horse, and there is something relatively single and salient you can do in response: you can form an image in your mind's eye, as we say, of a hexagon or a horse. The nature and ontological status of such a mental image is a fascinating and controversial topic in psychology and philosophy of mind, but that there is such a phenomenon as forming a mental image is not in dispute (Nelson Goodman discusses this in Chapter 22). If on the other hand I ask you not to imagine but to conceive of a horse, or a four-dimensional Moebius strip, or a molecule of human DNA, or the maximization of expected utility, there is no uniform, stable way for you to comply. 'Saying the words in one's mind' is, for instance, neither a necessary nor a sufficient condition for conceiving of something. There is no single act of the mind that counts as conceiving of something.

This is striking, since we rely so heavily on our judgments about what we can and cannot conceive. Consider the standard form of argument, exposed in reverse: such-and-such is impossible – why do you think so? – because it is inconceivable – how do you know? – I have tried to conceive of it, and failed. What is it that one has not succeeded in doing when one has tried to conceive of something and failed in the attempt? Many philosophers have considered this mental exercise to be the universal litmus test for logical possibility and truth, and yet, contrary to Descartes' vision, it is not a clearcut task made possible by releasing the mind from the shackles of brute imagination, but rather an indefinitely drawn-out and complex set of manipulations, shot through and through with mental imagery – not naked, but annotated, tagged with caveats and provisos. Berkeley was alluding to this, the fundamental tactic of 'conception', when he suggested that conceiving of the general triangle – the triangle that is neither definitely isosceles, right or scalene – was a matter of imagining some particular triangle and then noting parenthetically that the image had unintended features, reminding oneself not to use the image in certain ways when employing it in the course of thinking.

How do you know when you have succeeded in conceiving of DNA as the vehicle of genetic inheritance? Only when you have run through the story in your imagination, at many levels, with many variations, checking first this and then that, manipulating the details a thousand times, selectively ignoring now the woods, now the trees, now the branches. Conceiving of something complex – whether an abstract mathematical structure, a complicated physical process, or a system of rules and moves like chess or a grammar – is a matter of learning your way around in a 'space' you must construct in your mind. Only by actively exploring such spaces can we become familiar with them to the point of conceptual fluency, which is the point at which the Cartesian illusion is engendered of an act of direct conception. Getting to that level of fluency can be very difficult.

Primo Levi, in his magnificent personal odyssey through the space of chemistry[1] notes one of the difficulties:

> 'If to comprehend is the same as forming an image, we will never form an image of a happening whose scale is a millionth of a millimeter, whose rhythm is a millionth of a second, and whose protagonists are in their essence invisible.'

Yet certainly Levi himself comprehends these microscopic complexities. His lifetime as a chemist has made him adept at juggling his representations, with their well-worn and familiar handles and tags. They no longer have much power to mislead him with their oversimplifications. He no longer needs to read the warning on the rear-view mirror: CAUTION: OBJECTS APPEAR FARTHER AWAY THAN THEY ARE. Years of practice and hard thinking can bring an expert such as Levi to heights of conceptual virtuosity, but are there no short cuts, no ways of easing and speeding the apprenticeship?

Computer-enhanced conception

Here is where the computer comes in. Let us set aside for a moment the engrossing idea that we might make a computer that could really think. Let us attend instead to one of its more practical cousins: the idea that we might make a computer that expanded *our* capacity to think in much the way microscopes, telescopes, microphones, and cameras have expanded our sensory capacities. Many science fiction writers have imagined implanting electronic marvels in human brains to give their owners the vast and flawless memory or sheer computing prowess of a mainframe computer, but what I have in mind is, I think, more interesting and more useful. Looking up facts, or performing vast computations, are sometimes essential accompaniments to serious thinking, and sometimes even acceptable substitutes for serious thinking, but they do not by themselves do much to enable one to think about things one could not think about before. Is there some way of attaching a computer to a human mind so that the mind's *powers of conception* are enhanced?

I think that there is, and – somewhat out of character for a philosopher – I claim that this is not a mere possibility in principle, achievable in some distant science-fictional world, but something that is achievable right now, using existing technology. I will demonstrate some relatively simple devices that we have already developed for stretching the imagination, forerunners, I hope, of much more powerful systems.

Organic brains and electronic computers have very different architectures and modes of operation, but no miraculous brain-implants or novel 'interfaces' are required to yoke the two sorts of systems into powerful new configurations. Normal eyesight and hearing, if properly exploited, provide broad, swift avenues for the receipt of huge amounts of brain-usable information, and one's fingers on a keyboard, with perhaps a 'mouse' or other input gadget on the side, provide return channels capable of carrying back to the computer a greater volume of responses than a mind can modulate. Once these powerful channels have been exhausted we can begin to wonder about designing more intimate links, but we have scarcely begun to tax the resources already available.

Levi speaks of 'a happening whose scale is a millionth of a millimeter, whose rhythm is a millionth of a second, and whose protagonists are in their essence invisible' – if only we could make a *space-time microscope*, something that would enlarge and slow down such happenings by a factor of a million, and then go on to clothe the invisible features with visual metaphors! But we can. An ordinary microcomputer with the aid of color graphics and the right software can be turned into a space-time microscope, a vehicle for exploring those forbidding mind-spaces of science, a vehicle that even a novice can soon learn to drive.

Conceiving a computer

The computer itself will be our first *terra incognita*, a phenomenon of daunting complexity. The IBM-PC, for instance, contains several hundred thousand memory registers, linked to a central processing unit that steps through millions of elementary electronic processes each second, each 'in their essence invisible'. Who can conceive of how those billions of happenings somehow conspire to produce the visible, macroscopic magic we see on the screen? Computer scientists can, of course, thanks to their long apprenticeship. And so can you, in a few hours, with the aid of this space-time microscope.

First, let us look at a somewhat simplified computer, running about a million times slower than the PC that is simulating it (see Fig. 19.2).

This is AESOP, developed by Steven Barney at Tufts University, which has 256 memory registers – not 256 thousand – of which you are currently seeing the top 32. If you look closely – and if you know what you are looking at – you can see the individual instructions being brought, single-file, from the memory to the instruction register, decoded and executed, with the result appearing briefly in the accumulator. The program is generating the Fibonacci numbers. Primo Levi seems to be right; this is millions of times larger and slower than a real computer, and thousands of times simpler – and yet still it is too complex to take in at a glance! But that is only because you are unfamiliar with this particular system of landmarks and metaphors. Let us slow the system down further, and step through the process taking as much time as we need.

Focus, for instance, on a single memory register. It contains a 3-character string of symbols. In what language? The unfamiliar language of 'HEX' or hexadecimal notation. Each of these triplets can be understood to be a number, written in base-16 notation. It will help us understand why this is a

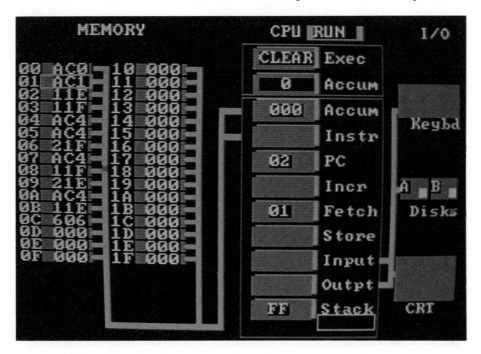

Fig. 19.2. AESOP, a simple computer whose operations are visible on the computer screen. Since AESOP's power depends on interactive animation, the 'stills' used to illustrate the printed version of the demonstration are almost guaranteed not to work for the reader, unfortunately, but are provided to help the reader imagine what the running program looks like.

natural and convenient way of representing happenings in a computer if we enlarge a register and see how it stores a number (see Fig. 19.3). Each hex digit is 'short for' four digits of binary arithmetic. There are 16 different permutations of four ONs and OFFs, so we can characterize the state of any group of 4 binary digits or BITS with a single character of hex. So the three hex digits we see in each AESOP register stand for 12 binary digits; AESOP is a 12-bit machine. (The IBM-PC is a 16-bit machine; some microcomputers are eight-bit machines, and larger computers are 32- and even 64-bit machines.)

Let's go back to AESOP and see what happens to one of these triplets when it arrives at the instruction register (see Fig. 19.4). It is translated and then executed. The first hex digit is the Op code or operation code; it tells the computer what to do – add, subtract, multiply, divide, compare, fetch, store,... or stop – there are only 16 possible moves for this simple computer to make; one for each hex symbol. The other two digits are for a memory address, to tell the computer which item to do its task on. There are 16^2 or 256 different addresses specifiable in two digits of hex; hence AESOP has a 256 register RAM or random access memory.

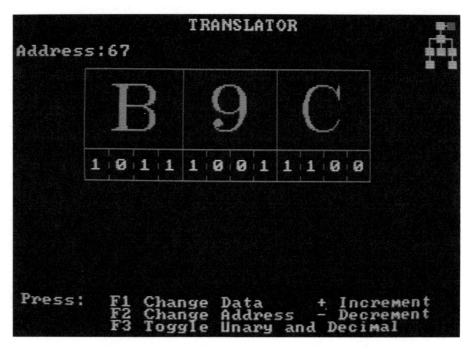

Fig. 19.3. An AESOP memory register, enlarged. It is hard to 'read' long strings of zeros and ones. Groups of 4 can be abbreviated into single symbols in hexadecimal notation. In this enlargement, it is possible to spin the numbers up and down, watching the binary and hexadecimal values change in unison. A decimal translation is also provided if the user wants it.

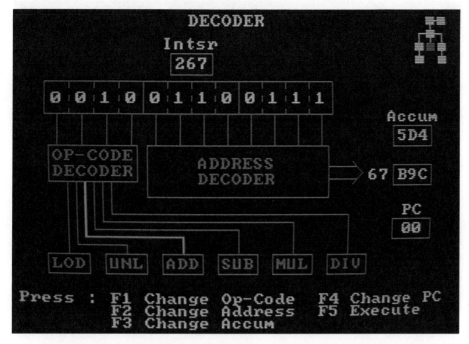

Fig. 19.4. The AESOP instruction register, enlarged: the first 4 bits are the Op code. Rather like a long-distance telephone area code, they open a line to one specialized circuit or another. The next 8 bits give the address of the item on which the specialized circuit is to do its work.

Why do computers use binary code – ONs and OFFs – to represent everything? We can literally see why if we descend a few more levels, magnifying our computer by another power of 10, and slowing down its operation still further. Here is the accumulator, a register with 12 bits, 12 ONs and OFFs, in a row (see Fig. 19.5). Each of those twelve boxes has to be designed to 'remember' its value (1 or 0, ON or OFF, red or green) until the computer does something to change it. If we zoom in on one box (see Fig. 19.6), we can see how this is accomplished, via a 'flip-flop' composed of simple 'logic gates' representing the logical functions AND, OR and NOT. Logic gates can be wired up differently to produce a circuit for performing an arithmetical operation on two different 12-bit numbers. Here is the circuit that is turned on by the ADD instruction (see Fig. 19.7): it too is composed of 12 boxes, each of which can add two digits and a 'carry' coming from the adjacent column if there is one. If we zoom in on one of them, we can see how they are composed of logic gates (see Fig. 19.8).

I have sped through this demonstration just to give you a brief glimpse of a world that can be endlessly explored. AESOP is a completely programmable, debuggable, runnable computer. If it strikes you as still too complicated a

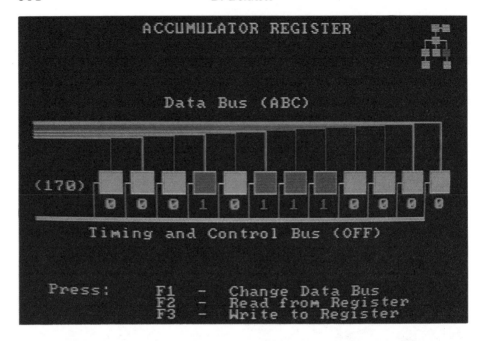

Fig. 19.5.   The AESOP accumulator register, enlarged. A register is made of 12
separate flip-flops, each of which must 'remember' what it has most recently been
'told': either 1 (ON) or 0 (OFF).

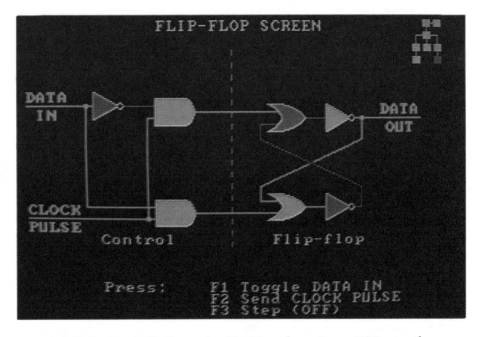

Fig. 19.6.   How a flip-flop works. The triangular units are NOT-gates; they
output the opposite of their input: if their input is 1, their output is 0, and vice
versa. The crescent-shaped units are OR-gates; they output 1 if *either OR both* of
their inputs are 1. The other units are AND-gates which deliver a 1 only when
both of their inputs are 1. Whenever a clock pulse arrives, the flip-flop gets a new
value to remember.

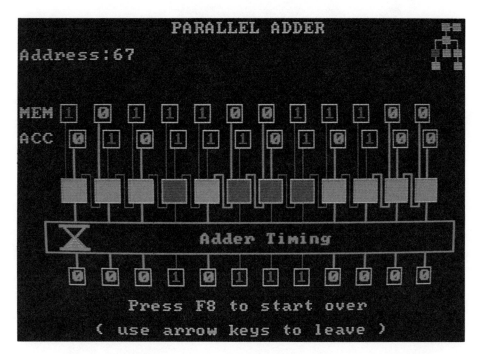

Fig. 19.7. The AESOP addition circuit, enlarged. When the number from the memory address and the number from the accumulator are fed into the parallel adder circuit, their sum is output. The time it takes to add the two numbers depends on how many 'carries' have to be performed, so there is a delay system, represented by the hourglass on the left.

starting point for a novice, you are in good company. Here is a still simpler world to explore, in an even friendlier vehicle: RodRego the Register Machine (see Fig. 19.9).

Here the registers are simple boxes, each of which can have beans in them – any number from zero on up. And there are only two operations the machine can perform: adding a bean to a box (INCrementing a register) and taking a bean out (DECrementing a register). What if the register in question is empty – has 0 in it? The Register machine must then Branch to another instruction, so we call the taking-away instruction DEB, for DEcrement or Branch). With INC and DEB our machine can compute anything AESOP can compute. In fact, it can compute any function any computer at all can compute – only very, very slowly! Teaching RodRego to add, subtract, multiply and divide, and to move or copy the contents of one register to another, is a pleasant and instructive exercise that is a vivid, memorable introduction to the fundamental principles of computer science: contents and addresses, subroutines, loops, commands as contents of registers, conditional branching and much more.

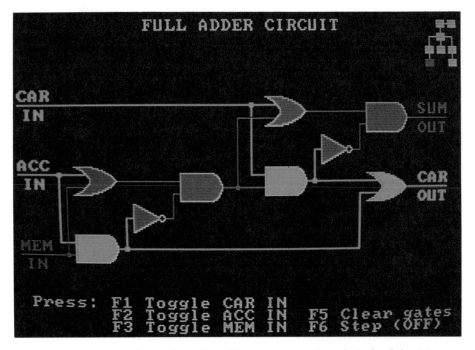

Fig. 19.8. A single box from the addition circuit, enlarged. Each of the 12 elements in the addition circuit shown in Fig. 19.7 has three inputs: one from the memory register, one from the accumulator, and a 'carry' line from its neighbor to the right. This circuit of logic gates does the actual binary addition. In binary arithmetic, $1 + 0$ is 1, and $1 + 1$ is 10, and $1 + 1 + 1$ is 11. If you work out the outputs for each input possibility in this diagram you will see that, for instance, when two of its three inputs are 1, it will 'put down' the 0 and 'carry' the 1 to its neighbor. The Space-Time Microscope performs all these operations for you, showing the flow through the logic gates in color.

Enhancing other concepts

Space-time microscopes are not the only instruments we can make for stretching the imagination. Consider how excellently suited a piano is to the task of exploring the complex space of musical harmony; it provides a swift, accurate response to the explorer's hunches and queries, and uses three different but easily inter-translated systems for displaying places, structures, and events in that space: two visual spaces – written musical notation and the keyboard array – and one auditory space. It is easy for the novice to use, but virtually inexhaustible. Imagine *concept pianos* for exploring other complex spaces.

In population genetics, for instance, one has to develop a feel for the relation between two different sorts of mathematical models: the very idealized models in which probability is allowed to reign supreme (thanks to the unrealistic assumption of unlimited population sizes) and more realistic

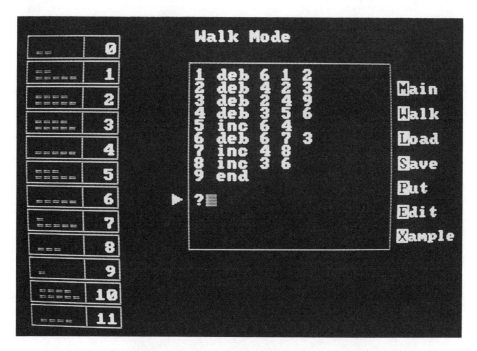

Fig. 19.9. The simplest computer: RodRego, a register machine. In this animated register machine, a cousin of the familiar Logo turtle (the little triangle) dashes back and forth, reading each instruction in turn, running to the appropriate register, and either removing or adding a 'bean' to the contents.

models in which the spread of genes is sensitive to population size, migration rates, and particular, local, 'random' factors. In the latter models, as in Nature, improbable trends can be tenacious and even victorious. GeneWright is a concept piano we have developed at the Curricular Software Studio for exploring in an efficient and satisfying way this huge space of possibilities. On it you can play all the standard textbook pieces, or create your own themes and watch to see if you understand the rhythms of change that develop before your eyes. You can refresh your understanding of the underlying mechanisms by zooming in on them or sit back and take a bird's eye view of generations swiftly succeeding each other (see Fig. 19.10). GeneWright is named in honor of Sewall Wright, the biologist who has perhaps done the most to expand biologists' appreciation of what is possible when there are a large number of small populations subject to stochastic phenomena, such as genetic drift. It is hard, even for experts, to imagine what can happen in small populations. GeneWright lets you *see the possibilities* unfold directly, and even experts find that there are ways they can use it to extend and sharpen their understanding.

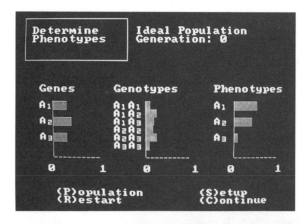

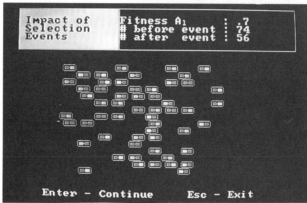

Fig. 19.10. Two views of GeneWright: top, Determining phenotypes; bottom, Impact of selection events. The graphs at the top show the frequencies of the alternative genes in a population of a species, and the frequencies with which they get expressed in individual phenotypes. At the bottom, one group of these phenotypes is seen being pruned by selection.

At Tufts we are now developing other devices for exploring other spaces: for studying the uptake of anaesthetics by mammalian respiratory systems, for internalizing the treacherous concepts of statistics, for learning to read the geological record, and one of my favorites: a dynamic, color-coded, functional architecture of the human brain, a space-time microscope I sometimes describe as the London Underground Map of the brain. Nearby at Harvard, Judah Schwartz and his colleagues at the Educational Technology Center have designed similar systems: the Geometric Supposer and its offspring in mathematics, and some elegant physics simulators.

The limits of these devices

I suppose there may be some complex objects of study that cannot be significantly tamed by such exploratory devices. The chaotic spaces and informal methods of philosophy itself have so far eluded us, perhaps because we cannot identify any *particular* powers of conception (aside from formal logic) that might be enhanced by the sort of apprenticeship experiences these devices can provide. Maybe we have just not given the matter the right sort of thought yet. In any event, the devices we have created to date are still fairly primitive, but I think they point in the right direction.

The most important feature of these prosthetic extensions of the mind is that they are designed not to replace your mind, but to strengthen it, to the point where you can drop the crutches and continue expanding your powers of imagination and conception of your own, less docile in the face of complexity, less dependent on the computer for the answers.

We are no match for computers in the memory and computation departments, which is just as well, since memorizing and computing are not much fun. Imagining, and the understanding that comes with it, is our strong suit, and if we can turn computers to the task of enhancing that strength, instead of just doing a crude and brittle job of mimicking it, we can increase our lead, maintain control over the technology, and experience the world's complexities more acutely in the bargain.

20

How do we interpret images?

RICHARD GREGORY

Most, though not all recent writers on perception follow the German Astronomer Johannes Kepler (1570–1630) in accepting that vision starts with optical images in the eyes; slightly different perspective pictures being projected optically on to each retina. But as pictures, retinal images are very odd – unique – for although they are indeed perspective pictures of the world, they are never seen, for there is no eye looking at them and so they are not objects of perception. They are, rather, just one cross-section of the visual pathway from objects to perceptions of objects. The retina does, however, have special importance; it is the interface from the optical projection of the world at the eye to the coded neural signals transmitted down the optic nerves to the brain, which are all the brain, in its dark chamber, receives from the eyes or indeed from the world of objects.

The key problem for perception is how meaning is read from neural signals from the senses. Vision presents problems of special interest, as especially for man visual perception is so rich, and yet – unlike the senses of touch, taste and smell – the optical images in eyes have no intrinsic biological significance, for they cannot directly monitor the presence of food or poison, or hot or cold. Organisms cannot eat images, or be eaten by them: to be useful they must, somehow, convey properties of objects which are not present in the image, which physically is but shadows or patterns of light. Though we see that a table is hard and a glass brittle, the eye's images are not hard or brittle. Somehow a wealth of such non-optical characteristics of objects are read from neural signals from retinal images – no doubt through inherited and learned interactive experience with objects and what they do in various situations. This is our starting point for considering the meaning of images; though as we shall see, this kind of account is not always accepted. For us vision starts with the optical images of the eye, but unlike the pictures of artists, visual perceptions are figments rather than pigments of imagination.

The role of retinal images is somewhat complicated by the fact that perceptions are built up from successive eye movements, which are necessitated in man by the concentration of optical resolution in the central *foveal* region of the retinae. But, as we learn from an after-image given by a bright flash of light, we can see an entire scene in a brief moment of time with a fixed eye. So, for simplicity, we may refer to static retinal images as the pictures – though unseen as pictures – whose meaning we are considering when we try to explain visual perception. Here we will ignore movements of the eyes, and also motions of objects. And we may also ignore the small but important differences between the images of the eyes which give stereoscopic depth, for the world of objects is generally seen in convincing and fairly reliable depth with a single stationary eye (and distances and form in three dimensions are seen quite well in flat perspective paintings and photographs), which shows that much is read from a single retinal image, though *it* is not seen as a picture or object is seen.

Passive and active theories of perception

Theories of perception, and explanations of how depth for example is read from the signals from a single stationary eye, stand on either side of a Great Divide which separates '*Passive*' and '*Active*' accounts of perception. On a Passive account, meaning is supposed to be in the world, to be picked up by a passive observer, whose brain has little or nothing to do beyond some selection of what may be needed. On an Active account, the observer (or listener, feeler, taster or whatever) is seen as creating rich meanings from limited and only indirectly related data available from the senses. These active brain processes are supposed to involve a great deal of stored knowledge, for inferring or 'reading' objects from scarcely adequate sensory signals.

Passive theories in some form have generally been favoured by philosophers. For the notion that perceptions are *directly* related to the perceived world (or even are *samples* of surfaces of objects) offers a secure base to epistemology – for perceptions to give undoubtedly true premises for reason to build upon. This is traditionally appealing to philosophers who seek certainty; but it is hardly a plausible paradigm for scientists, who are all-too-used to hard-won data turning out to be inadequate and sometimes misleading. No doubt because this is their life-work, scientists see interpreting data as a highly creative activity for making sense of the world, which is the essence of Activist accounts of perception. So perhaps it is not surprising if Active accounts appeal more to scientists than to philosophers. But there are exceptions; the well-known psychologist, the late James J. Gibson[1, 2], robustly defended a Passivist account, in which visual perception is supposed to be by 'direct pick-up of information, from the ambient array of light'. Very differently, on the 'Active' side of the Great Divide, the modern originator of

Activism, the nineteenth century polymath Hermann von Helmholtz[3], described perception as 'Unconscious Inference', from data and subtle cues available to the senses.

Modern Passivist accounts of perception start with the Idealist philosopher George Berkeley (1685–1753) in his celebrated discussions[4] of the status of visual sensations and objects. Berkeley held that what exists is what is perceived (*esse est percipi*), and that 'ideas' arise essentially passively from habitual associations of tactual, auditory, visual and other sensations. But as he could not conceive how retinal images could be meaningfully related to external objects by the mind, he rejected the commonsense notion that objects exist in their own right, independently of perception. In particular, he could not conceive how the sizes of retinal images could indicate or represent object sizes or distances – for any given retinal image, or subtended angle at the eye, might arise from a large distant object or equally from a nearer, smaller object. The geometer, or the surveyor can stand outside to measure distances and sizes, but this is not possible for perception by a single stationary eye; so for Berkeley neither sizes nor shapes of retinal images could possibly provide valid evidence of external objects. For him God comes to the rescue, as Ronald Knox put it:

> There was a young man who said 'God
> Must think it exceedingly odd
> if He finds that this tree
> continues to be
> When there's no one about in the Quad'

To which was added:

> Dear Sir:
> Your astonishment's odd:
> I am always about in the Quad
> And that's why the tree
> Will continue to be,
> Since observed by
> Yours faithfully GOD

The Activistic psychologists took on Berkeley's problem, though not his Idealism, by supposing that vision works from various subtle cues, used for deriving sizes and distances and so on with cognitive processes of inference. They held, in effect, that Berkeley demanded over-certainty of vision, and that although retinal images are essentially ambiguous, they convey sufficient information for usually reliable inferences to external objects, though the process is not infallible. My preference here is to consider perceptions as *hypotheses*, somewhat similar to the predictive hypotheses of science[5, 6, 7]. A striking difference, however, and it is not clear how important this is, is that perceptions are associated with awareness or consciousness, but hypotheses of science (we assume) lack the vital richness, such as colour or brightness, of the sensations that are our immediate reality.

For Berkeley, and indeed for virtually all philosophers, perceptions are supposed to be made of the experienced 'sense data' of perceptual awareness. But, due to later developments by psychologists, the status of sense data has changed dramatically, for the evidence is that we are seldom if ever aware of the data for perception in consciousness; so we cannot know by introspection just what features of objects, as signalled by the senses, are accepted for perceptions. Thus Helmholtz spoke of perceptions as 'conclusions of unconscious inferences' from various 'clues', or 'cues', available to the senses; but as introspection is not available, it requires experiments to establish what these may be. Thus Helmholtz took the study of perception several steps away from experience, and so away from the founder of what we are calling Activism, the empiricist philosopher John Locke (1634–1707), who wrote[8]: 'All knowledge is founded on and ultimately derives itself from sense . . . or sensation'. But since Helmholtz's denial of sensation as the stuff and basis of perception, the emphasis has been on neural signals, and the information they convey, with, it must be confessed, sensation left as utterly mysterious and with no causal or any other role to play. How are sensations related to perceived objects? Locke, who was much concerned with this question, distinguished between 'Primary' properties of objects which are important for physics, and 'Secondary' properties which are sensations of perception. But just where this distinction can be made has never been established, and it changes, both with changes of physics and of accounts of perception. This is the problem of what is 'subjective' and what is 'objective'. It is usually held, with Locke, that experience of colours, shapes, motion and so on are in the *observer* and so 'subjective'; but there is generally some physical basis to experienced colour and brightness, as well as for shapes and movements of objects, which have clear causal effects apart from perception. Locke's difficult-to-define distinction between Primary and Secondary characteristics may be denied by philosophers trying to hold that what we experience resides in the object world; but they meet the difficulty that perception, in some degree, depends on states of the nervous system and on where and who we are. Also illusions, perceptual errors, are evidence for the essential separateness of perceptions from objects. For Activists, illusions are seen as highly suggestive evidence for various kinds of inferences in perception, many illusions being seen as fallacies of perceptual inference. So, illusions of many kinds are grist to the mill for Activists, but embarrassing chaff for Passivists, who have a hard time explaining how any illusions are possible if perceptions are directly related to object reality.

On the other side of the Great Divide, Gibson[1] tried to deny illusion altogether; for if perception is direct pick-up-of-information how can illusions occur? Gibson suggested, most daringly, that there is a surprising *lack* of illusions – which he sees as *evidence* against what we are calling cognitively 'Active' theories (!) Thus, he writes (his italics):

> *For the visual worlds of different observers are more alike than they ought to be if the doctrine* (Helmholtzian perceptual inference) *were the complete truth.* The evidence accumulates that men, and moreover even animals, appear to react to the spatial environment with an accuracy and precision too great for any known theory of space perception to be able to explain. . . If space perception is a subjective process then why are we so seldom misled by illusory perceptions?

Gibson sums up his 'Passivist' position:

> According to the present argument, however, the objective world does not require for its explanation a process of construction, translation, or even organisation. The visual world can be analysed into impressions which are object-like, and these impressions are traceable to stimulation.

So for Gibson, meaning is in the world, to be picked up by passive perception. He does allow, though, that Active cognitive processes are involved in language perception[1(a)].

> When this ('Active') doctrine of perception is applied to such abilities as the apprehension of meaning – to the understanding of language for instance – it works very well and accounts for most of the experimental facts . . .

For at least the Passivist Gibson, meaning in visual perception and language are very different; but for Activists they are similar, visual data being accepted as tokens and clues by which the world is 'read', with active intelligence by eye and brain. Language structure and understanding may reflect, and be derived from, cognitive processes of (especially visual) perception. Activists might well expect many perceptual illusions to correspond, at least roughly, to errors of language. Thus visual ambiguities; distortions; paradoxes; fictions, and effects of context, are indeed found in perception (or misperception) and in language. They may be seen as evidence for Active intelligent processes for seeking, though not always finding, stable and true meaning.

Algovists

It is far less clear how Passivists can make use of the concepts of sensory data, and stimulus clues or 'cues'; for how can effective use of data be made without some kind of active intelligence? A recent suggestion is, effectively, to stress the importance of fairly simple and generally applicable rules – algorithms – for deriving perception from signalled features. While the *Passivists* support mainly 'bottom-up' stimulus-driven accounts of perception, the *Activists* support largely 'top-down' knowlege-based accounts; it might be held that algorithmic rule-following can generate perceptions 'sideways' – without either strictly adequate stimuli or detailed knowledge of objects. Being less dependent on stimuli or knowledge, computational algorithms fall into a middle position: the advocates of algorithms we will call *Algovists*, and they may occupy the Great Divide between Passivists and Activists.

The present emphasis on following algorithms by real-time neural comput-ing[9] follows recent technical developments in high-speed machine computa-tion. So far, however, success in object recognition is not impressive compared with perception even in simple organisms. Is this because algorithms are over-used, with corresponding under-use of knowledge, applied top-down, for interpreting sensory signals in terms of objects? It is suggestive that a cartoonist, using a few lines, can convey familiar objects quite easily; though unlikely objects are far harder to represent effectively (see Pearson, *et al.*, Chapter 3). Thus, the artist has no problem showing a nose seen sticking *out* of a face – because once recognised as a nose (by top-down inference) it almost certainly sticks out, as this is the way noses are. For very familiar objects the cartoonist does not need to provide specific depth-cues, such as perspective, shadows or shading; though unfamiliar objects (or even worse, familiar objects with atypical features) are extremely difficult to draw convincingly. It is interesting that very familiar objects, such as faces, which are virtually never reversed in depth, are exceedingly hard to see correctly when they *are* depth-reversed – as with a hollow mask, which looks like a normal face – in spite of stereoscopic evidence from the two eyes. Even strong depth-cues are not sufficient to override the knowledge that noses virtually always stick out, not in. This demonstration gives strong support for a knowledge-based Activist paradigm; for knowledge of objects clearly can override (bottom-up or sideways) texture, perspective, stereoscopic or motion parallax depth cues, and such object knowledge is too specific to be described in terms of algorithms.

But there is plenty of evidence that cues, such as perspective, texture, shadows and the rest are important. How are cues read to give meaning and, we suppose, select 'perceptual hypotheses' of objects?

Cues for meaning

The words 'cue' and 'clue' are used interchangeably, though 'clues' more strongly suggest the need for perceptual intelligence. *Passivists* can hardly accept 'clues' in this sense, as for them perception is not intelligent: so Passivists are always clueless and generally cueless. For cognitive *Activists* following Helmholtz, cues are important premises for perceptual inferences, perceptions being conclusions of unconscious inferences. The status of 'cues' is not so clear for the *Algovists*, who stress running computations rather than inferences. For them restraints on what are likely object shapes are more important than evidence of specific features of objects. Thus David Marr[9] stressed that the immense computational problem can be made tractable by accepting restraints such as that the parts of animals and humans are approximately cylinders. Adopting restraints on what is possible or likely for typical objects limits what needs to be computed. Thus, considering perspective-based cues, algorithms can work from general geometrical laws of perspective; for provided the perceived objects have typical shapes, the rules should be effective though working on very *general* restraints and applying to a very wide range of typical objects. We should, however, expect perception to fail in reliability and show some wild illusions with odd-shaped objects, when the rules are inappropriate. Or, at least, perception should drastically slow down, as the computational problem is far greater for atypical objects. Here it is well worth considering the Ames demonstrations[10] in which objects having markedly 'built in' perspective shapes (such as the Ames Window) are exceedingly hard to see correctly. This, indeed, is a converse case to the difficulty of seeing a hollow mask as hollow (as hollow faces are unlikely), which shows the importance of specific object knowledge – for the Ames demonstrations show how very *general* assumptions, such as perspective convergence, mislead when they are inappropriate.

The distinction between general and specific knowledge clearly provides a crucial distinction between Activists and Algovists. Further, it suggests experimental tests of these paradigms as more-or-less general claims of how perception works, and also for how illusory phenomena may be explained. So we will look now in some detail at a depth 'cue', chosen with these questions in mind: *occlusion*. This takes us to the wonderful phenomena of Illusory Contours and to ghostly Fictional Surfaces.

Testimony from fictional contours and ghostly surfaces

Among the most intriguing illusions of all are visual fictions of clearly visible yet non-existent illusory contours and surfaces. These occur, for virtually all observers, in a variety of simple line figures. They continue to be seen even though recognised as fictional.

Illusory contour figures, such as Schumann's early example[11] (Fig. 20.1), or the Kanizsa triangle (Fig. 20.2), elicit illusory contours bounding an illusory surface, which always appears slightly darker or lighter than its background. There are, however, illusory contour figures (such as Fig. 20.3) which do not produce illusory surfaces – but only contours. These have not been studied in such detail; isolated contours seem to have identical characteristics to the boundary edges of illusory surfaces, though the isolated contours evidently have a somewhat different origin.

I suggested in 1972[12] that the illusory surfaces of the Kanizsa triangle and other examples may be *postulated surfaces*, accounting for unlikely gaps as due to eclipsing or occlusion by some nearer object or opaque surface.

> The cognitive paradigm of perception regards perceptions as hypotheses selected by sensory data, but going beyond available data, to give 'object hypotheses'. This paradigm would be satisfied by supposing that the illusory object is 'postulated' as a perceptual hypothesis to account for the blank sectors and the breaks in the triangle[5].

This very often happens in normal object perception, for nearer objects

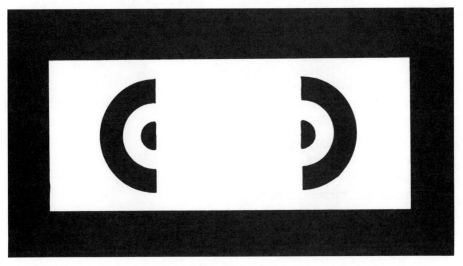

Fig. 20.1. Schumann's figure. This is the first known cognitive contour figure (1904).

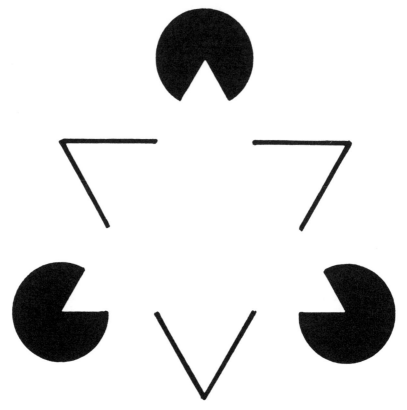

Fig. 20.2.   Kanizsa's triangle. This is the most famous example of an illusory surface bounded by illusory contours. It is suggested that the illusory surface is a postulated occluding surface to account for the gaps, perceptually.

usually partly hide further objects – though these are still recognised, and are assumed to be complete. If this requires knowledge of particular shapes of objects occlusion must be a sophisticated depth-cue, requiring cognition.

This continues:

> As these features are removed from the figure, the hypothesis becomes weaker, until the postulated masking object is no longer seen. Is this because the *evidence* is weaker?

But is this a weakening of evidence for inference of an object or surface, or is it weakening of evidence for applying an algorithm? Or on a 'Passive' view, could it be a relatively simple interactive effect, perhaps at the retinal level (this point is carefully argued by Dumais & Bradley[13])?

Stanley Coren[14] suggested that the illusory surfaces are due to depth-cues. The interesting question is whether, and if so how, object-shaped-gappiness,

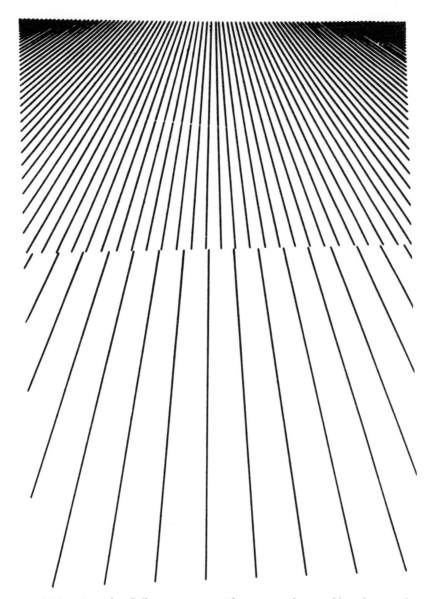

Fig. 20.3. An isolated illusory contour. This is given by a sudden change of
depth.

as a basis for postulating an eclipsing surface, should be thought of as a depth-
cue. Is occlusion essentially different from other depth-cues, such as perspective which follows simple general rules? Is the postulation of an occluding
surface derived from specific object knowledge, top-down or 'sideways',
Algovistically – by following general rules applying to almost all objects?

Illusory surfaces are rather clearly associated with 'gappy' figures. Inspection of many figures evoking illusory surfaces suggests that they occur when:

(a) the gaps are *unlikely*; (b) they form a *likely* object shape. This is a prediction of the postulated-surface account, which inspection of a wide variety of examples seems to confirm. But is the implication plausible that the visual system computes probabilities of whether gaps are more likely to occur by chance, or are probably due to eclipse by some nearer object or surface? This probability-balancing must be in terms of what are likely object shapes. The *probability* of objects having parallel sides, or right-angular corners, is also essential for perspective-depth – but this is simpler and more readily implemented with general algorithms. On this basis, perspective as a cue fits the less cognitively demanding Algovist paradigm very plausibly; but perhaps postulation-of-occluding-surfaces by gappiness demands too much special knowledge of object shapes. Whether this is based on *particular* knowledge of objects, or on *generally* likely object shapes, is clearly the key question for deciding whether illusory surfaces are top-down inferences or are derived by general rule-following.

The first question to answer is whether the visual system does select nearer from further surfaces on the basis of shapes. This should be closely linked to the classical *figure-ground* phenomena.

Surprisingly, from his Passivist position, Gibson gives an interesting discussion of occlusion and Figure-Ground, in which he concedes that occlusion can hardly be a simple direct cue to depth[1(b)].

> Natural scenes, however, do not divide up neatly into figures and background. In most of them it is a relative matter whether a given area be regarded as a figure or as a background. One object may be the background for another nearer object, and another larger object may be the background of the first. . . Seen as a field, with the head and eyes fixed, one area can be described as *eclipsing* the other, to use an astronomical term. Seen as a world, however, one object lies *in front* of another.

Gibson[1(c)] proceeds to discuss the status of occlusion as a depth cue:

> The phenomenon of the superposition of objects is actually not a clue to the depth of objects but a perception which requires explanation. A man knows that a near object can partially obscure a far object but his retina does not, and the retinal explanation should be sought first . . . There is no texture, double imagery (stereopsis), or relative motion in these drawings. They suggest the principle that the more complete, continuous, or regular outline tends to be the one which looks near. Is completeness, then, a sign or clue for distance?

Using the examples of Fig. 20.4, Gibson goes on to give remarkably non-Passivistic suggestions to account for selection of object over ground: that a nearer object tends to have the more *regular*, *complete* and 'closed' contours.

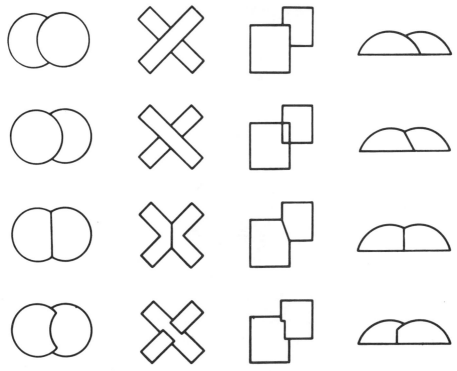

Fig. 20.4. Occluding surfaces. These, surely, show something of the rules by which the perceptual system decides what is hiding and what is hidden, in an overlap situation (from[1]).

These, he thinks, are best described not as 'stimuli for perceptions of space', but as special 'probable signs, secondary to the others'. Or as 'having doubtful status'. This seems an eminently reasonable account; though it is not in the Gibsonian Passivistic tradition, as evidently he realizes.

Figure-Ground effects

Most figure-ground effects can be handled with the minimal cognition of Algovism; but consider cases such as Rubin's vase-face figure. Here one might think the balanced probabilities of the vase and the face as objects is the crucial point; but perceptual effects from specific knowledge of vases and faces would clearly be top-down and so would fit the Activist paradigm. An Activist's account of a postulated masking surface would suggest special object knowledge[15] working top-down to set probabilities. This would predict that for people unfamiliar with vases the Rubin's faces-vase (Fig. 20.5) would not be ambiguous, but would simply be a pair of faces, looking at each other. It may be noted that clearly knowledge-induced contours can be seen, if

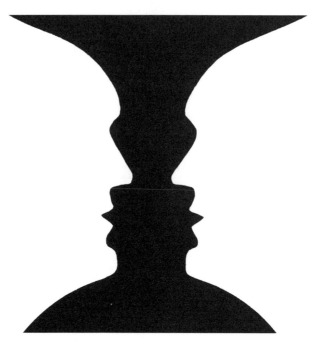

Fig. 20.5.   Perhaps the most famous object-ambiguous figure: Rubin's faces/
vase. Does knowledge of faces and vases affect which is seen; setting up a roughly
equal appearance-time for each?

faintly, as in the form of the dalmatian dog (Fig. 12.7). This surely depends on
knowledge of dogs. But it is not clear that its seen edge is the same as the
illusory contours we are considering. An even purer 'cognitive' example is
the bear-behind-the-tree (Fig. 20.6). But does one actually *see* the bear? – it is
only 'seen' conceptually. Evidently there is a gold mine here for experiments
to investigate the claims of Passivism, Algovism, and Activism from visual
ambiguities.

An Algovistic account demands that illusory contours should always be
simple, smooth curves, and should only be induced by or follow smooth
closed curves. The demonstrations with adjustable wires[16] shown in Fig.
20.7 suggest that this is so, for when the ends of the wires form a simple
smooth shape (a circle) there is a strong illusory disk; but when the wires are
individually pushed in and out, to give a more and more jagged edge, the
illusion is diminished and finally disappears. Also, a single wire pushed inside
or outside the circle is ignored; though several wires forming a gradual
distortion of the circle drag the contour with them – to form a distorted figure,
with all the wires touching its illusory contour. When the wires are displaced
in *depth* (seen by stereoscopic vision) the illusory surface becomes correspond-

ingly three-dimensional – its edges remaining attached to the wires – provided they form a smooth curve in the third dimension. A wire that is too near or too distant from the others is rejected, just as for discontinuities in a plane; but now the shift at the retina is very small, for stereoscopic depth dislocation, so the (Algovistic) rules evidently apply to perceptual space in three dimensions rather than simply to the retinal projection. This strongly suggests a

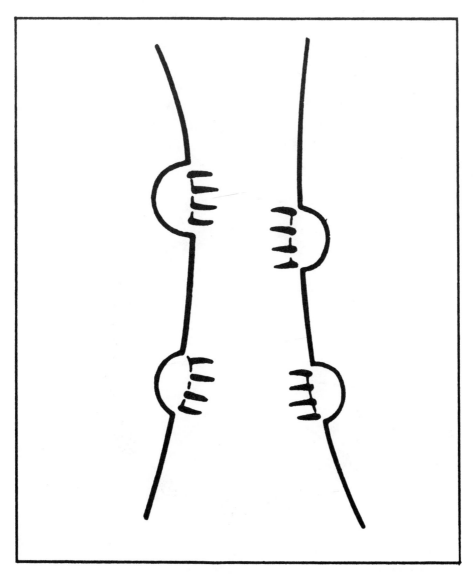

Fig. 20.6. A Bare Bear. Here the evidence is enough to elicit a 'conceptual' hypothesis of a bear; but perhaps not sufficient for actually *seeing* it perceptually.

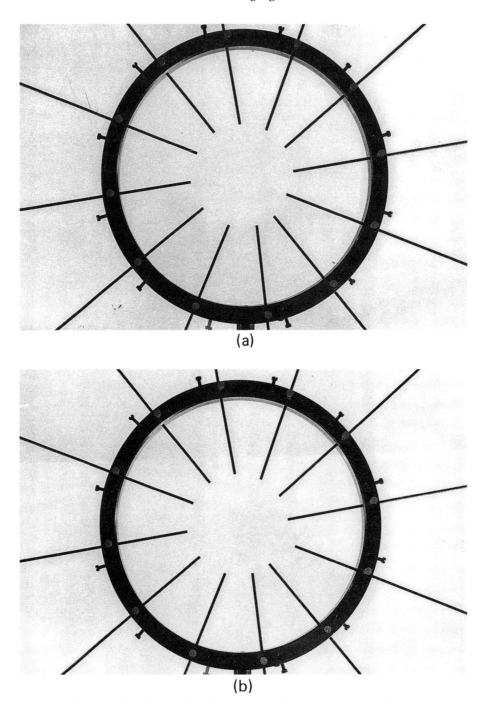

(a)

(b)

Fig. 20.7.   Spokes that speak of meaning. (a) The converging wires forming a
circle are seen as touching an illusory surface with a faint but distinct illusory
contour. (b), (c) The contour will follow a displaced wire – up to a certain point –
then 'reject' the aberrant wire. (d) When the wires are randomised, the contour

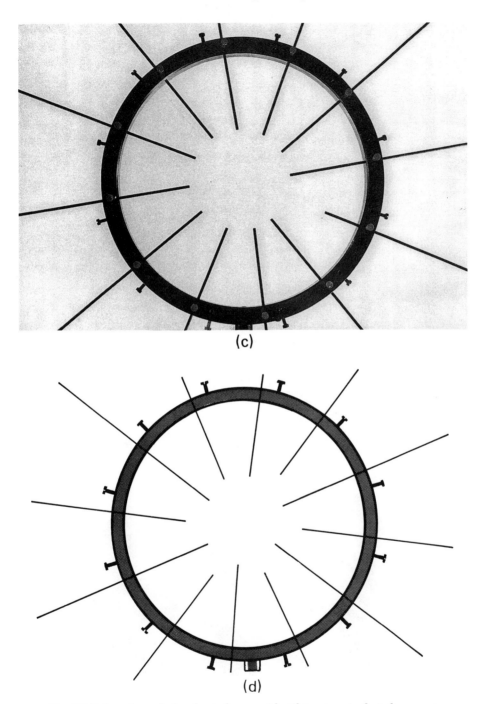

(c)

(d)

Fig. 20.7. (*cont*)   and ghostly surface vanish. This suggests that they must represent a likely (smooth-edged) object. How far this is given by an algorithm (like graph fitting) and how far knowledge of specific objects, is an important question as to how images convey meaning.

post-retinal origin for the phenomena. Further evidence for this will be given below, and also evidence that the phenomena originate fairly early in the visual system, though not at the retina.

A somewhat surprising finding[12, 17, 18] is that illusory contours can occur through *binocular fusion* of parts of the figures – though neither eye alone has sufficient features to produce the phenomenon, indicating that it occurs in the brain, not the eyes[19]. For example, the illusory surface of the Kanizsa triangle is seen by binocular fusion. These findings are compatible with an Activist or an Algovist account.

In 1973 John Harris and I[20] presented pairs of figures giving differently curved illusory contours to each eye. We found that not only would they fuse but – just as for true contours of these curvatures – they fused into a single contour lying in *stereoscopic depth*. As stereo depth requires different contours in each eye for stereo fusion, it follows that each eye system must be capable of generating its own illusory contours. But, as this must take place *before* the coming together of the signals from the eyes, the illusory contour generation must take place before (or perhaps at) stereo fusion. It follows that illusory contours can be produced by processes lying before the combining of the signals from the eyes giving stereopsis. From another experiment with John Harris[21] it seems clear that illusory contours must be post-retinal. This means that illusory contours can be produced by processes which occur not right at the start, but quite early on in the visual system. But if they occur in the early stages of processing, how can these be cognitive knowledge-based phenom-

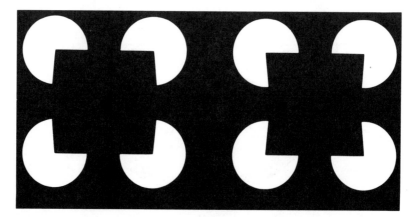

Fig. 20.8.   This stereo-pair evokes a three-dimensional illusory contour (on the side coming out), by stereopsis. (The inward-going side tends to give double vision, or lack of fusion.) The outgoing contour shows that each eye system is capable of generating its own illusory contour – for fusion into depth (from[20]).

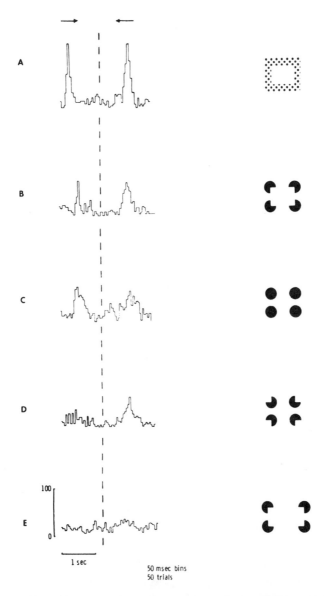

Fig. 20.9. The images on the right were moved up and down across the receptive field of a nerve cell recorded in the visual cortex of an anaesthetized cat, producing the responses plotted, on the left, as histograms showing the frequency of impulses. This cell, typical of those in the primary visual cortex (see Chapter 17), responded well to a non-illusory contour, such as that formed by a white patch on a background of dots (A), moving in either direction. It also responded a little to other patterns with black-white boundaries that just fell within the receptive field as they moved across it (B,C,D). However, it did not respond at all to a strong illusory contour in which the inducing components were far enough apart not to touch the receptive field (E). No responses to illusory contours were found in the primary visual cortex (from Note 25).

ena? In particular, how can it be supposed that they are as subtle as *postulates*, based on the evidence of *unlikely gaps* forming shapes of *probable objects*? For probabilities based on knowledge of objects can hardly be assessed so early in the visual system. On the other hand, simple algorithms applying to virtually all objects might be computed early in the visual system.

Inspection suggests that these phenomena are not produced by surprising absence of *particular* objects or features, but rather by breaks or losses of *typical* object characteristics. Thus a missing nose, though unlikely, does not evoke a fictional nose. The ghostly shapes that are produced seem, rather, reasonably shaped *kinds* of objects and not *particular* objects, or parts of objects; so this could be minimally knowledge-based probability decision-taking, compared with what is surely required for full object recognition. If, indeed, we do not have to suppose that the illusory surfaces are postulated for *specific* objects, or specific classes of objects, the neural origin of illusory surfaces could well be early in the visual system, and even in each eye system – prior to binocular fusion – before the parietal cortex, in which knowledge of objects may be stored[22].

Is there positive evidence that illusory surfaces are postulated (though only by algorithms without special object knowledge) to account for otherwise surprising gaps? An obvious prediction is that they must, as they generally appear to do, lie perceptually *in front* of the gaps. So a test of any *occlusion* account of illusory surfaces is to see whether there is an asymmetry between *nearer* and *further* surfaces – as a surface cannot produce gaps by occlusion unless it is in front of the gaps. So we presented a simplified Kanizsa triangle figure, of three dots, in a stereoscope (Fig. 20.10) using a specially designed stereoscopic shadow projector[23]. We found that when the three dots were forced by stereopsis behind the broken-line triangle the illusory surface disappeared, or was very weak. After some minutes, however, it could reappear; but in a curious form, for its central region would pop up in front of the gaps of the broken-line triangle, bending so that its corners touched the dots behind the gaps, but the gaps were still occluded. The conclusion was that the critical region of the surface must indeed lie in front of the gaps – which is necessary for the gaps to be due to an occluding surface. (When the stereoscopic disparity was reversed the surface was clearly seen lying well in front of the gaps.) This asymmetry is predicted from this account; but it seems bizarre on any other account so far suggested, and so is good evidence for a postulated occluding-surface explanation of the ghostly phenomena.

We should look more carefully for illusory contours that are clearly being produced by *particular* object knowledge, such as the border of the dalmatian dog. They must surely be generated further up the visual system, surely

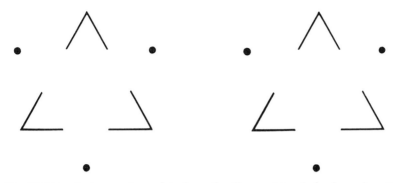

Fig. 20.10. A stereo-pair used to force the illusory triangle back – when it disappears. Or forward – when it is clearly seen in front of the gaps. The experiment used a range of disparities (from[21]).

beyond stereo fusion. So we should experiment on these contours – expecting some different results.

Another fact to be considered is the finding[24] that, in a suitable figure-ground ambiguous figure, the illusory surface switches (or disappears in one perceived configuration) according to which parts of the figure are accepted as figure or rejected as ground. This clearly fits a fully cognitive account; the alternatives being, in our terms, rival perceptual hypotheses. Being predictive, they may carry probabilities which may be very different, though there is but a single stimulus input. But, on the other hand – perhaps figure-ground reversal switches algorithms!

Perceptual and conceptual meaning

A disturbing feature of all illusions is that we can be *perceptually* illuded while at the same time knowing this – so we are not *conceptually* deluded. While studying illusory phenomena we experience an illusion while knowing it is illusory. This strange fact of illusion is hardly if at all considered by philosophers; yet it is highly significant that perception can easily and dramatically depart from belief and knowledge. It can be unfortunate for philosophy and science, and dangerous that knowledge cannot correct mis-perception, or perception correct mis-belief. This demands some explanation.

Why should *perception* and *conception* be so separate? In the first place, if perception were *driven* by knowledge it would be almost impossible to perceive anything highly unusual. But unusual objects and events do occur; and may threaten danger, or be potential opportunities requiring action. Separateness of perception allows sensed novelty to overcome the inertia of wisdom. We may note that perception and conception serve somewhat different purposes – and certainly work on very different time-scales. Perception serves to ensure survival into the next few seconds; but conceptual understanding works over a far longer time-scale. We perceive objects in a fraction of a second, which is essential for moment-to-moment survival; but it takes a long time, even many years, to generalise experience and organise ideas for planning and for expression in words. Consider this in computational terms; it would be strictly impossible to access all our knowledge in the short time allowed for recognising surrounding objects, therefore it must, for an essentially engineering reason, be impossible to check what we see by all we know. So the intelligence of perception is necessarily a specialised intelligence, which cannot access all our knowledge and understanding because it must work fast. Perception and conception are, and have to be, essentially separate; they cannot completely check each other, and we should expect this division also in perceiving intelligent robots. When we study illusory contours and ghostly surfaces, we see what we know is illusion. Could this separation between perception and conception be the distinction between 'subjective' and 'objective', and so divide art and science, so that we live with two kinds of meanings?

PART 6

Images and meaning

MARGARET DRABBLE

Throughout the sessions of the symposium which I was able to attend, my mind kept turning to the question of 'thinking in imagery', and of the differences that are traditionally held to distinguish the 'scientific' from the 'artistic' thinker, or the 'analytic' from the 'creative' mind. I use inverted commas to remind myself that these distinctions are by no means generally accepted, and the symposium itself reminded us that we do not know what a mental image is, or even whether it exists, and have at present little access to the mental pictures that occupy the minds of others. One or two of the final speakers from the floor appeared to be attempting to assert the validity of artistic as opposed to scientific perception, and I myself had the temerity to introduce the penultimate speaker, Jon Darius, with a garbled quotation or two from William Blake. Blake deeply distrusted the scientific and analytic mind, wrote satirically of Newton, Locke, the Royal Society itself, and of the philosophy of the Enlightenment, insisting instead that 'If the doors of perception were cleansed, everything would appear to man as it is, infinite.' He also declared, when asked if the sun did not appear to him as a round disk of fire somewhat like a guinea, that on the contrary he saw 'an Innumerable company of the Heavenly host crying "Holy, Holy, Holy is the Lord God Almighty".' Imagine my delight when Dr Darius, far from repudiating this vision, showed as one of his first slides a representation of (Fig. 21.1) a comet perceived as a flaming sword in the heavens.

The paper moved on to discuss misapprehensions of the eye and misinterpretations of the brain, and included the example of the famous 'canals' on Mars, an optical illusion probably verbally reinforced by the choice of the word 'canals' (or *canali*) instead of the more neutral, natural 'channels'. In the second paper of the afternoon, and the final one of the whole symposium, Professor Nelson Goodman invited us to a philosophical consideration of what we mean by mental pictures. What do we see, he asked, when told to picture a horse? Do we see an ideal Platonic horse, an Aristotelian general horse, a particular remembered horse from infancy, a Landseer horse, a computer-designed horse, a Jungian horse of the subconscious? He went on to ask how we would recognise a centaur if we saw one. We had moved, in the space of an hour, from the outer limits of outer space, where the eye as an organ is unable to penetrate, and can be helped only, in the words of Dr Darius, by 'superior statistics', a region where puzzles and paradoxes abound, to the extreme depths of inner space, where no certain ties prevail, and no scientific comparisons are possible. A surreal journey, and a very stimulating one.

Many questions remain with me from those three days, as I am sure they do with all who attended. I certainly received much valuable new food for one of my own obsessions, which is to do with the nature of metaphoric or imagistic thinking, and the use, in the thought process, of the visual image. Writers, like painters, tend to think in pictures. We know that Freud considered image-thinking, in or out of dreams, a primary process – and by primary he meant primitive, rather than essential, or superior. If he made a value judgement, it was in favour of 'secondary', 'analytic', or 'philosophic' thinking. And we know also that Freud himself admitted that his dreams were probably 'less rich in sensory elements than I am led to suppose is the case in other people' – which may have been one of the reasons why he undervalued symbols, and the thought processes that are set in motion by symbolic juxtaposition.

We are now, as we saw in Chapter 3, within reach of enabling the deaf to speak by cartoon image in sign language over the telephone. But as yet there is no way of direct communication of those private, interior mental images that for many of us constitute, waking or dreaming, so much of what we fondly call our thoughts. Art, poetry, film, can suggest these images, can use them in their own form of discourse. Are the modes of thought of the scientist and the artist radically different, as Blake believed? Is one mode superior to the other, as Freud, in his desire for scientific recognition for his own discipline, was led to assert? We do not really know how others think: many of us are unaware of our own thought processes. It is good to be given a chance to consider these matters, and to draw comparisons from such an interesting range of thinkers.

My final comment is an expression of gratitude to the symposium for enabling me to listen to and watch the presentations of scholars and artists from very different spheres from my own. It is not often that one has such opportunities. The Royal Society provided a meeting place for the two cultures, and my stock of images, and my understanding of some of them, has been greatly increased. All I need now is for someone to invent a machine that can record my dream pictures as they occur, so that, on waking, I can retrace the narrative.

21

Scientific images: perception and deception

JON DARIUS

No one doubts that there is a science of optical illusions, but not everyone appreciates the role of optical illusions in science. That is not to say that physicists and biologists are regularly confounded by the illusions of Hering, Müller-Lyer, Ponzo and Zöllner. Errors of visual judgement far more subtle and pervasive can nevertheless affect scientific observations and the inferences drawn from them.

Their protestations of objectivity notwithstanding, scientists are quite as susceptible to quirks of visual perception, including illusions, as anyone else – perhaps more so than their peers in other fields. The reason for this heightened susceptibility is straightforward enough. The researcher testing his theory against fresh observations has something in common with the oil baron forecasting prices for a barrel of crude: vested interest. That is putting it perhaps too strongly, but the myth of scientific objectivity and rationality has been effectively punctured by Imre Lakatos among others[1].

Selective vision, both metaphorically and perceptually, is nothing new; its practice in early observations of natural phenomena accounts for some of the curious drawings which have come down to us of anatomy and zoology, of atmospheric phenomena like aurorae and celestial phenomena like comets. These earlier philosophers and writers need not be accused of falsifying their observations. Those who saw the latest apparition of Comet Halley, especially in the northern hemisphere before perihelion, will readily concur that it appeared as a blur of light in the sky; apart from preconceptions all too easily imposed, there was little to choose between the medieval image of a glittering celestial sword (Fig. 21.1) and the contemporary view of coma-shrouded nucleus and tail.

Illusions gain credibility, then, from false expectations and from misinterpretation of the data – not that these two are independent. On the contrary,

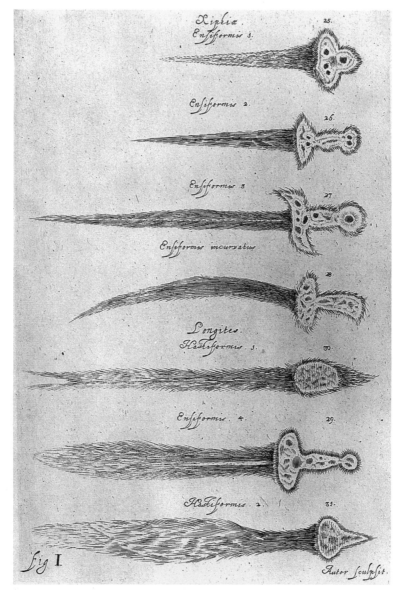

Fig. 21.1. Sword-like shapes of comets classified by Johannes Hevelius in his *Cometographia*, published in Danzig (now Gdansk) in 1668.

the first affords a slippery slope to the second. As a simple example, look at the image of the Araguainha Dome in Brazil, obtained from the remote sensing satellite Landsat with its multispectral scanner in 1972 (Fig. 21.2). Corroborative evidence from field expeditions on the ground[2] confirms that it is an

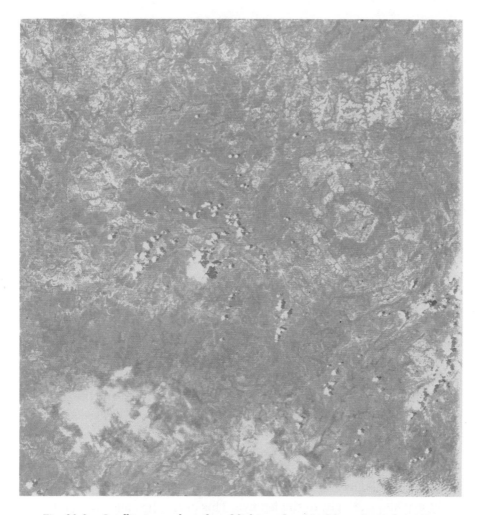

Fig. 21.2. Satellite image by infrared light rendered in false colour, showing concentric rings round the Araguainha Dome at right.[43] Clouds and their shadows are clearly discernible. North is at top. Source: National Oceanic and Atmospheric Administration.

impact structure owing its origin to the fall of a prehistoric meteorite which left a characteristic scar in the Mato Grosso region. You can see what appears to be a pattern of concentric shock waves. But wait a moment! The 'ground truth' tells a different story: the first two rings are structural features of the impact, all right. The outer ring is simply a band of vegetation which has sprung up in the rich soil at the foot of the 'dome'. Our quite reasonable expectations are deceived.

It is only fair to add by way of a caveat that, the substance of this review notwithstanding, all scientists are not duped all the time. They are accus-

tomed to building in conceptual safeguards, treating their observational
evidence with a healthy dose of scepticism and taking the evidence of others
with even bigger grains of salt. Peer review tends to maintain researchers'
vigilance: they will hardly want to parade in public their susceptibility to
illusions of any variety. Reputations are too hard won and too easily lost. On
the other hand, no one studying the evidence marshalled here can deny that
illusions do distort even scientifically trained perceptions on occasion – and it
is to these odd occasions that this review is devoted.

Innocent illusions

Illusions in science can be considered in three not wholly distinct categories.
Although categories can be conceptual straitjackets, they will be useful if
slightly arbitrary constructs for our purposes. The simplest category is the
innocent illusion, where perceptual confusion, sometimes enhanced by false
expectation, leads to interpretative ambiguity or error. (Richard Gregory
discusses perceptual illusions in Chapter 20). The classic optical illusions are
of this type, but only a few fall within our purview. The most pernicious is
undoubtedly the pseudoscopic illusion by which relief is inverted, troughs
becoming crests and protuberances cavities. The brain is the more readily
fooled for not knowing what to expect, and it is not surprising that the effect
works best when the source of light is not explicitly shown and the surface, be
it pinhead or planet, is unfamiliar. Indeed, a certain worthy science journal
published a note on the subject, complete with a careful assessment of a
photograph in fact reproduced the wrong way round.

In the last century Charles Wheatstone realized that inversion of relief
could be effected by converting a stereoscope to present the left image to the
right eye and the right to the left eye. This device he called a pseudoscope;
there are several examples on display in the new Optics Gallery at the Science
Museum, London. But the visual cues from familiar objects can be so
compelling as to make inversion difficult to attain, and a teacup viewed
through a pseudoscope (Fig. 21.3) is reluctant to present itself inside out. The
forking pattern to the east of the plains of Lunae Planum on Mars, on the
other hand, is perceived by some naive observers – naive in the sense of the
experimental psychologist – as a network of dry gullies where rivers must
once have flowed; to others, as tongues of lava or the like spreading over the
land (Fig. 21.4a). Simply inverting the photograph (Fig. 21.4b) can sometimes reverse the perceived relief. Examples could be multiplied[3], but I would
draw attention just to the etched surface of a diamond, as illustrated in the
admirable book by Tolansky[4], where rectangular projections can be converted to recesses through the simple expedient of rotating the photomicro-

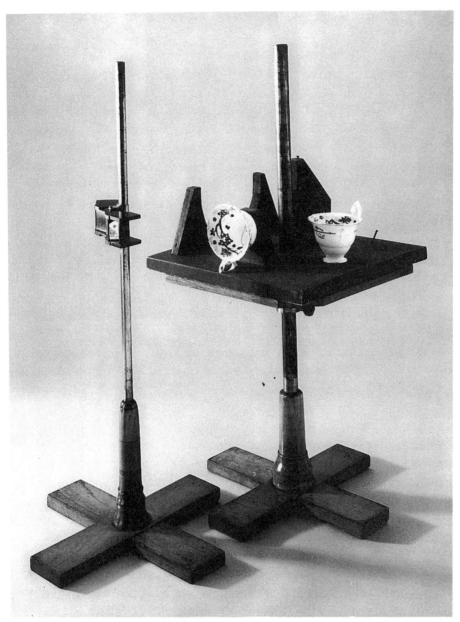

Fig. 21.3. Wheatstone's pseudoscopic apparatus used to view a teacup. Reproduced by permission of the Trustees of the Science Museum.

graph. Amateur telescope makers experience a related type of confusion when applying the Foucault test to their half-ground mirrors: one person's hollow is another's hillock.

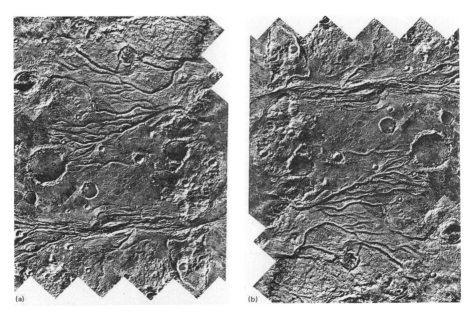

Fig. 21.4a,b. Furrows or ridges? Craters or domes? The brain tends to perceive relief differently according to orientation and illumination. This mosaic of images showing Maja Valles and Vedra Valles was prepared from observations by the Viking 1 orbiter in August 1976.[44] North is at top in Fig. 21.4a. Source: National Aeronautics and Space Administration.

Many other examples of the innocent illusion can be found in planetary observations, where tricks of vision can so easily trap unwary observers[5]. Once upon a time there was a putative lunar bridge which, through press coverage rife with hyperbole, became better known to the world at large than the crater Tycho or the dry lunar 'sea' Mare Serenitatis – for all that these features are visible to the naked eye from the Earth. In 1953 the discovery of the natural bridge was reported in good faith by the science correspondent of the *New York Herald Tribune*, John J. O'Neill[6]. Near the northwest limb of the Moon lies the great basin Mare Crisium, Sea of Conflict or Discord, and at one point there is a pass running from the floor of an old crater to the surrounding plain. The pass is flanked by two bluffs or promontories, part of the old crater wall, once known as Olivium and Lavinium (names no longer officially endorsed). O'Neill thought he saw evidence for a 20-km natural bridge spanning the two bluffs. Veteran lunar observers lost no time in trying to confirm the sighting of this lunar wonder, with contradictory results. The bridge figures in the gazetteer *The Moon*[7] by H. Percy Wilkins and Patrick Moore, respectively Director and Secretary of the Lunar Section of the British

Astronomical Association at the time. 'It certainly exists,' asserted Wilkins in 1954; 'This bridge, natural or artificial, is one of the most interesting features yet revealed by the telescope on any planetary body.'[6] Weighing up the evidence in *Sky and Telescope*, Joseph Ashbrook was more cautious: 'In my opinion while the existence of the bridge is quite unlikely, this area deserves careful study.'[8] At the November 1954 meeting of the British Astronomical Association, F.J.T. Maloney stated categorically that 'the O'Neill bridge has no existence and . . . the topographical features described . . . on radio and in the press have no counterpart in reality.'[9] Patrick Moore, having first espoused the cause, later repudiated it: 'O'Neill's sketch was hopelessly inaccurate, but later observations made by Wilkins indicated that some sort of arch did in fact exist nearby. This may be so: but at best it is a tiny natural feature of no interest or importance whatsoever.'[10]

The moral of this little fable was drawn by Leland Copeland[9]:

> Changes in the angles of illumination and observation alter the appearance of lunar scenery somewhat as a kaleidoscope redesigns its patterns. Mountain walls that tower tonight may appear insignificant tomorrow. Small craters that dot floors of larger rings under one illumination may be absent under others. Long clefts, clearly marked at times, vanish with the shifting of light and shadow. A further complication comes from handicaps in the Earth's atmosphere – air currents, dust, mist, wisps and veils of cloud. Obscure or unsteady seeing has a major influence on the aspect of lunar detail. . . Among the oddities reported are snow, hoarfrost, vanishing craterlets and light streaks, grey or black areas of vegetation, and shadowy masses of moving animals. Most of these must have been fancies, evoked by imperfect viewing.

O'Neill's bridge was just such a fancy, but all the same it is rather a shame that the Ranger and Surveyor probes failed to confirm the lunar counterpart to Utah's Landscape Arch and Rainbow Bridge.

Inferential illusions among stars and galaxies

The most pervasive of scientific illusions constitute a second category, which I shall call the inferential illusion. (It is cognate with, but not identical to, Helmholtz's 'unconscious inferences'.) Here the visual evidence, Othello's 'ocular proof', is solid enough; it is the interpretation placed on that evidence which justifies branding it an illusion. An apposite if slightly facetious illustration of the inferential illusion is reproduced in Fig. 21.5.

Let us carry on with the night sky. Anyone accustomed to studying plates from a photographic atlas of the sky, such as the Palomar Observatory Sky Survey, is bound to have stumbled over many weird configurations of stars, nebulae and galaxies. The omnipresent question posed by these configura-

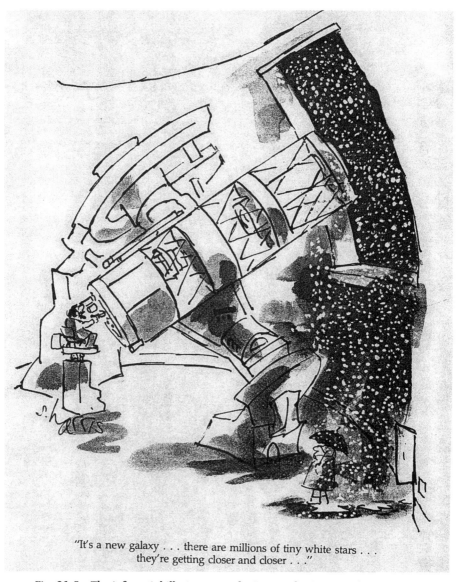

"It's a new galaxy . . . there are millions of tiny white stars . . .
they're getting closer and closer . . ."

**Fig. 21.5   The inferential illusion at work. Cartoon by S. Harris for *American
Scientist*.**

tions is to figure out what is physically significant and what the fortuitous
impact of blind chance. Dismissing various anthropocentric fantasies is easy
enough. No one will pause to write an academic paper explaining why
galaxies in the Virgo Cluster group themselves into a gargantuan question
mark or what the face of an owl or an Eskimo is doing in a planetary nebula or
how stars manage to create cross-like constellations in northern and south-

ern hemispheres. After all, these configurations, even at their most conspicuous, exist very much in the eye of the beholder: within our own culture the Big Dipper has also been Arthur's Wain (for King Arthur), Charles' Wain (for Charlemagne) and even King David's Chariot (for an early Irish ruler). To the Egyptians it was the Foreleg, to the Greeks the Great Bear (Ursa Major), to the Syrians the Wild Boar and to the Chinese the Government.

Other, simpler configurations present more of a conundrum. Stars disposed in a nearly perfect circle or line tempt the astronomer to infer some causal mechanism. Surely it is asking too much of the random scattering of stardots round the sky to conjure up so many rings and chains; surely they cannot be freaks attributable to the superposition of unrelated stars at different distances from the Earth and in roughly the same line of sight; surely they must reflect certain conditions of star formation or gravitational interaction (see Fig. 21.6). Perhaps the first astronomer to claim a physical connection between stars in an apparent chain was V. Oberguggenberger, who in 1938 tabulated over 300 such objects[11]. Noting chains of stars in the North America Nebula, the American physicist S.O. Kastner commented[12] in the early 1950s, 'It is obvious that this lining-up could not have occurred by chance alone'. It may be 'obvious' but is it true?

Persuasive, if not quite compelling, arguments for the formation of stars in

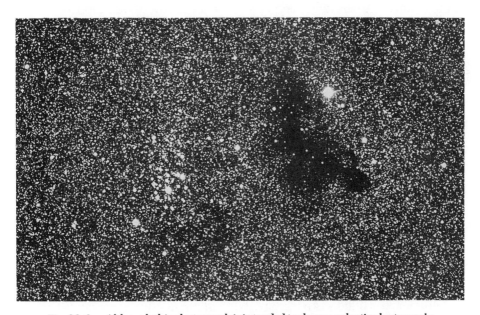

Fig. 21.6.   Although this photograph is intended to show a galactic cluster and a dark cloud, centre left and right respectively, it also displays many star chains and rings under closer scrutiny. Photographed with the Anglo-Australian Telescope by David Malin.

chains have been advanced. In the first place a region of undisputed star formation like the Orion Nebula displays a great deal of filamentary gaseous material. Forty years ago K.E. Edgeworth calculated[13] just how a rotating disk of gas would form from a primordial galaxy, parallel filaments from instabilities in the disc, and finally stars from fragments of filaments. In the following decade Soviet astronomers V.G. Fessenkov and D.A. Rojkovsky purported to find stellar chains associated with nebulosity in the Veil Nebula in Cygnus. Their claims were undermined, however, by other photographs at higher resolution and by theoretical arguments setting a lower limit on the density at which a star will form. Reviewing the situation with a healthy degree of scepticism, Otto Struve could see how a first star would form from the filament but suspected the limiting density for the formation of a second and subsequent stars to be unreasonably high; and one star, be it said, does not make a chain. In the face of the visual evidence, however, Struve concluded tentatively that 'we are tempted to accept as real some. . . star chains'[12].

Statistical arguments for and against the existence of chains have been aired, but there have also been photometric and low-dispersion spectroscopic studies. In 1975 G. Hahn and H.F. Haupt, Austrian astronomers working at the Observatoire de Haute-Provence, examined in detail ten typical examples of the chains in Oberguggenberger's list. They found that in most cases the component stars formed nothing like a chain in 3-dimensional space and that 'for star chains as a whole we draw the conclusion that they happen to be a projection effect produced by pure chance'[14].

The question can also be approached by the converse route: instead of looking at star chains and asking whether they are random, one can simulate random fields and check for 'star' chains. J. Meurers conducted experiments at Bonn with suspended solid and liquid particles. Lines and loops certainly occurred, but critics subsequently questioned the randomness of his experimental conditions. So in 1975 E. Lindemann and G. Burki at the Geneva Observatory used random numbers to generate artificial star fields.

Once again accidents of alignment produced chains and rings just as in the real sky. An example is shown in Fig 21.7. (The eye may not at once descry the phantom chains and rings and they are therefore shown explicitly below). The problem with all such features, comments the veteran American observer Walter Scott Houston, can be likened to trying to see a polar bear on an iceberg in the middle of a blizzard. Lindemann and Burki conclude that 'at least a large part of the stellar rings and chains could be due to random arrangements of stars.'[15]

Astronomers became even more excitable and prolific on the subject of star

(a)

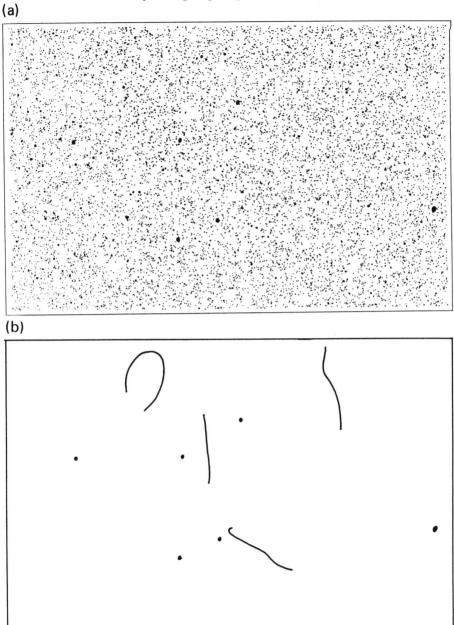

(b)

Fig. 21.7. Simulated star field (a): by E. Lindemann & G. Burki of the Observatoire de Genève[15]. (b): Some chains and the arc of a ring are picked out.

rings. Announced at a meeting in Prague by J. Isserstedt in 1967, stellar rings have always carried more weight than stellar chains.[16] In the first place Isserstedt found that in the majority of cases their linear minor diameter tended towards the same absolute value of seven parsecs whereas the apparent angular diameter will differ according to the distance. (1 parsec = 3.26 light-years or about 30 million million km.) Groups of stars not too densely clustered, called open or galactic clusters, sometimes display shell structure in the distribution of their stars and dust, especially among younger clusters. The diameter of the shell lies between five and ten parsecs, entirely consistent with the size of stellar rings. So it is not unreasonable to expect a true physical link between rings and shell-type stellar aggregates.

The proof of the pudding must lie in observing claimed rings and asking: (1) whether the stars lie at the same distance and represent a real configuration rather than an accident of projected geometry; and (2) whether the stars are young enough not to have dispersed. Now for many rings the answer is indisputably 'no'; but however bullet-riddled the target, it is not easy to kill it altogether. For one thing, even the staunchest champion of stellar rings would concede that *some* must be attributable to chance. For another, it is difficult to decide how much latitude to allow in the spectral types and in the intrinsic or 'proper' motions of the component stars. Even within a group there is bound to be a good deal of variation, and judging the point at which the deviations become too great to maintain credibility as a group is not straightforward.

However, the weight of evidence does not favour stellar rings. Studies of putative rings by a dozen observers have failed to confirm the physical reality of any ring save the one in Orion, which happens to be a special case.[17] The stars in the rings examined in depth were not coeval, nor do they occur at the same distance: rings, like chains, are most probably random phantoms.

Illusory alignments are no less familiar on terra firma. There are still those who will draw extravagant conclusions from the observation that Glastonbury Tor, Stonehenge and Druid's Grove all lie on the same straight line. Alignments with the cardinal points will sometimes be a structural feature, as in the west-facing naves of churches, and sometimes fortuitous. Not all such patterns deserve short shrift, and if it is healthy to be sceptical about apparent alignments it is no less so to be sceptical about the virtues of instant and automatic scepticism!

A case in point is the subject of fierce controversy and speculation at present. The scale is the grandest; the issue, the structure of the Universe. We know that stars and star clusters are grouped into galaxies, galaxies into clusters, and clusters of galaxies in turn into superclusters. Where does the hierarchy stop? What would be a god's-eye view of the array of clustered galaxies in the present and future Universe? Even granted that our penetration in space is lamentably shallow, we can at least muster the available evidence to seek structure on the largest scale. In 1967 C.D. Shane and C.A. Wirtanen[18] published galaxy counts based on the Lick Catalogue of Galaxies, in its day the deepest survey of its type. Shane and Wirtanen tabulated galaxy counts binned into one-degree squares, but they actually worked with 10-minute squares. To recover the valuable extra resolution, the Princeton group under P.J.E. Peebles reperformed the analysis a decade later and then published a computer map of the results.[19]

Two conclusions could seemingly be drawn from that analysis and map (Fig. 21.8). First, although galaxies cluster together in a continuum of scales above 10 megaparsecs until one reaches the realm of the supercluster, there is a break at 2.5 degrees. Second, the map exhibits persuasive visual evidence for filamentary structure. Valérie de Lapparent, Margaret Geller and Michael Kurtz have now cast doubt on the reality of both characteristics. Vignetting, plate-to-plate variations, differences in counting between Shane and Wirtanen and changes in their counting ability with time conspire to create artificial structures in the data.[20] In a sense, of course, these artefacts are not illusions: they are genuine but incorrect.

Another inferential illusion – if it is one – ought to be raised here: the infamous observations at the root of the whole redshift controversy. Redshift refers to the displacement towards longer wavelengths of spectral lines in distant galaxies and quasars – a redward shift – produced by the expansion of the Universe, first announced by Edwin Hubble in 1929. In a nutshell the controversy pits protagonists of the consensus view that redshifts act as cosmological distance indicators against the few but vociferous antagonists who assert that some intrinsic contribution to redshifts undermines their validity as cosmic yardsticks.[21] Quasars would consequently be closer and less energetic than they would if the entire redshift were ascribed to speed of recession.

Where does illusion enter the picture? There are quite a few cases of quasars and galaxies with *different* redshift very close to each other. The antagonists argue that the chances that such proximity would arise by accident are vanishingly small and that they must share a physical association or at least a common distance. Indeed, evidence of bridges between two bodies of discrepant redshift has been presented, but the claims are far from incontrovertible. The majority view, which may be wrong, is that the doubting Thomases like Halton Arp are suffering from an inferential illusion. As with star chains, the phenomenon looks real in projection on the sky but

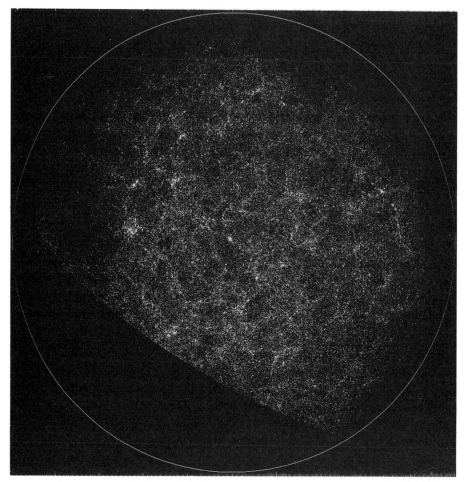

Fig. 21.8.   Maps plotting counts of more than a million galaxies were made on
the basis of the Lick catalogue of galaxies. Counts for the northern hemisphere are
shown here, summed in cells 10 arcminutes square with brighter dots for higher
counts[19]. Source: P.J.E. Peebles, Princeton University.

falls apart on closer probing. Recourse to statistical arguments is valid up to a
point but hardly conclusive; there is no point in telling the winner of the Irish
Sweepstakes that his chances were negligibly low. If ever it could be convincingly shown that two objects at the same distance truly displayed inconsistent redshifts, minor differences due to proper motion apart, it would smash
the cosmological speedometer and bring down the temple of redshift
believers.

To pay heed to the dangers of the inferential illusion is only prudent, but we
must be careful not to err too much on the side of scepticism, as suggested

earlier. Let us return briefly to what is currently one of the hottest topics in observational cosmology: the structure of the Universe on the grand scale. Discoveries of superclusters, consisting of tens of clusters each containing hundreds, even thousands, of galaxies apiece, have continued to multiply. Unexpectedly, these superclusters often turn out to be separated from each other by 'supervoids', great holes of more or less spherical shape apparently devoid of galaxies. With his Harvard colleagues Valérie de Lapparent and Margaret Geller, John Huchra thoroughly surveyed distant galaxies in a strip of sky 117 degrees by 6 degrees and plotted their redshifts (Fig. 21.9). The resulting map of some 1100 galaxies reveals huge shells or bubbles, typically 25 parsecs in diameter.[22] (Unthinking comparison of Figs. 21.8 and 21.9 may imply the resurrection of filamentary structure, but the two maps are fundamentally different: we must distinguish between physical filaments and arcs of shells.) The Universe resembles the suds of a bubble bath with galaxies clustered around voids. The odd 'bubble' has been observed previously but there was no hint that the whole Universe could be frothy.

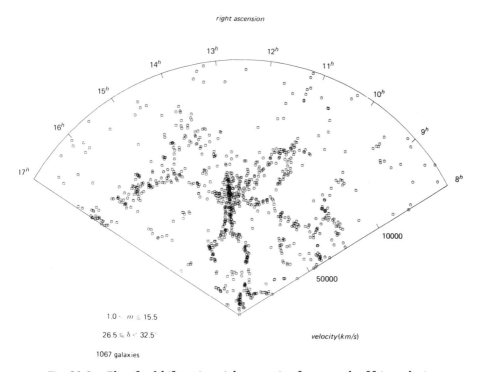

Fig. 21.9. Plot of redshift against right ascension for a sample of faint galaxies near the north galactic pole[22]. The stick figure, an innocent illusion of the Rorschach variety, represents the Coma cluster of galaxies! Source: Valérie de Lapparent, Harvard-Smithsonian Center for Astrophysics.

Could these giant bubbles, outlined by strings of clusters of galaxies, not be inferential illusions analogous to star chains? Statistical arguments have not yet burst the bubbles.[23] The plot of Fig. 21.9 does need to be treated with some caution, however. Since no correction has been made for the galaxies' *intrinsic* velocities relative to the expansion of the Universe, the fact that they tend to lie on lines pointing towards the Earth – the so-called fingers-of-God effect – must be discounted. Moreover, there is bound to be a selection effect in that only the brightest of the more distant galaxies will have been observed. But otherwise the sample is exceptionally complete and homogeneous, and it looks increasingly unlikely that the bubbles are illusory. Explaining their existence may not be easy, but astronomers have made a start.[24] Strong philosophical arguments favour a Universe which, however clumpy it might be on smaller scales, is smooth on the largest scales. But evidence from galactic redshifts seems to indicate otherwise. One is reminded of Michael Land's droll remark that from 1955 to 1975 scampi could not see[25]; in much the same way the Universe has had a uniform distribution of superclusters for decades and now, to the dismay of some, it turns out to be a vast celestial sink of soapsuds.

Other inferential illusions

To the inferential illusions attaching to data, especially in graphic form, only lip service will be paid. Linear regression has been used to fit more straight lines to plotted data points than Procrustes ever found visitors for his famous bed. (You will recall that he 'adjusted' his customers to fit the bed.) Normal distribution curves are regularly applied where they have no business at all. But the abuse is so widespread and the subject so vast that for the purposes of this contribution I must content myself with drawing attention to the malady without further diagnosis.

In nuclear physics great play is made of the ionization trails of charged particles traversing a Wilson cloud chamber or the later bubble chamber. The interpretation of patterns of droplets can be no less delicate and deceptive an issue than that of patterns of stars in the sky. In 1969 a group of physicists led by C.B.A. McCusker at the University of Sydney were studying air showers of cosmic rays in the quest for the quark. The quark is a hypothetical component of elementary particles called baryons and mesons and it would possess a fractional charge. Now R.K. Merton made much of what he called the Matthew Principle, 'Unto him that hath shall be given'; but for the laboratory scientist St Matthew offers a more relevant and more hazardous alternative: the principle 'Seek and ye shall find'. McCusker and Cairns sought – among the tracks of over 55,000 particles – and they did indeed find.[26] Two young ladies who must have been cross-eyed by the time they had scanned 55,000 tracks brought to the attention of McCusker and Cairns just four whose ionization trails were markedly weaker than the others. That is to say, they manifested fewer drops per unit length. Could these be the elusive quarks of 2/3 unit charge?

Logically, of course, a lesser charge would indeed produce lower ionization, but the converse does not necessarily hold. Nevertheless, McCusker, Cairns and their colleagues considered and dismissed alternative explanations and, were they right, could have laid claim to the first observations of free quarks. For various reasons physicists maintain that free quarks, like monopoles, do not occur. So it must have been a disappointment but also a relief when Adair & Kasha[27] and Rahm & Louttit[28] published papers soon afterwards debunking the quark discovery. If not a quark, what was this strange quarry? High-energy particles from the core of the shower generate lower-energy particles through cascade processes. That the quark candidates do not belong to the core of the air shower in the most promising of the photographs can be inferred from the fact that all the tracks are perfectly parallel save the suspect track. This slight deviation was overlooked in the heat of 'discovery'.

Redshifts aside, spectroscopy is probably more rife with inferential illusion than any other branch of science. The nub of the problem lies in distinguishing both signal from noise and true signal from phantom signal. For a spectroscopist taking his vows, the most solemn of them must be to distrust coincidence, for that way illusion lies. Astronomers working on data provided by the International Ultraviolet Explorer satellite began a column in their NASA *Newsletter*, 'Science Fiction with IUE'. For instance, the ultraviolet spectrum of the variable star RW Aurigae (Fig. 21.10) shows two strong emission features, a sharp one at 280 nm attributed to singly ionized magnesium and a diffuse one at 270 nm to singly ionized vanadium. Examination of the corresponding 'photowrite' suggests that the magnesium line is genuine but blows the whistle on the diffuse feature: it results from nothing more than an energetic cosmic ray striking the detector, according to a variant of Murphy's Law, at just the right time and place to cause maximum confusion[29].

Spectral lines result from transitions among energy levels of molecules, atoms and ions, and ideally they serve as 'identikits' for the substances emitting or absorbing them. But there are so many hundreds of thousands of substances, each capable of manifesting so many lines, that the identity parade cannot always be trusted to provide quick and reliable answers. The relative line intensities and profiles depend on excitation conditions and their wavelengths on the motion of the source. In consequence spectra are excel-

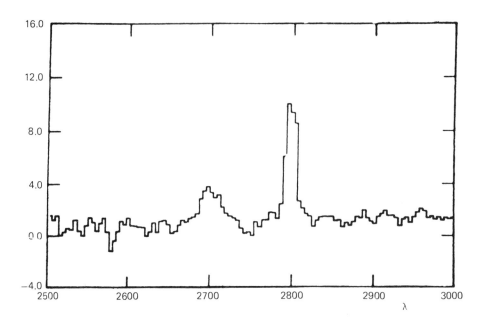

Fig. 21.10. Ultraviolet spectrum at low resolution in the long-wavelength camera of the International Ultraviolet Explorer satellite[29]. Of the two apparent emission lines, the sharp one is real and the other, more diffuse, an artefact.

lent breeding grounds for inferential illusion and indeed for the last category, prejudicial illusion.

Prejudicial illusions

From the rationalist standpoint, the prejudicial illusion is not merely unfortunate; it is odious. The illusion, deception, misinterpretation is motivated, often unconsciously, by preconceptions as to what *ought* to be perceived. With the injection of a remarkably mild degree of preconception, the innocent and the inferential illusion can be impelled to rush headlong into the category of the prejudicial illusion. As Einstein succinctly put it, 'It is the theory which decides what we can observe'.

Perhaps scientists would like to think that they are somehow above suspicion, that their reputation for detachment and disinterest will safeguard them from prejudicial illusions. It is all very well that a von Däniken should look at an old Japanese sculpture and infer a terrestrial stopover by alien astronauts, that a Midwest farmer should peer up at a lenticular cloud and see a flying saucer, that believers in some spiritual leader should convert unaccountable sores into saintly stigmata. The scientific mind, on the other hand, ought to be proof against the power of expectation over perception.

But scientists, as we have seen, are human and fallible, not acolytes of 'most sovereign reason'. One of the most durable illusions of the scientific world was that of the Martian canals. During the opposition of Mars in 1877 Giovanni Virginio Schiaparelli began to study in depth the markings on the surface of the red planet. With a telescope of 22-cm aperture at Brera Observatory in Milan, he noted the existence of a network of apparent channels, which he had the misfortune to call 'canali' (echoing P.A. Secchi a decade earlier), along with promontories, peninsulas and seas. His purpose was to provide a set of rigorous observations leading to a map of the planet. Some preliminary efforts by Father Secchi and by Wilhelm Beer in the 1830s notwithstanding, no one had properly charted Mars.

Schiaparelli was not given to fantasy, and nowhere did he try to ascribe the *canali* to an artificial source. He was alert to the tricks of vision which scrutiny of the planets can inflict on unwary observers. Seeing at one point what appeared to be two parallel straight lines (a phenomenon called gemination), he wrote, 'At first sight I believed it was an illusion, caused by fatigue of the eye and some new kind of strabismus, but I had to yield to the evidence'.[30]

Others were less circumspect, and within the decade the notion that the *canali* might be artificial conduits constructed by Martian civil engineers had taken root. Canals, a false friend for *canali*, are rather more evocative than grooves or channels. The French popularizer Camille Flammarion was inspired to speculate about Martians and their civilization, but no one was to make such capital out of the *canali* as Percival Lowell[31], an American observer whose family fortune funded the construction of an observatory at Flagstaff, Arizona. Inspired by Schiaparelli, Lowell was determined to study Mars at the next favourable opposition, in 1894. (Oppositions occur every 26 months; favourable ones, when the Earth lies further and Mars nearer in their elliptical orbits about the Sun, every 15 years.)

Lowell was convinced that no naturally occurring process could account for the *canali* because 'the lines exceed in regularity any ordinary regularity of purely natural contrivance' and because they form 'not a single network, but one whose meshes connect centres directly with one another'. Rivers, fault patterns, the grooves of meteorites at grazing incidence and other alternative explanations were summarily dismissed. The prejudicial illusion was bound to triumph and from his hundreds of drawings of Mars Lowell was able to distil over 700 *canali* and related features and to adduce evidence of seasonal variation (Fig. 21.11). He polevaulted with ease from the conviction that the markings could not be attributed to known natural causes to the belief that they testified to the presence of intelligent life on Mars. Nor was he abashed by objections that the surface temperature of Mars was low, that the polar ice

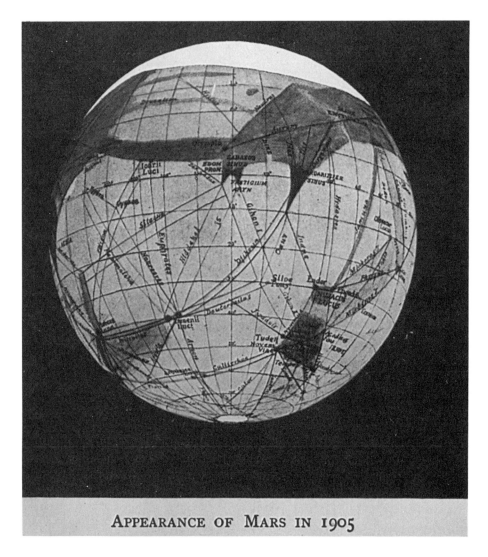

APPEARANCE OF MARS IN 1905

Fig. 21.11.   A map of Mars by Percival Lowell, the surface traversed by illusory
canals. Reproduced by permission of the Trustees of the Science Museum.

caps could be more readily explained by dry ice (solid CO_2) than by water ice
and that the atmosphere was highly rarefied. Lowell retorted, 'To argue that
life of an order as high as our own, or higher, is impossible because of less air
to breathe than that to which we are locally accustomed is, as Flammarion
happily expresses it, to argue not as a philosopher but as a fish.'

Nor was Lowell's observational prowess without its adherents; indeed,
many planetary observers for the greater part of the 20th century have seen

features similar to those he described. When we consider the assertion that they must represent irrigation channels set up by intelligent Martians, however, the band of the faithful dwindles somewhat. Prejudicial illusions may be influential in the way that any well publicized claim can sway fashion, but they are not necessarily contagious. The character of the prejudicial illusion is summed up perfectly in a remark by Edward Holden, first director of the Lick Observatory: 'It is suggested that the conclusions reached by Mr Lowell at the end of his work agree remarkably with the facts he set out to prove before his observatory was established at all.' Charles Young of Princeton University concurred: 'It is easy to see what one expects and wishes to find, especially on a disc so small and delicately marked as that of Mars.'

For all that, Martian canals are not to be consigned to the scrapheap of fraudulent discoveries like Piltdown man and the transfer factor. The gross features of Schiaparelli's observations and to a lesser extent Lowell's could be trusted insofar as they did represent 'albedo' markings (that is, patches of different brightness) on the planet's disc. But were they 'canals'? Even the thousands of photographs taken at successive favourable oppositions failed to settle the matter. In the first place, the prejudicial illusion can operate quite as effectively on the photographic emulsion as it can at the focus of a telescope eyepiece. More importantly, the photographic plate, which in any case suffers from reciprocity failure at low light levels, would record not only the light of the planet but also the blurring influence of the Earth's atmosphere. The eye of a dedicated observer, in contrast, can scan the image hour upon hour, alert for that split second of better seeing which briefly sharpens the smeared features. I am reminded of Colin Blakemore's comment on the dolphins in the queen's bathroom at Knossos: 'Perception is like inspired archaeological reconstruction.' Some planetary observers have let their inspirations run riot.

In the astronomical literature, but more especially in the popular press, the argument simmered for decades. It was not until the first fly-by by Mariner 4 in 1965 that a very different picture began to emerge.[32] A world pockmarked with ancient craters, not crisscrossed with waterways, greeted the vidicon cameras of Mariner 4, then 6 and 7, and finally 9 – this time an orbiting mission.[33] Our best images of Mars were transmitted by the two Viking orbiters and landers from 1976 to 1982, and they afford discoveries spectacular enough – but no canals.

So what were the *canali*? In the light of the Mariner and Viking orbiters, they are patently not waterways or associated riverbank vegetation. They are not Martian motorways or other artefacts of an advanced civilization. They are not crater rays. Apart from Valles Marineris, which correlates well with Agathodaemon, they do not correspond with faults or with ridges as Carl Sagan and James Pollack hypothesized following the first Martian fly-by mission.

The classic explanation for the canals was advanced by E. Walter Maunder and his wife Annie as the result of a series of experiments[34] using as subjects students at the Royal Hospital School in Greenwich. They found several conditions under which fictitious straight lines, or 'pseudolines', can be generated: two or more spots at the limit of resolution can appear to be joined by a line; so can a wavy line and an extended surface irregularity. It is true that the odd canal can be correlated with craters lying along a roughly straight path – such as Oxia – but on the whole the Maunders' explanation seems to be no less illusory than the lines it purports to explain. Altogether the traditional albedo features do not match the close-up images, and Peter Millman concluded[35] that 'we must be pessimistic about learning anything definite concerning planetary geology . . . where we have only low-resolution information on surface detail.' The canals had been deceptively laid to rest many times before; in 1909 E.M. Antoniadi, whom Maunder called 'an architect by training and an astronomer by genius', concluded following many years' observations that 'the spider's webs of Mars are doomed to become a myth of the past'.[36] But it was not until the advent of the Mariner spacecraft that a stake was driven through the heart of the Martian vampire.

If Antoniadi deserves credit for the early puncturing of one prejudicial illusion, he must be castigated for foisting another one upon us. For many years his map of Mercury (see Note 37) was, if not unique, certainly *primus inter pares*. It was compiled with the 83-cm refractor of the Observatoire de Paris at Meudon between 1920 and 1929, and subsequent maps by H. Camichel and A. Dollfus and by C. Chapman confirmed its major features. Unfortunately, these maps were drawn at a time when it was believed that Mercury was locked into a 1:1 spin-orbit resonance such that its period of rotation equalled its period of revolution about the Sun. Radar measurements have since disclosed a 2:3 spin-orbit resonance, 59 days and 88 days respectively. Somehow, even when different faces of the planet were being observed, Mercurian cartographers managed to compile mutually consistent maps! It must be said, however, that they would have seen the same face each time the planet was best placed for observation. But in the course of its three fly-by encounters Mariner 10 revealed a crater-scarred surface which resembled the best prior maps as the Yorkshire Dales resemble the Gobi Desert.

Prejudicial illusions are not the exclusive province of planetary observers although it is only to be expected that staring at fluctuating markings at low light levels for long periods can induce many tricks of visual perception. Let us now turn to an example drawn from another field, cytology. Knowing how the eukaryotic cells of plants and animals reproduce by dividing into two in the process known as mitosis, a biologist of just a few decades ago must have been sorely tempted to speculate that essentially the same process takes place in the smaller and simpler prokaryotic cells. Edward DeLamater made an intensive study of various strains of bacteria with the optical microscope and new staining and dehydration techniques, and he concluded that 'classical mitosis' as observed in higher organisms occurs in more primitive cells as well. 'It is felt,' wrote DeLamater, 'that the evidence presented for the occurrence of mitosis in bacteria clearly demonstrates that (1) the structure of the nucleus is comparable to that which is known in larger organisms, and (2) the divisional process follows essentially the same mitotic pattern as has already been established in these larger forms. The only essential difference appears to be one of size. We are dealing with essentially the same structures and cyclic story, except that they occur in miniature.'[38] What is more, DeLamater published many photographs to prove his point.

The biology student of today will recoil from this blatant untruth, knowing for one thing that eukaryotic cells have by definition a nucleus, lacking in bacteria, and will question the authenticity of the photographs. One interpretation would be that the pictures are genuine although their content is deceptive. DeLamater might have had literally thousands of photos of bacteria from which to choose and in good if misguided faith would have selected those pictures which fitted the story he had to tell. Just as given enough time, monkeys tapping at a keyboard are supposed to type out the works of Shakespeare – in fact a mathematically fatuous notion properly derided by Dawkins[39] – colonies of bacteria are bound to generate all the simulacra of mitosis that a vigilant cytologist could want. On the other hand, the work of DeLamater and his colleagues has been severely criticized in terms of both procedure and interpretation by Kenneth Bisset[40], who pointed out amongst other things that the claimed centrioles of mitotic spindles are nothing more than developing septa on the periphery of dividing cells. When DeLamater realized that excessive zeal in proving his case had let him into serious error, he published a frank retraction[41] in *Nature*. Bacteria do split by binary fission, but the observation that they undergo true mitosis in the same fashion as higher cells was but a prejudicial illusion.

Our discussion of illusions and deceptions, especially the inferential and prejudicial varieties, smacks woefully of the benefit of hindsight. When one 'knows' that matter is composed of atoms, it is easy to say that Democritus and Leucippus were 'right' with their indivisible particles and Aristotle 'wrong' with his five elements. Partly to redress the balance, let us consider a case of illusion where the verdict is, in Scottish parlance, not proven. For the past decade Harold Hillman and Peter Sartory of the University of Surrey have contended[42] that the fine structure of the living cell, as it has been taught to biologists since the advent of electron microscopy as a research tool in the 1940s, is little more than an artefact of preparation of the specimen. They accept the existence of the nucleolus, the nuclear membrane, granules and mitochondria; they dispute the endoplasmic reticulum, the Golgi apparatus, the cristae of mitochondria, nuclear pores and the trilaminar appearance of cell membranes. They do not go so far as to deny lysosomes, crudely speaking the cell's digestive system, but they still criticize the observations.

The source of the bewilderment of this quixotic pair lies in the suspicious uniformity of cell structure seen in scanning electron micrographs. If pores are genuine circular holes, for example, then electron microscopists ought to be generating a range of eccentricities from the ellipse to the circle. I think the problem might reside not in the electron micrographs but in too strict an interpretation of the holes. Yes, if the holes were perfectly cylindrical and rigid in cross-section, then Hillman & Sartory's expectations would be justified. But if the walls of the hole were bowed, such that the hole formed part of a hollow sphere with opposite ends guillotined – rather like a bottomless but otherwise typical olivewood salad bowl – then the puzzle vanishes. Slice a sphere in *any* direction and the result is a circle or circular disc. In fact the channel is neither cylindrical nor subspherical; it is filled with irregular strands. That the organism should relax into circles in the course of preparation I do not find unpalatable.

It is to the preparation, indeed, that Hillman & Sartory attribute the genesis of artefacts. 'During electron microscopy,' they write, 'whether by transmission, scanning or freezing techniques, the tissue is dehydrated. Dehydration of any aqueous solution or suspension causes precipitation of solutes. We believe that the endoplasmic reticulum and the cristae of the mitochondria are the crystal pattern of the cytoplasmic and mitochondrioplasmic solutes, respectively.' Whether the whole argument stands up is open to question – professional cytologists must pronounce – but it is certainly true that the electron microscope is not a tool for *in vivo* study. Indeed, it pays to bear in mind that the observed subject (what Stoney[5] liked to call the eidolon) and the actual subject cannot be expected to coincide completely. This rather Berkeleian view was adumbrated by Feng-shen Yin-Te when he wrote, 'With a microscope you see the surface of things. It magnifies them but does not show you reality. It makes things seem higher and wider. But do not suppose you are seeing things in themselves.'

Conclusion

To conclude from all this evidence that the truism 'seeing is believing' is false would be extremely naive. I am sure that we have witnessed enough card tricks, screen deaths and innocent optical illusions to be convinced already that seeing is not believing. In fact, my contention is that, on the contrary, believing and seeing are all too closely related even among those supposed to be the possessors of a 'marvellous newtrality', as John Dee put it. Scientific literature, especially where it utilizes graphed data, is rife with questionable claims based on illusory perceptions. Impartiality is no friend of the visual cortex, and it would be prudent to distrust that which one can see at least as much as that which one cannot. Perception is always skirting the brink of deception, and tumbles in more often than scientists care to acknowledge[45].

22

Pictures in the mind?

NELSON GOODMAN

Dilemma

In characterizing cognitive psychology, Howard Gardner writes 'in talking about human cognitive activities, it is necessary to speak about mental representations.'[1] The present conference and the other literature of cognitive psychology offer an abundance of such fascinating talk, including circumstantial reports of encounters with and experiments upon mental imagery. Yet cognitive psychology has been engaged from its beginnings in a life-and-death struggle over the very existence of pictures in the mind. Sometimes a psychologist's most assiduous accounts of phenomena of mental imagery have the flavor of tracts by impassioned believers in flying saucers. And the flames of controversy feed on the stubborn resistance of behaviorists, physicalists, and acidulous philosophers. [Roger Shepard replies in a Postscript, p. 365.]

Before going further, I should explain that in this chapter the term 'mental images' applies to images of memory and imagination as distinguished both from material images such as paintings and from optical and other sensory images. However, I shall often shorten 'mental image' to 'image', taking 'mental' as understood. Mental images, although they include 'pictures in the mind', are not all pictorial; some, for example, are musical and some are verbal[2].

On the one hand, we talk quite confidently of the mental images we have, of their clarity or vagueness, of details present or missing, of manipulating and experimenting on such images. We can describe them, picture them, compare them with other images or with their objects. We know what it is to succeed or fail in trying to conjure up an image, and can compare our own experience of images with that of other people. Indeed, discourse about images is in this sense hardly less intersubjective than discourse about objects. And our talk of images, so central to cognitive psychology, seems surely not to consist of fairy-tales but to be serious, significant, and at its best scientific. That we have images and can report on them with reasonable reliability is incontestable, isn't it?

And yet – and yet – on the other hand, what *are* these pictures in the mind? They are pictures not painted, drawn, engraved, photographed – not in any material medium. And they are invisible, intangible, altogether insensible. A visual image cannot be seen (for seeing requires looking at something before the eyes); an auditory image makes no noise; and the pain in my toe I can now imagine does not hurt. Again, whatever mental images may be, where are they? There is no small theater in the head where these images are projected on a screen, and there is nobody there to look at them anyway. When we are asked what or where mental images are, we falter. Our answers are negative and self-defeating. When the mental image goes on trial, testimony for the defense is itself enough for conviction. The mental image seems to be unimaginable, a mere figment of the imagination! Or, in words less minced, the inevitable conclusion seems to be that there are no mental images.

How shall we resolve this dilemma? Shall we, deciding that the talk of mental imagery in everyday life and cognitive psychology is indispensable and veridical, simply suffer in silence the embarrassing questions asked by philosophers and other troublemakers? Or shall we, deciding that no one in his right mind could ever find any pictures there, just dismiss all talk of mental images as so much vacuous verbiage? I think we are stuck with both horns of the dilemma: that we can talk significantly about mental images but that there are none.

Psychology and mythology

Having painted myself into that corner, I think it is time to change the subject. Let's talk of centaurs or of Don Quixote. A centaur has a man's head and torso and a horse's rear; has four legs, not two or six, and no horns. Don Quixote wears a beard, and is Spanish not Greek. He is heroically and pathetically and delightfully daft, rides a horse named Rosinante and has a servant named Sancho Panza. We can distinguish centaurs from unicorns and mermaids, and Don Quixote from Winston Churchill and Rip van Winkle. In short, we know a good deal about centaurs and about Don Quixote. And yet, and yet, there are no centaurs, there is no Don Quixote.

How then can I know about them? To begin with, while there are no centaurs, there are descriptions, stories, pictures of them[3]. And we know something about centaurs to the extent that we can judge or produce descriptions or pictures of centaurs, sort out descriptions and pictures that are of centaurs from those that are not, accept right ones and reject or criticize or revise wrong ones. But isn't this begging the question? For if there are no centaurs, how can there be pictures *of* them? Our language misleads us here. A picture said to be of a centaur, or a description said to be of Don Quixote does not, strictly, depict or describe anything, since there is nothing for it to describe or depict. Rather, it is a picture or description of a certain kind; and to block seductive wrong inferences, we may do better to call it a centaur picture, Don Quixote description, etc. We classify fictive pictures and descriptions not through having examined anything they depict or describe but – just as we classify furniture into chairs, tables, desks, etc. – through having learned the application of the predicates in question.

What we say ostensibly about centaurs or Don Quixote thus has to be interpreted in terms of discourse about centaur (or Don Quixote) pictures or descriptions. When we say that centaurs differ from unicorns and from Don Quixote we don't mean to be taken at our word; for strictly, since none of these exists, all centaurs are unicorns, all unicorns are centaurs, and Don Quixote is both unicorn and centaur. To know that centaurs differ from unicorns and from Don Quixote is to know that centaur pictures and descriptions differ from unicorn pictures and descriptions and from Don Quixote pictures and descriptions. What we ordinarily call knowledge about centaurs or Don Quixote is, speaking more carefully, centaur-knowledge or Don Quixote-knowledge.

By now, of course, the point of my fabulous digression has been obvious for some time. If we can talk sensibly and responsibly about (i.e. ostensibly about) centaurs although there are none and Don Quixote who never was, can we perhaps talk likewise about mental images although there are none?[4] Can I say that there are no mental images and yet say quite intelligibly and truly that I now have in my mind a picture of Capri? Yes, if having that image is construed in terms of my ability to describe or picture or sort out descriptions of pictures of the image – though any descriptions or pictures I produce or encounter will not be *of* the image but rather image-descriptions and image-pictures.

If we here seem headed toward absorbing cognitive psychology into mythology or fiction, that may be an unwelcome prospect for some, though hardly inappropriate for a conference that includes novelists and opera-directors along with psychologists. But let's postpone bemoaning or rejoicing until we have looked a little more closely into what is involved.

Notice first that in likening psychology to fiction, I am no more denying the genuineness of image-knowledge than I am denying the genuineness of centaur-knowledge or Don Quixote-knowledge. Centaur descriptions or Don Quixote pictures, etc. may be right or wrong. In checking on them we go back to classical literature and iconography[5] or to the works of Cervantes and his commentators and illustrators, and so on. In checking on talk of images, we have no Greek fables or Spanish tales, but something more like a continuing soap-opera or several of them – a growing corpus of our own and others' verbal and pictorial discourse and the reports of psychologists. Thus in all these cases there are standards of rightness – not comprehensive, absolute, fixed standards, but standards with some stability. And that, indeed, is all we have for discourse about absent actual objects[6]. Even for present objects, usually a rather small part of what we know results from direct examination. Questions about Don Quixote's life are as open to investigation as questions about Napoleon's; and whether proposed answers are right or wrong can be legitimately debated in both cases. Psychology and mythology are distinguished from each other by such a difference in basis. Neither need feel demeaned by its affinity with the other.

Images and action

Translation of talk about nothing into talk about something often takes some trouble. I said a moment ago that centaurs differ from unicorns in that centaur pictures and descriptions differ from unicorn pictures and descriptions. To 'centaur pictures and descriptions and unicorn pictures and descriptions' we may well add 'and centaur images and unicorn images' since centaur images and unicorn images also differ. But then we must remember that since there are no such images (or any other images), talk ostensibly about them must be treated in the same way as talk of centaurs and unicorns, so that the expanded statement will read: 'Centaurs differ from unicorns in that centaur pictures and descriptions differ from unicorn pictures and descriptions, and centaur-image pictures and descriptions differ from unicorn-image pictures and descriptions.'

This brings up the question how an image picture, say a certain centaur-image picture or a horse-image picture can be told from a centaur picture or horse picture. A blurry horse picture is surely not a picture of a blurry horse; the blurriness belongs to the picture or the image. But is the picture before us a blurry picture of a horse, or a blurry picture of a horse-image or a picture of a blurry horse-image? That is, is it a blurry horse picture or a blurry horse-image picture or a blurry horse-image-picture? Sometimes that will be doubtful, and we may have to look to descriptions, to verbal reports and answers to questions. But these cannot always be taken at face-value. A request to describe a given image as such is easily confused with a request to say what it is an image of. Furthermore we seldom take due account of such oddities of depiction as that a picture of a horse-picture is not always a horse-picture, that a picture of a picture need not be a copy of it, that some (i.e.

abstract) pictures are not even fictively pictures of anything, and that a picture of a picture of nothing is still a picture of something. Such complications are not peculiar to our present discussion but arise in the underlying general theory of representation. I mention them here only to illustrate how the tightening of loose talk about images can call for a good deal of care.

In view of all this, what is to be done? Perhaps, weary of such sophistry, we may be inclined simply to jettison all talk of nothing as worth nothing, to condemn as nonsense all talk ostensibly about mental images. But that would be to condemn an indispensable part of ordinary and psychological discourse on grounds such as would serve, no less plausibly, for condemning the works of Cervantes and Shakespeare.

In contrast, the cognitive psychologist may be glad to hear that there is a way of making sense of talk about mental images, and take comfort in the thought that the availability of an automatic process for purifying talk of images leaves him free to go on exactly as before, and refer all queries to the philosopher. But the treatment of image-talk I have been suggesting is not a quick and easy excision of some pseudo-entities; it does not amount to translation by routine application of a simple formula. Indeed, although I have spoken loosely of it as translation, it is hardly that; for translation of nonsense would presumably still be nonsense. Rather, what goes on is replacement of statements ostensibly about images by statements about objects and events. That cannot complacently be left until after the psychological investigations have been carried out in ordinary parlance; for our image-talk raw and unprocessed is a terrible tangle. To accept at face-value both the statement that there are no mental images and the statement that I have one in my mind is to forego all consistency. If we give up the former statement and say that there *are* mental images, we face innumerable unanswerable questions about what and where they are. Thus I have been proposing that we replace the second statement by statements concerning image pictures and descriptions[7].

We no longer need to go hunting for images any more than we need to go hunting for centaurs. Yet if a centaur happens to pass by some day we can easily accommodate to that without much trouble, though if a mental image liberated itself and fell on the desk before me, I doubt if I could recognize it as such. What really matters is that we are not committed to there being any centaurs or images; but neither are we committed to there being none.

Finally, interpretations of image-talk along lines here suggested throw a different light on cognitive psychology. Having an image amounts not to possessing some immaterial picture in something called a mind but to having and exercizing certain skills – a matter of producing, judging, revizing certain material pictures and descriptions. To Howard Gardner's statement that 'in talking about human cognitive activities, it is necessary to speak about mental representations' perhaps we should add a clause: 'but talk of mental representations turns out in the end to be talk of cognitive activities'.

Cognition without pictures in the head

Ironically, the final chapter in a book on images and understanding calls in question the whole notion of mental images as pictures in the mind. And despite my rather emphatic assurances that much ordinary and scientific discourse that is ostensibly about mental images can be significant and valid, the physiologist, neurologist, and psychologist working on cognition may be somewhat dismayed. As a philosopher long allied with cognitive psychology, I am by no means condemning all that cognitive scientists say and do, but rather seeking clarification of some of it. Since talk of 'pictures in the mind' taken literally is nonsense, and taken metaphorically needs careful interpretation, it can be highly misleading.

An analogy may help here. We all have responsibilities, some of them more pressing than others. But to suppose that there are such things, such entities, as responsibilities is to risk utter confusion that can be avoided if we speak rather of being responsible for doing so-and-so, for acting in a certain way, and ask what this involves. Likewise, in an earlier paper[8], I suggested that having a mental image may be construed in terms of ability to perform certain activities; for instance, that I may be said to have a horse-image in my mind to the extent that I can describe or draw a horse, sort descriptions and pictures into those that are of horses and those that are not, criticize or revise faulty descriptions and pictures of horses.

When a physiologist says in effect that a certain image consists of a certain pattern of firings of cells in the cerebral cortex, he is reporting on painstaking scientific investigation. But how has he validated this formulation? Surely, by checking it not against pictures he finds and examines in the brain but against verbal reports and other behavior of the subject. [See Chapters 1, 6, 8, 17 and Postscript for neurobiological methods of validation – eds.] Such a physiological account and the sort of philosophical account I have outlined are complementaries. Putting them together we get, with some ellipsis, something roughly like this: when firings of the required kind occur in certain cells, the subject can to some extent produce, sort out, criticize, revize descriptions or pictures of a horse. The 'image' and the 'picture in the mind' have vanished; mythical inventions have been beneficially excised. Of course, in less formal discourse we may speak loosely of mental images or pictures so long as we remain aware that such talk is dangerous and needs careful interpretation. Its dangers and the difficulties of interpreting it increase when, as in talk of the rotation and other manipulation of mental images, the context becomes more complex. As Roger Shepard fully recognizes in the penultimate paragraph of his Postscript (see pp. 369–70), we must construe informal talk of rotating images in some way that does not imply that there are images twirling in the head.

Thus while a conviction that literally there are no pictures in the head may challenge some work in psychology, it is entirely compatible with the pursuit of cognitive science[9].

POSTSCRIPT

On understanding mental images

ROGER SHEPARD

Many different things that we call images have an objective, physical existence: paintings, drawings, bas-reliefs, rubbings, wax impressions, photographs, television images, retinal images, reflections, shadows, and holograms. Although their understanding requires, in some cases, technical knowledge of physics, optics, electronics, or chemistry, they present no troubling philosophical or conceptual puzzles. More problematic are images that have only a subjective, mental existence: the so-called *mental images* of memory, imagination, dreams, and hallucinations. Because no physical object or process has been identified within the brain that resembles the images we experience, some would conclude with Nelson Goodman [see Chapter 22] that although we can talk about a mental image, just as we can talk about a centaur, there really is no such thing. As a cognitive psychologist who has devoted some years to the scientific study of what appears, on this view, to be the nonexistent, I would like to indicate how some cognitive psychologists propose to understand mental imagery.

We assume that mental imagery, like any other mental phenomenon, corresponds to a physical process in the brain (compare the Chapters by Barlow (1), Blakemore (17), Movshon (8), and Perrett (6)). However, the correspondence is one of causal connection, not of resemblance. When an individual reports imagining St Paul's Cathedral (see Fig. P.1), for example, we suppose that some particular neurons are firing within that individual's brain. Those particular neurons do not themselves resemble St Paul's in spatial configuration or, certainly, in colour, sound, or smell. We presume that their firing is, however, a necessary condition for the individual's truthful report of imagining St Paul's.

Of course, the individual imagining St Paul's need not know anything about which neurons are firing in his or her brain or even of the existence of such neurons. (Aristotle, who understood more than most about mental phenomena, reportedly did not realize that they were mediated by the brain.) How, then, does it happen that an individual, upon the occurrence of neural activity that is unknown to him or her and that bears no resemblance to St

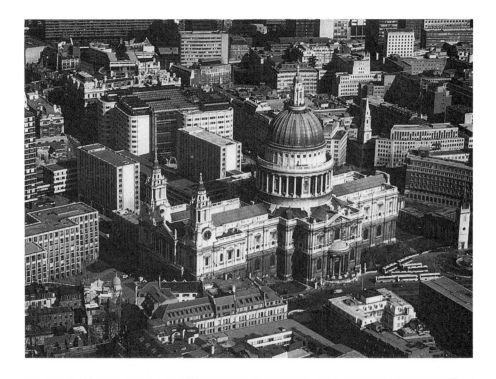

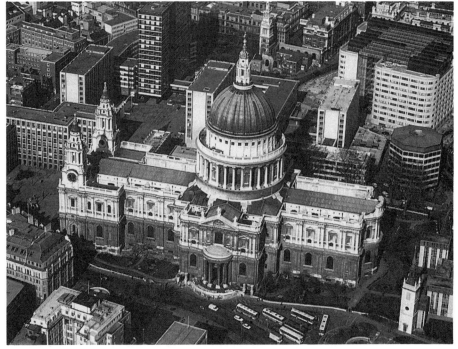

Fig. P.1.   St Paul's is St Paul's, however you look at it. Photographs courtesy of
the Central Electricity Generating Board.

Paul's, reports that he or she is imagining St Paul's? Very simply: it happens because whatever neural activity is going on his or her brain overlaps sufficiently with the neural activity that has previously been elicited in that same brain by the physical presence of St Paul's itself, or of a picture of St Paul's.[1] Thus, although it is the causal connection of the neural activity with the verbal report that informs us that someone is imagining something, it is the causal connection of that neural activity with a previously encountered external object that defines what is being imagined. When we imagine St Paul's what we imagine is the external object, St Paul's; it is not the internal neural activity that causally mediates our imagining of St Paul's. The imagining of a thing is, on this view, no more mysterious than the perceiving of that thing.

Does this conceptualization help us in the scientific study of mental imagery? Indeed it does! By relating mental imagery to perception we convert what appeared to be a purely subjective phenomenon into an objective one. To illustrate: Podgorny and I had subjects look at a square 5×5 grid under two conditions. In a perceptual condition, certain squares of the grid were shaded to form a particular object, say a block capital letter 'F'. In an imaginal condition, the grid remained empty and we instructed the subject to imagine the corresponding squares as shaded to form that same object. We then tested the subject, in either condition alike, by flashing a small coloured dot in one of the 25 squares of the grid and recording the speed and accuracy of the subject's response indicating whether the probe dot fell on a figural or nonfigural square of the grid. The data from the two conditions were identical: all reactions were fast and accurate, and the detailed pattern of reaction times depended in a highly regular way on the spatial relation of the probe to the figural pattern – even when that pattern was only imagined and not physically present in the grid[2]. Such results provide objective evidence that the same processes underlie perception and imagery; they also place some significant constraints on the nature of those processes.

Not only the imagination of objects, but the imagination of the transformations of objects can be investigated in this way. Here, too, the crucial step is to require subjects to choose, on the basis of what they are imagining, between two responses of which one, only, is objectively correct. For example, in our first experiment on 'mental rotation'[3] we presented the subjects on each trial with perspective views of two three-dimensional objects (see Fig. P.2) and recorded the times they took to decide whether the two objects, though differing in orientation, were inherently identical in shape or were mirror images (enantiomorphs) of each other. Decision times increased as a remarkably linear function of the angular difference between the objects in

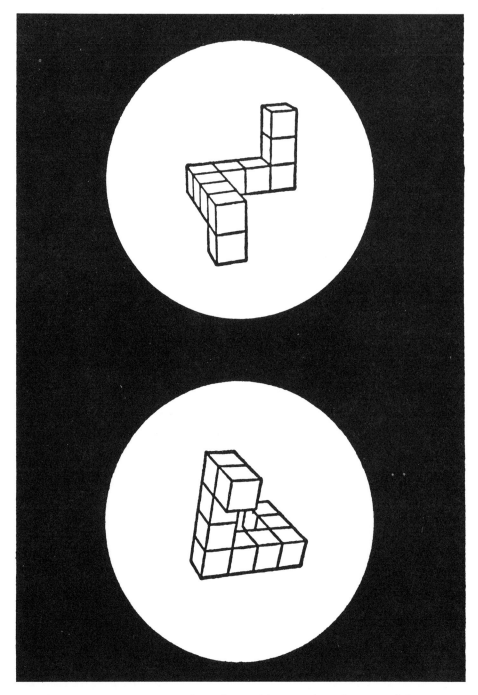

Fig. P.2.   Perspective views of two objects of the same three-dimensional shape,
but oriented differently in space. Shepard & Metzler (1971)[3] measured the times
people required to determine that two such objects were, as in this pair, of the
same shape.

three-dimensional space (see Fig. P.3) – just as if the subjects were having to imagine one object rotated into congruence with the other and could only do so at a rate of about 60° per second. Subsequent experiments, in which we probed subjects with variously rotated stimuli during the course of mental rotation, provided still more compelling evidence that the subjects were mentally representing an object in successively more and more rotated orientations during the process[4].

In describing research of this kind, we can avoid philosophical perplexities by exercising care in talking about mental imagery. To speak of the subject as 'rotating the image of an object' is to suggest that the image itself, like a physical object, can literally be rotated somewhere. (Where? In the subject's brain?) But to talk this way is quite unnecessary and probably inappropriate.

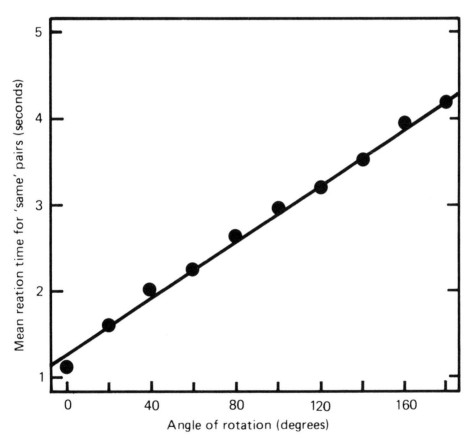

Fig. P.3.   A plot of the results obtained by Shepard & Metzler (1971)[3]. The time required to determine that two three-dimensional objects were of the same shape increased linearly with the angular difference in the portrayed orientations of the objects.

As noted by Michael Kubovy[5], we can just as well speak of the subject as 'imagining the rotation of an object' and, thereby, avoid all the puzzling issues raised by the former formulation. Moreover, the latter, more careful reformulation brings out the essential feature of mental imagery as I recommend we understand it: mental imagery is of external objects, and is therefore to be defined and studied not as some strange, non-material 'picture in the head' but in relation to potential test stimuli that are both external and physical.

In short, whether or not we wish to subscribe to the ontological claim that mental images, as such, 'exist' (whatever may be meant by that claim), *mental imagery* is quite real and quite susceptible to quantitative scientific investigation[6].

Notes

Notes to Chapter 1

1. Herrick, C.J. (1928). *An Introduction to Neurology*, W.B. Saunders Co., Philadelphia.
2. Craik, K.J.W. (1943). *The Nature of Explanation*. University Press, Cambridge.
3. Marr, D. (1982). *Vision*, W.H. Freeman, San Francisco.
   Poggio, T., Torre, V. & Koch, C. (1985). Computational vision and regularization theory. *Nature*, **317**, 314–19.
4. Geschwind, N. (1974) Selected papers on language and the brain. *Boston Studies in the Philosophy of Science*, vol. XVI (ed. R.S. Cohn & M.W. Wartofsky), Reidel, Boston.
5. Daniel, P.M. & Whitteridge, D. (1961). The representation of the visual field on the cerebral cortex in monkeys. *J. Physiol.*, **159**, 203–21.
6. Hubel, D.H. & Wiesel, T.N. (1962). Receptive fields, binocular interaction and functional architecture in the cat's visual cortex. *J. Physiol.*, **160**, 106–54.
7. Hubel, D.H. & Wiesel, T.N. (1977). Ferrier Lecture: Functional architecture of macaque monkey visual cortex. *Proc. Roy. Soc.* B **198**, 1–59.
8. Blasdel, G.G. & Salama, G. (1986). Voltage sensitive dyes reveal a modular organization in monkey striate cortex. *Nature*, **321**, 579–85.
9. Kuffler, S.W. & Nicholls, J.G. (1976). *From Neuron to Brain*. Sinauer Associates, Sunderland, Mass.
10. Barlow, H.B., Blakemore, C. & Pettigrew, J.D. (1967). The neural mechanism of binocular depth discrimination. *J. Physiol.*, **193**, 327–42.
11. Cajal, S.R. (1899, 1952). *Histologie du Système Nerveux de l'Homme & des Vertébrés*. Instituto Ramon Y Cajal, Madrid, 1952.
12. Van Essen, D. & Kelly, J. (1973). Correlation of cell shape and function in the visual cortex of the cat. *Nature*, **241**, 403–5.
    Gilbert, C. & Wiesel, T.N. (1979). Morphology and intracortical projections of functionally characterised neurones in the cat visual cortex. *Nature*, **280**, 120–5.
    Martin, K.A.C., Somogyi, P. & Whitteridge, D. (1983). Physiological and morphological properties of identified basket cells in the cat's visual cortex. *Exp. Brain Res.*, **50**, 193–200.
13. Barlow, H.B. (1985). Cerebral cortex as model builder. In *Models of the Visual Cortex*, pp. 37–46. Ed. D. Rose & V. Dobson. John Wiley, Chichester.
14. Zeki, S. (1978). Functional specialization in the visual cortex of the rhesus monkey. *Nature*, **274**, 423–8.
    Livingstone, M.S. & Hubel, D.H. (1984). Anatomy and physiology of a color system in the primate visual cortex. *J. Neuroscience*, **4**, 309–56.
15. Barlow, H.B. (1981). Critical limiting factors in the design of the eye and visual cortex. The Ferrier Lecture, 1980. *Proc. R. Soc.* B **212**, 1–34.
    Barlow, H.B. (1985) Why have multiple cortical areas? *Vision Research*, **26**, 81–90.

Notes to Chapter 2

1. An example is a view of Breslau after F.B. Werner, c.1750, in Heinrich Höhn, *Alte Deutsche Städte*, Leipzig, 1935.
2. Sancti Gregorii Magni *Epistolarum Libri XI*, Epist XIII, Migne, *Patrologia Latina 77*, Col.1128.
3. Claus Nissen, *Die botanische Buchillustration*, 2 vols., Stuttgart, 1951.
4. Now in the Louvre, Paris; Wilhelm Gundel, *Dekane und Dekansternbilder*, Hamburg, 1936, pl.XI.
5. Loren Mackinney, *Medical Illustrations in Medieval Manuscripts*, Wellcome Historical Medical Library, 1965, Chapter VI, pp. 48–50.
6. Translated and edited by Casey A. Wood and F. Marjorie Fyfe, Stamford USA/ Oxford, 1943.
7. Bagrow, Leo, *History of Cartography* (revised R.A. Skelton), London, 1964.
8. Windsor, Royal Library, Nos.12683, 12277 and 12278, see A.E. Popham, *The Drawings of Leonardo da Vinci*, London, 1946, pp. 264–6.
9. Compare his Study of muscles, Windsor, 12640 (Popham, *op.cit.* p. 237) or his many studies of wave motions illustrated in my *The Heritage of Apelles*, Oxford, 1976, especially Fig. 86.
10. Lehmann-Haupt, Hellmut, *The Göttingen Model Book* (Facsimile and translation), Columbia, Mo, 1972.
11. See Gerardus Mercator, *On the Lettering of Maps*, as illustrated in Svetlana Alpers, *The Art of Describing*, Chicago, 1983, Fig. 80.
12. Bascetta, Carlo, *Sport e Giuochi, Trattati e Scritti del 15 al 18 secolo* (2 vols.) Milan, 1978.
13. Arbeau, Thoinot, *Orchésographie*, 1589, translated and edited by Julia Sutton, New York, 1967.
14. A facsimile of the English edition is included in Nicholas Orme, *Early British Swimming 55 B.C. to A.D. 1719*, Exeter, 1983.
15. Compare Emilio Faccioli, *Arte della Cucina, Libri di ricette dal 14–19 secolo*, Milan, 1966.

Notes to Chapter 3

1. Harmon, L.D., 'The recognition of faces', in *Image, Object and Illusion, Readings from Scientific American*, pp. 101–12. W.H. Freeman and Co., San Francisco, 1974.
2. Sutcliffe, T.H., *Sign and Say*, Royal National Institute for the Deaf, London, 1981.
3. Pearson, D.E., 'Visual communication systems for the deaf', *IEEE Trans. Commun.*, vol. COM-29, pp. 1986–92, 1981.
4. Pearson, D.E. & Six, H., 'Low data-rate moving image transmission for deaf communication', *Proc. IEE Conference on Electronic Image Processing*, York, England, pp. 204–8, 1982.
5. Robinson, J.A. & Pearson, D.E., 'Visual teleconferencing at telephone data rates', *Proc. Internat. Teleconference Symp.*, London/Sydney/Tokyo/Toronto/Philadelphia, pp. 386–93, 3–5 April 1984.

6. Pearson, D. E. & Robinson, J. A., 'Visual communication at very low data rates', *Proc. IEEE*, **73**, No. 4, 795–812, 1985.

7. Pearson, D.E., 'Transmitting sign language for the deaf', *National Electronics Review*, 65–8, 1986.

8. Robinson, J.A., 'Low data-rate visual communication using cartoons: a comparison of data compression techniques', *Proc. IEE*, **133**, Pt. F, No. 3, 236–56, 1986.

9. Sperling, G., Pavel, M., Cohen, Y., Landy, M.S. & Schwartz, B.J., 'Image processing in perception and cognition', in *Physical and Biological Processing of Images*, Proc. of an International Symposium organized by the Rank Prize Funds, ed. O.J. Braddick, & A.C. Sleigh, 27–29 September 1982, London, England, pp. 359–78, Springer-Verlag, 1983.

10. Letellier, P., Nadler, M. & Abramatic, J-F., 'The telesign project', *Proc. IEEE*, **73**, 813–27, 1985.

11. Ono, H., Seki, H. & Deguchi, T. (Tokyo Gakugei University, Japan), 'Animated TV telephone system for deaf people', oral presentation at the *International Congress on the Education of the Deaf*, University of Manchester, England, 1985.

12. Hanna, E., Pearson, D.E. & Robinson, J.A., 'Low data-rate coding using image primitives', *Proc. 2nd International Technical Symposium on Optical and Electro-optical Applied Science and Engineering*, **594**, 138–41, 4–6 December 1985.

13. Attneave, F., 'Some informational aspects of visual perception', *Psych. Rev.*, **61**, 183–93, 1954.

14. Green, R.T. & Courtis, M.C., 'Information theory and figure perception: the metaphor that failed', in *Psychology and the Visual Arts*, ed. J. Hogg, Penguin, 1969.

15. It is also possible to state the postulate in terms of the stereographic projection of the Gaussian sphere (Horn, B.K.P., *Robot Vision*, M.I.T. Press, 1986). Cartoon lines should be drawn wherever the surface of an object maps into a narrow annulus at the outer extremity of the projection of the Gaussian sphere. It is interesting to note that the human form is well approximated by a cluster of egg-shaped solids (ovoids) and that there are few concave surfaces (Hale, R.B., *Drawing Lessons from the Great Masters*, Watson-Guptill Publications, New York, USA, 1964; Koenderink, J.J. & van Doorn, A.J., 'The shape of smooth objects and way contours end', *Perception*, **11**, pp. 129–37, 1982). The theory locates the extremities of these ovoids, if they are sufficiently prominent for their bounding surfaces to be parallel or nearly parallel to the line of sight. The reader is referred to the following contributions for some interesting geometrical insights (Enomoto, H. & Katayama, T., 'Structure lines of images', *Proc. 3rd International Conference on Pattern Recognition*, pp. 811–15, 1976; Koenderink, J.J., 'What does the occluding contour tell us about solid shape?', *Perception*, **13**, pp. 321–30, 1984).

16. Witkin, A.P., 'Scale-space filtering', *Proc. 8th International Joint Conference on Artificial Intelligence*, vol. 2, pp. 1019–22, Karlsruhe, West Germany, 8–12 August 1983.

17. Robinson, J.A., 'Low data-rate visual communication', Ph.D. thesis, University of Essex, England, 1985.

18. Both valley detectors and radio receivers can alternatively be described in the frequency domain as bandpass filters with narrow or broad responses as a function

of frequency. In the image case, the filter is followed by a peak detector to locate the valleys.

19. Martinez, K. & Pearson, D.E., 'Algorithmic complexity, speed and architectural parallelism in low data-rate visual communication', *Proc. IERE Conference on Digital Processing of Signals in Communications*, Loughborough, England, IERE Conference Publication No. 62, 22–25 April 1985.

20. Gombrich, E.H., *Art and Illusion*, Phaidon Press, London, England, 1959.

21. Gombrich, E.H., Hochberg, J. & Black, M., *Art, Perception and Reality*, The Johns Hopkins University Press, Baltimore, USA, 1972.

22. Robson, J.G., 'Neural images: the physiological basis of spatial vision', in *Visual Coding and Adaptability*, ed. C.S. Harris, pp. 177–214, Lawrence Erlbaum Associates, Hillsdale, N.J., USA, 1980.

23. Barlow, H.B., 'Understanding natural vision', in *Physical and Biological Processing of Images*, ed. O.J. Braddick & A.C. Sleigh, Springer-Verlag, Berlin, 1983.

24. Marr, D., *Vision*, W.H. Freeman & Co., San Francisco, USA, 1982.

25. Watt, R.J. & Morgan, M.J., 'Spatial filters and their localization of luminance changes in human vision', *Vision Research*, **24**, pp. 1387–97, 1984.

26. Campbell, F.W. & Robson, J.G., 'Application of Fourier analysis to the visibility of gratings', *J. Physiol.*, **197**, pp. 551–66, 1968.

27. In these experiments we have been concerned only with that part of the human visual system which recognizes faces. It is possible, however, that the sensitivity to valleys applies to other recognition tasks; it is known, for example, that dark letters on a light background are easier to read than the reverse (G.W., Radl, 'Experimental investigations for optimal presentation-mode and colours of symbols on the CRT-screen', in *Ergonomic Aspects of Visual Display Terminals*, ed. E. Grandjean & E. Vigliani, pp. 127–42, Taylor and Francis Ltd., London, 1980).

28. We are grateful to John Robson of the University of Cambridge, UK, for suggesting this experiment.

Notes to Chapter 4

1. Gautier D'Agoty, J., *Observations sur l'Histoire Naturelle, sur la Physique et sur la Peinture*, **1**, 106–9 (1752).

2. Le Baron Roger Portalis & Béraldi, Henri, *Les Graveurs du dix-huitième siècle*, vol. 1.2, (Paris, Damascène and Charles Fatout, 1880).

3. Gautier D'Agoty, J., *Anatomie générale des viscères* (Paris, 1753).

4. Gautier, J., *Mercure de France*, March, 1750, pp. 158–60.

5. Gage, J., *Journal of the Warburg and Courtauld Institutes*, **44**, 1–26 (1981); Lang, H., *Colour Research and Application*, **8**, 221–31 (1983).

6. Anonymous *Traité de la Peinture en mignature* (La Haye, 1708).

7. Castel, Louis-Bertrand, *L'Optique des Couleurs* (Paris, Briasson, 1740). As the 18th century advanced, experiments on colour mixture became more sophisticated and more quantitative. Particularly striking, though now little known, are those of S. Galton, which were published in the *Monthly Magazine*, **8**, No. 48, 1799, but had been demonstrated to the Lunar Society of Birmingham some years earlier.

8. Lilien, O.M. *Jacob Christoph Le Blon 1667–1741* (Stuttgart, Anton Hiersemann, 1985); Gage, J., *Print Quarterly*, **3**, 65–7 (1986); Melse, E., *Antiek*, October, 144–51

(1984). An account of Le Blon's method of weaving tapestries is given by C. Mortimer, *Philosophical Transactions of the Royal Society*, **37**, 101 (1731).

9. See, for example, Newton, I., *Opticks*, 4th edn (London, William Innys, 1730) Queries 12, 13; M. [Gautier] Dagoty, Père, *Exposition anatomique des organes des senses, jointe à la neurologie entière du corps humain* (Paris, Demonville, 1775).

10. Young, T., *Philosophical Transactions of the Royal Society*, **92**, 12–48 (1802).

11. For a general introduction to the retina and visual processes see Barlow, H.B. & Mollon, J.D., *The Senses* (Cambridge, Cambridge University Press, 1982). Among reviews of colour vision, the following may be especially recommended: Gouras, P., *Progress in Retinal Research*, **3**, 227 (1984); Lennie, P. & D'Zura, M., *CRC Critical Reviews in Clinical Neurobiology*, in press.

12. Dartnall, H.J.A., Bowmaker, J.K. & Mollon, J.D., *Philosophical Transactions of the Royal Society, London*, **B220**, 115–30 (1983). Technically, the ordinate of the graph is the logarithm of the factor by which light is attenuated as it passes through the outer segment of an individual receptor cell. Very recently, direct electrical recordings have been obtained from 2 of the 3 types of human cone: Schnapf, J.L., Kraft, T.W. & Baylor, D.A., *Nature*, **325**, 439–41 (1987).

13. Sperling, H.G., in *Colour Vision Deficiencies V*, ed. G. Verriest (Hilger, Bristol, 1980).

14. Pokorny, J., Smith, V.C., Verriest, G. & Pinckers, A.J.L.G., *Congenital and Acquired Colour Vision Defects* (Grune & Stratton, New York, 1979). Although the short-wave cones are genetically more stable, they appear to be more vulnerable to diseases and toxins that affect the receptor cells.

15. Liebmann, S., *Psychologische Forschung*, **9**, 300–53 (1927); Koffka, K. & Harrower, M.R., *Psychologische Forschung*, **15**, 145–275 (1931). There has not been published a modern contrast-sensitivity-function for an equiluminous grating in which the bars are distinguished only by the short-wave cones. Mullen, K., (*J. Physiol.*, **359**, 381–400 (1985)) gives results for a blue-yellow grating, but cells of the type shown in Fig. 4.5b would respond well to such a grating.

16. Tansley, B.W. & Boynton, R.M., *Science*, 1976, **191**, 954–7; Boynton, R.M., 1978, in J.C. Armington, J. Krauskopf & B.R. Wooten, eds., *Visual Psychophysics and Physiology* (New York, Academic Press, 1978).

17. Mollon, J.D. & Polden, P.G., *Journal of Physiology*, **254**, 1–2P (1975).

18. Nathans, J., Thomas, D. & Hogness, D.S., *Science*, **232**, 193–202 (1986); Nathans, J., Piantanida, T.P., Eddy, R.L., Shows, T.B. & Hogness, D.S., *Science*, **232**, 203–10 (1986); Nathans, J., *Ann. Rev. Neurosci.*, **10**, 163–4 (1987). For an introductory account of the molecular biology, see Mollon, J.D., *Nature*, **321**, 12–13 (1986).

19. As early as 1892, on the basis of the facts of colour blindness, Christine Ladd-Franklin proposed a successive differentiation of the photosensitive molecule underlying daylight vision (in *International Congress of Psychology*, London 1892, Kraus Reprint, 1974).

20. Jacobs, G.H., *Comparative Color Vision* (New York, Academic Press, 1981). In proposing that there remains a clear distinction between an ancient and a more recent subsystem of colour vision, I draw particularly on the physiological work of Derrington, A.M. & Lennie, P., *J. Physiol.*, **357**, 219–40 (1984) and Derrington, A.M., Krauskopf, J. & Lennie, P., *ibid*, 241–65, who concurrently studied the chromatic and spatial properties of cells in the parvocellular layers of the lateral geniculate nucleus of the macaque monkey and who make a firm distinction

between the 2 types of cell represented schematically in Fig. 4.5. I have also been guided by the review of Gouras, P., *Progress in Retinal Research*, **3**, 227–61 (1984). But it should be mentioned that some authors have distinguished more than 2 major groups of chromatically opponent cell at early stages of the visual pathway: see, for example, de Monasterio, F.M., in G. Verriest *Colour Vision Deficiencies VII*, pp. 9–28 (The Hague, Dr W. Junk, 1984). Figure 4.5 is modified from the classical paper of Wiesel, T.N. & Hubel, D.H., *J. Neurophysiology*, **29**, 1115–56 (1966).

21. Livingstone, M. & Hubel, D. (*Journal of Neuroscience*, 1984, **4**, 321) have written: 'We assume that the point of opponency is to render ineffective things like diffuse light or white light, rather than to permit a cell to have two kinds of response.' For the specific case of colour vision, the point was made early by Gouras, P., in an article in *Investigative Ophthalmology*, **11**, 423–34 (1972).

22. Derrington, A.M. & Lennie, P., *J. Physiol.*, **357**, 219–40 (1984); Derrington, A.M., Krauskopf, J. & Lennie. P., *J. Physiol.*, **357**, 241–65 (1984).

23. Doht, E. & Meissl, M., *Experientia*, 1982, **38**, 996–1000.

24. For an introduction to colour constancy, see Land, E., *Scientific American*, 1977, **237** (No. 6), 108–28; and Mollon, J.D., *The Listener*, 1985, **113** (No. 2891), 6–7. A group of recent technical papers on the subject will be found in the *Journal of the Optical Society of America* for October, 1986.

25. The relationship between coloured shadows and colour constancy was grasped as early as 1789 by the brilliant geometer, Gaspard Monge. The text of his lecture, given to the Académie Royale on the eve of the Revolution, was printed in *Annales de Chimie*, **3**, 131–47.

26. Schmidt, I., *Klinisches Monatsblatt für Augenheilkunde*, 1934, **92**, 456–7; Verriest, G., *Die Farbe*, **21**, 7–16 (1972).

27. Estévez, O., Spekreijse, H, van Dalen, J.T.W. & Verduyn Lunel, H.F.E., *American Journal of Optometry and Physiological Optics*, **60**, 892–901 (1983); Cavonius, C.R. & Kammann, J., in 'Colour Vision Deficiencies VII', ed. G. Verriest (W. Junk, The Hague, 1984).

28. Lyon, M., *Biological Review*, 1972, **47**, 1–35; Gartler, S.M. & Riggs, A.D., *Annual Review of Genetics*, 1983, **17**, 155–90.

29. This hypothesis requires that the visual system of the carrier should be plastic enough to take advantage of the extra class of cone, so as to allow new discriminations. This possibility is lent some plausibility by recent studies of South American squirrel monkeys (Mollon, J.D., Bowmaker, J.K. & Jacobs, G.H., 1984, *Proc. Roy. Soc.*, **222B**, 373–99): this species of monkey is basically dichromatic, having apparently only one genetic locus (on the X-chromosome) for a photopigment in the red–green range; but those female monkeys who inherit different versions of the photopigment from their two parents do become behaviourally trichromatic, being able to discriminate colours in the red–green region of the spectrum.

30. Mollon, J.D., in 'Frontiers of Visual Science', Committee on Vision (National Academy of Sciences, Washington, 1987).

31. I am grateful to Susan Astell and Gabriele Jordan for preparation of figures. The experimental work on heterozygotes was supported by a grant from the Medical Research Council.

Notes to Chapter 5

1. Wiley, Roland John (1978), *Two Essays on Stepanov Dance Notation*, New York, CORD Inc.
2. Benesh, Rudolf and Joan (1977), *Reading Dance: The Birth of Choreology*, London, Souvenir Press Ltd. (Reprinted 1983). *Benesh Movement Notation*, © Rudolf Benesh, 1955.
3. *Das Lied von der Erde* was created in 1965 for the Stuttgart Ballet.
4. *Different Drummer* was created in 1984 for The Royal Ballet, Covent Garden, London.
5. *Swan Lake* was created in 1895 for the Mariinsky Theatre by Marius Petipa and Lev Ivanov.
6. Goodman, N. (1968). *Languages of Art*, London, Oxford University Press.

Further reading

The Benesh Institute (1986). *Benesh Movement Notation Score Catalogue*, London.

Dail-Jones, Megan (1984). *A Culture in Motion: A Study of the Interrelationship of Dancing, Sorrowing, Hunting and Fighting as Performed by the Warlpiri Women of Central Australia*, M.A. thesis, University of Hawaii.

Eshkol, Noa (1984). *Tomlinson't Gavot*, Tel Aviv University.

Feuillet, Raoul Auger (2nd edn, 1701), *Choregraphie, ou L'art de De'crire la Dance*. Paris.

Grau, Andrée (1983). *Dreaming, Dancing, Kinship: The Study of Yoi, the Dance of the Tiwi of Melville and Bathurst Islands, North Australia*, Ph.D. thesis, Queen's University of Belfast.

Jones, Julie (1980). *The Sega of Mauritius*, M.A. thesis, Queen's University of Belfast.

Kipling-Brown, Ann & Parker, Monica (1984). *Dance Notation for Beginners*, London, Dance Books Ltd.

McGuiness-Scott, Julia (1983). *Movement Study and Benesh Movement Notation*, Oxford, Oxford University Press.

Pilkington, Linda (1984). *Syllabus of Professional Examinations of the Cecchetti Method Recorded in Benesh Movement Notation*, London, The Benesh Institute.

Ralov, Kirsten (1979). *The Bournonville School*, New York, Marcel Dekker Inc.

The Royal Academy of Dancing (1982). *The Royal Academy of Dancing Children's Examination Syllabus in Benesh Movement Notation*, 1982 revision by Julie Jones, London, The Royal Academy of Dancing.

Notes to Chapter 6

1. Chapters by H. Barlow, C. Blakemore, J. Mollon and A. Movshon, this volume, provide a general background and details of orientation, colour and movement processing respectively.
2. Bruce, C.J., Desimone, R. & Gross, C.G., *J. Neurophysiol.*, **46**, 369–84 (1981). Rolls, E.T., *Human Neurobiology*, **3**, 209–22 (1984).
3. Area TPO and PGa of Seltzer, B. & Pandya, D.N. (1978), *Brain Research*, **149**, 1–24 (1978).
4. In a sample of 35 unidirectional cells recorded in area TPO the mean preferred directions calculated for each cell (K.V. Mardia *Statistics of Directional Data* N.Y.

Academic Press 1972) were found to be highly clustered (P < < 0.0001, Binomial Test) around the 6 principal directions: A.J. Chitty, D.I. Perrett, A.J. Mistlin & M. Harries (in prep.).

5. Perrett, D.I. *et al. Human Neurobiol.* (1984), **3**, 197–208. Perrett, D.I. *et al. Proc. Roy. Soc.*, B **223**, 293–317 (1985). Perrett, D.I. *et al.*, in: H. Ellis, M.A. Jeeves, F. Newcombe & A. Young (eds.) *Aspects of Face Processing*. Martinus, Nijhoff, Dordrecht (1986).

6. Not 3 or 5 as we have suggested earlier Perrett, D.I. *et al.*, *Behav. Brain Res.*, **16**, 153–70 (1985).

7. Binford, T.O., Paper presented to IEEE Conference on Systems and Control, Miami, (1971). D. Marr, *Vision: A Computational Investigation into the Human Representation and Processing of Visual Information*. Freeman, San Francisco (1982). Marr, D. & Vaina, L., *Proc. Roy. Soc.* B **214**, 501–24 (1982).

8. Cutting, J.E. & Kozlowski, L.T., *Bull. Psychophys.*, **14**, 201–11 (1977). Johansson, G., *Percept. Psychophys.*, **14**: 201–11 (1973). Runeson, S. & Frykholm, G., *J. Exp. Psych.*, **112**, 585–615 (1983).

9. Chitty, A.J., Perrett, D.I., Mistlin, A.J. & Harries, M. (in prep.)

10. Marr, D. & Nishihara, H.K., *Proc. Roy. Soc. Lond.* B **200**, 269–94. (1978).

11. Chitty, A.J. *et al.*, *Perception*, **14**, A14 (1985).
    Perrett, D.I., Mistlin, A.J., Harries, M.H. and Chitty, A.J., in M. Goodale (ed.) *Vision and Action: The Control of Grasping*, Ablex Pub. (in press) (1988).

12. Leslie A.M., *Perception*, **11**, 173–86 (1982). Michotte, A., *The Perception of Causality*, Methuen, London (1963).

13. Paillard, J., *Phil. Trans. Roy. Soc.* B **298** 111–34 (1982).

Notes to Chapter 7

1. Fast, J. (1970). *Body Language*. New York: Evans & Co.

2. Brazil, D., Coulthard, D. & Johns, C. (1980). *Discourse Intonation and Language Teaching*. Longman.

3. Bull, P.E. & Connelly, G. (1985). Body movement and emphasis in speech. *Journal of Nonverbal Behaviour*, **9** (3), 169–87.

4. Bull, P.E. (1987). *Posture and Gesture*, Oxford: Pergamon Press.

5. Freedman, N. & Hoffman, S.P. (1967), Kinetic behaviour in altered clinical states: approach to objective analysis of motor behaviour during clinical interviews. *Perceptual and Motor Skills*, **24**, 527–39.

6. Bull, P.E. (in press). The use of hand gesture in political speeches: some case studies. *Journal of Language and Social Psychology*.

7. Atkinson, J.M. (1983). Two devices for generating audience approval: a comparative study of public discourse and text. In K. Ehlich *et al.* (eds.), *Connectedness in Sentence, Text and Discourse*, pp. 199–236. Tilburg, Netherlands: Tilburg Papers in Linguistics.
    Atkinson, J.M. (1984*a*). *Our Masters' Voices: The Language and Body Language of Politics*. London: Methuen.
    Atkinson, J.M. (1984*b*). Public speaking and audience responses: some techniques for inviting applause. In J.M. Atkinson & J. Heritage (eds.), *Structures of Social Action: Studies in Conversation Analysis*, pp. 370–409. Cambridge: Cambridge University Press.

8. Heritage, J. & Greatbatch, D. (1986). Generating applause: a study of rhetoric and response at party political conferences. *American Journal of Sociology*, **92**, 110–57.

9. Cohen, A.A. & Harrison, R.P. (1973). Intentionality in the use of hand illustrators in face-to-face communication situations. *Journal of Personality and Social Psychology*, **28**, 276–9.

10. Duncan, S. Fiske, D.W. (1977). *Face-to-face Interaction: Research, Methods and Theory*. Hillsdale, New Jersey: Lawrence Erlbaum.

11. Duncan, S. (1972). Some signals and rules for taking speaking turns in conversations. *Journal of Personality and Social Psychology*, **23**, 283–92.

12. Mehrabian, A. & Williams, N. (1969). Non-verbal concomitants of perceived and intended persuasiveness. *Journal of Personality and Social Psychology*, **13**, 37–58.

13. Kiritz, S.A. (1971). Hand movements and clinical ratings at admission and discharge for hospitalised psychiatric patients. Unpublished doctoral dissertation, University of California, San Francisco. Cited in Ekman, P. & Friesen, W.V. (1974), Non-verbal behaviour and psychopathology. In R.J. Friedman & M.M. Katz (eds.), *The Psychology of Depression: Contemporary Theory and Research*, pp. 203–32, New York: Wiley.

Notes to Chapter 8

1. Purkinje, J. (1825). *Beobachtungen und Versuche zur Physiologie der Sinne*, Bd. II, 60.

2. Barlow, H.B. & Brindley, G.S. (1963). Inter-ocular transfer of movement after-effects during pressure blinding of the stimulated eye. *Nature*, **200**, 1346–7.

3. For example those by G. Wertheimer (1912). Experimentelle Studien uber das Sehen von Bewegung. *Zeitschrift fur Physiologie*, **61**, 161–265.

4. For example those proposed by Adelson, E.H. & Bergen, J.R. (1985). Spatiotemporal energy models for the perception of motion. *Journal of the Optical Society of America*, A **2**, 284–99.

5. See for example Barlow, H.B. & Levick, W.R. (1965). The mechanism of directionally selective units in the rabbit's retina. *Journal of Physiology*, **178**, 477–504.

6. Movshon, J.A., Thompson, I.D. & Tolhurst, D.J. (1978). Receptive field organization of complex cells in the cat's striate cortex. *Journal of Physiology*, **283**, 79–99.

7. Ungerleider, L.G. & Mishkin, M. (1982). Two cortical visual systems. In *Analysis of Visual Behaviour*, ed. D.J. Ingle, M.A. Goodale & R.J.W. Mansfield. Cambridge, MA: MIT Press.

8. Maunsell, J.H.R. & Newsome, W.T. (1987). Visual processing in monkey extrastriate cortex. *Annual Review of Neuroscience*, **10**, 363–401.

9. Livingstone, M.S. & Hubel, D.H. (1984). Anatomy and physiology of a color system in the primate visual cortex. *Journal of Neuroscience*, **4**, 309–56.

   Shipp, S. & Zeki, S.M. (1985). Segregation of pathways leading from area V2 to areas V4 and V5 in the macaque monkey visual cortex. *Nature*, **315**, 322–5.

   DeYoe, E.A. & Van Essen, D.C. (1985). Segregation of efferent connections and receptive field properties in visual area V2 of the macaque. *Nature*, **317**, 58–61.

10. Van Essen, D.C. & Maunsell, J.H.R. (1983). Hierarchical organization and functional streams in the visual cortex. *Trends in Neurosciences*, **6**, 370–5.

    Van Essen, D.C. (1985). Functional organization of primate visual cortex. In *Cerebral Cortex Volume III*, ed. A. Peters & E.G. Jones. New York: Plenum Press.

11. Van Essen, D.C. & Maunsell, J.H.R. (1980). Two-dimensional maps of the cerebral cortex. *Journal of Comparative Neurology*, **191**, 255–81.

12. Enroth-Cugell, C. & Robson, J.G. (1984). Functional characteristics and diversity of cat retinal ganglion cells. *Investigative Ophthalmology and Visual Science*, **25**, 250–67.

13. Hubel, D.H. & Wiesel, T.N. (1968). Receptive fields and functional architecture of monkey striate cortex. *Journal of Physiology*, **195**, 215–43.

14. Kaplan, E. & Shapley, R.M. (1982). X and Y cells in the lateral geniculate nucleus of the macaque monkey. *Journal of Physiology*, **330**, 125–43.

15. Zeki, S.M. (1974). Functional organization of a visual area on the posterior bank of the superior temporal sulcus of the rhesus monkey. *Journal of Physiology*, **236**, 549–73.

16. Adelson, E.H. & Movshon, J.A. (1982). Phenomenal coherence of moving visual patterns. *Nature*, **300**, 523–5.

17. Movshon, J.A., Adelson, E.H., Gizzi, M.S. & Newsome, W.T. (1986). The analysis of moving visual patterns. In *Pattern Recognition Mechanisms*, ed. C. Chagas, R. Gattass & C.G. Gross. Rome: Vatican Press. (Reprinted in Supplementum 11 to *Experimental Brain Research*, 1986.)

18. Motter, B.C. & Mountcastle, V.B. (1981). The functional properties of the light-sensitive neurons of the posterior parietal cortex studied in waking monkeys: foveal sparing and opponent-vector organization. *Journal of Neuroscience*, **1**, 3–26.

19. Saito, H., Yukie, M., Tanaka, K., Hikosaka, K., Fukada, Y. & Iwai, E. (1986). Integration of direction signals of image motion in the superior temporal sulcus of the macaque monkey. *Journal of Neuroscience*, **6**, 145–57.

20. See for example, Lisberger, S.G., Morris, E.J. & Tychsen, L. (1987). Visual motion processing and sensory-motor integration for smooth pursuit eye movements. *Annual Review of Neuroscience*, **10**, 97–129.

21. Nakayama, K. (1985). Biological image motion processing: a review. *Vision Research*, **25**, 625–60.

22. The preparation of this chapter and some of the work it describes were supported in part by grants from the National Institutes of Health (EY2017) and the National Science Foundation (BNS 82–16950). Other support was provided by a Senior International Fellowship from the Fogarty International Center of the National Institutes of Health, and by a Guest Research Fellowship from the Royal Society.

Notes to Chapter 9

(Place of publication London unless otherwise indicated.)

1. Lévi-Strauss, Claude, 'The Structural Study of Myth', in *The Structuralists*, ed. Richard & Fernande DeGeorge (New York, 1972), pp. 169–94.

2. Kermode, Frank, *The Sense of an Ending* (1966).

3. *Great Dialogues of Plato*, trans. W.H.D. Rouse (New York, 1956), p. 190. I am indebted to Gérard Genette's discussion of this passage in *Narrative Discourse* (Oxford, 1980).

4. See Browne, Roger M., 'The Typology of Literary Signs', *College English*, **XXXIII** (1971), p. 6.

5. Amis, Martin, *Money* (Penguin edn 1986), p. 168.

6. Woolf, Virginia, *Mrs Dalloway* (1947 edn), p. 8.
7. See Bakhtin, Mikhail, *Problems of Dostoevsky's Poetics*, (Manchester, 1984), p. 181 ff.
8. Fielding, Henry, *The Adventures of Joseph Andrews* (World's Classics edn. 1929), p. 26.
9. Conrad, Joseph, Preface to *The Nigger of the Narcissus*, (Everyman edn, 1945), p. 5.
10. Hardy, Thomas, *The Woodlanders* (New Wessex edn. 1974) p. 43.
11. Isherwood, Christopher, *Lions and Shadows* (Signet edn, 1968) pp. 52–3.
12. Eliot, George, *Scenes of Clerical Life* (Penguin edn, 1973), p. 53.
13. Iser, Wolfgang, 'The Reading Process: a phenomenonological approach', *New Literary History*, III (Winter 1972), pp. 287–8.
14. Flaubert, Gustave, *Madame Bovary*, transl. Alan Russell, (Penguin edn, 1950), p. 16.
15. See Jakobson, Roman, 'Two Aspects of Language and Two Types of Linguistic Disturbances', in Jakobson & Halle, *Fundamentals of Language* (The Hague, 1956), and the present writer's *The Modes of Modern Writing: metaphor, metonymy and the typology of modern literature* (1977).
16. Greene, Graham, *The Heart of the Matter* (1948), p. 1.
17. Uspensky, Boris, *A Poetics of Composition* (1973).

Notes to Chapter 10

1. Krebs, J.R. (1978), *New Scientist*, June 3, **70**, 534–6.
2. When evolutionary biologists talk about 'interest' or 'benefit' they are using shorthand. It is generally accepted that behaviour and other aspects of living organisms have evolved by natural selection: some individuals pass on more copies of their genes than do others, and this leads to evolutionary change. The individuals that are successful at passing on their genes (i.e. at surviving and reproducing) are those that are best 'adapted' or suited to their environment. When evolutionary biologists talk about 'benefits' of a behaviour or other trait, they mean the contribution of the trait to increasing the individual's success in passing on its genes. Thus, for example, the ability of rabbits to run rapidly away from foxes is 'beneficial' to the individual that escapes. The fox and the rabbit do not share a common 'interest' in the interaction because the fox's chance of surviving and reproducing is increased if it catches the rabbit while the reverse is true for the rabbit. For a good general account of modern evolutionary theory see Dawkins, R. (1986), *The blind watchmaker*, Longman.
3. Stern, D. (1977), *The first relationship. Infant and mother*. Fontana.
4. Krebs, J.R. & Dawkins, R. (1984), In J.R. Krebs & N.B. Davies (eds.) *Behavioural Ecology*, 2nd edn, pp. 380–402. Blackwell Scientific Publications.
5. Krebs, J.R. (1977), *Anim. Behav.*, **25**, 475–8.
6. Borgia, G. (1986), *Sci. Amer.*, **254** (6), 70–9.
7. Dennett, D.T. (1983). *Behav. Brain Sci.*, **6**, 343–90.
8. I do not include in my article the debate about chimpanzees and other apes using sign language (see Weiskrantz, L. (ed.) (1984), *Animal Intelligence*, Royal Society) because I am restricting myself to naturally occurring animal communication systems.

9. Isack, H., *Proc. 19th Int. Orn. Congr.* (in press).

10. Lloyd, J. (1981). *Sci. Amer.*, **245** (1), 110–17.

Notes to Chapter 11

1. I am grateful to Trevor Pateman for helpful comments on an earlier draft of this chapter.

2. Saussure, F. de (1959). *Course in General Linguistics.* Glasgow: Fontana. (First published in French in 1916).

3. Hockett, C.F. (1960*a*). The origin of speech. *Scientific American*, **203**, 88–96.

4. Hockett, C.F. (1960*b*). Logical considerations in the study of animal communication. In W.E. Lanyon & W.N. Tavolga (eds.) *Animal Sounds and Communication*, Washington, D.C.: American Institure of Biological Sciences, 392–430.

5. See for example Deuchar, M. (1984). *British Sign Language*, chapter 2. London: Routledge and Kegan Paul; and Lane, H. (1984). *When the Mind Hears: A History of the Deaf.* New York: Random House.

6. Stokoe, W. (1960). *Sign Language Structure: An Outline of the Visual Communication System of the American Deaf.* University of Buffalo: Studies in Linguistics Occasional Paper no. 8.

7. For more details see Deuchar, M. (1987) Sign language research. In J. Lyons, R. Coates, M. Deuchar & G. Gazdar (eds.), *New Horizons in Linguistics 2.* Harmondsworth: Penguin.

8. Woll, B. (1984). The comparative study of different sign languages. In F. Loncke, P. Boyes-Braem & Y. Lebrun (eds.), *Recent Research on European Sign Languages.* Lisse: Swets & Zeitlinger, 79–91.

9. See for example Klima, E.S. & Bellugi, U. (1979). *The Signs of Language*, chapter 3. Cambridge, Mass.: Harvard University Press.

10. See for example Tervoort, B. (1961). Esoteric symbolism in the communicative behaviour of young deaf children. *American Annals of the Deaf*, **106**, 46–80; and Feldman, H., Goldin-Meadow, S. & Gleitman, L. (1978). Beyond Herodotus: the creation of language by linguistically deprived deaf children. In Lock, A. (ed.), *Action, gesture and symbol. The emergence of language*, pp. 351–414.

11. See for example Bonvillian, J. (1983). Early sign language acquisition and its relation to cognitive and motor development. In Kyle, J. & Woll, B. (eds.), *Language in Sign: An International Perspective on Sign Language.* London: Croom Helm, pp. 116–25.

12. Brown, R. (1977). Why are signed languages easier to learn than spoken languages? Paper presented at the National Symposium on Sign Language Research and Teaching, Chicago, Illinois.

13. Mandel, M. (1977). Iconicity of signs and their learnability by non-signers. *Proceedings of the First National Symposium on Sign Language Research and Teaching*, pp. 259–66.

14. For discussion see Baron, N. (1981). *Speech, Writing and Sign*, pp. 248–62, Bloomington: Indiana University Press.

15. Bates, E. (1979). *The Emergence of Symbols. Cognition and Communication in Infancy.* New York: Academic Press.

16. Klima, E.S. & Bellugi, U. (1979). *The Signs of Language*. Cambridge, Mass.: Harvard University Press.
17. Bellugi, U. & Klima, E. (1976). Two faces of sign: iconic and abstract. *Annals of the New York Academy of Sciences*, **280**, 514–38.
18. See Eco, U. (1976). *A Theory of Semiotics*, p. 192. Bloomington: Indiana University Press.
19. See for example Lewis, D. (1969), *Convention: a Philosophical Study*. Cambridge, Mass.: Harvard University Press; Pateman, T. (1982). David Lewis's theory of convention and the social life of language. *Journal of Pragmatics*, **6**, 135–57; and McGinn, C. (1984). *Wittgenstein on Meaning*. Oxford: Basil Blackwell.
20. Andersen, H. (1986). Iconicity in language: a map of the landscape. Unpublished manuscript, Copenhagen: Institut for lingvistik.

Notes to Chapter 12

1. Lessing, Gotthold Ephraim (1766). *Laŏcoon*.
2. Scharf, Aaron (1968). *Art and Photography*.

Suggested further reading

Kolers, Paul Aram (1972). *Aspects of Motion Perception*.
Marek, Kurt Wilhelm (or Ceram) (1965). *Archaeology of the Cinema*.

Notes to Chapter 13

1. Frisch, K. von (1967). *The Dance Language and Orientation of Bees*. Cambridge Mass., Harvard University Press.
2. Land, M.F. (1981). Optics and vision in invertebrates. In: *Handbook of Sensory Physiology*, vol. VII/6B (ed. H. Autrum), pp. 471–592. Berlin, Springer.
3. Hurley, A.C., Lange, G.D. & Hartline, P.H. (1978). The adjustable 'pin-hole camera' eye of *Nautilus*. *J. Exp. Zool.*, **205**, 37–44.
4. Land, M.F. (1965). Image formation by a concave reflector in the eye of the scallop, *Pecten maximus*. *J. Physiol.*, **179**, 138–53.
5. Hartline, H.K. (1938). The discharge of impulses in the optic nerve of *Pecten* in response to illumination of the eye. *J. Cell. Comp. Physiol.*, **11**, 465–77.
6. Vogt, K. (1980). The optical system of the crayfish eye. *J. Comp. Physiol.*, **135**, 1–19.
7. Leeuwenhoek, A. (1695). Quoted in: Wehner, R. (1981). Spatial vision in arthropods. In: *Handbook of Sensory Physiology*, vol. VII/6C (ed. H. Autrum), pp. 287–616. Berlin, Springer.
8. An account of the way this elegant arrangement works in flies is given by Kirschfeld, K. (1972). The visual system of *Musca*: studies on optics structure and function. In: *Information Processing in the Visual Systems of Arthropods* (ed. R. Wehner), pp. 61–74. Berlin, Springer. The water boatman eye probably works in the same way.
9. Wiese, K. (1974). The mechanoreceptive system of prey localization in *Notonecta*. II. The principle of prey localization. *J. Comp. Physiol.*, **92**, 317–25.

10. Schwind, R. (1980). Geometrical optics of the *Notonecta* eye: adaptations to optical environment and way of life. *J. Comp. Physiol.*, **140**; 59–68.

11. Munk, O. (1970). On the occurrence and significance of horizontal band-shaped areas in teleosts. *Vidensk. Meddr. dansk naturh. Foren.*, **133**, 85–120.

12. Schwind, R. (1983). Zonation of the optical environment and zonation in the rhabdom structure within the eye of the backswimmer, *Notonecta glauce*. *Cell Tissue Res.*, **232**, 53–63.

13. Schwind, R. (1984). The plunge reaction of the backswimmer *Notonecta glauca*. *J. Comp. Physiol.*, A **155**, 319–21.

14. Bristowe, W.S. (1958). *British Spiders*. London, Collins.

15. Land, M.F. (1972). Mechanisms of orientation and pattern recognition by jumping spiders (Salticidae). In: *Information Processing in the Visual Systems of Arthropods* (ed. R. Wehner), pp. 321–47. Berlin, Springer.

16. Forster, L. (1985). Target discrimination in jumping spiders (Araneae: Salticidae). In: *Neurobiology of Arachnids* (ed. F.G. Barth), pp. 249–74. Berlin, Springer.

17. Drees, O. (1952). Untersuchungen über die angeborenen Verhaltensweisen bei Springspinnen. *Z. Tierpsychol.*, **9**, 169–207.

18. Walls, G.L. (1942). *The Vertebrate Eye and its Adaptive Radiation*. Michigan, Cranbrook Institute.

Notes to Chapter 14

1. Barzel, Ronen & Barr, Alan H. 'Dynamic Constraints', *Proc. SIGGRAPH '88*, Atlanta, 1988.

2. Kass, Michael, Witkin, Andrew & Terzopoulos, Demetri. 'Snakes: Active Contour Models,' *Proc. International Conference on Computer Vision*, London, 1987. *Int. J. of Computer Vision*, **1** (4), 1987.

3. Kass, Michael & Witkin, Andrew. 'Analyzing Oriented Patterns', *Computer Vision Graphics and Image Processing*, **37**, pp. 362–85, 1987.

4. Platt, John. 'An elastic model for interpreting 3D structure from motion of a curve,' to appear.

5. Terzopoulos, Demetri. 'Regularization of inverse visual problems involving discontinuities,' *IEEE Trans. Pattern Analysis and Machine Intelligence*, **8**, pp. 413–24, 1986.

6. Terzopoulos, Demetri, John, Platt, Barr, Alan & Fleischer, Kurt. 'Elastically Deformable Models', *Proc. SIGGRAPH '87*, Anaheim, 1987.

7. Terzopoulos, Demetri, Witkin, Andrew & Kass, Michael. 'Symmetry-seeking models for 3D object reconstruction', *Proc. International Conference on Computer Vision*, London, 1987. *Int. J. of Computer Vision*, **1**(3), 1987.

8. Terzopoulos, Demetri, Witkin, Andrew & Kass, Michael. 'Energy constraints on deformable models: recovering shape and non-rigid motion', *Proc. AAAI-87*, Seattle, 1987.

9. Witkin, Andrew, Fleischer, Kurt & Barr, Alan. 'Energy constraints on parameterized models', *Proc. SIGGRAPH '87*, Anaheim, 1987.

10. Witkin, Andrew, Terzopoulos, Demetri & Kass, Michael. 'Signal matching through scale space', *Proc. AAAI-86*, Philadelphia, 1986. *Int. J. of Computer Vision*, **1**(2), 1987.

Notes to Chapter 15

1. The 'eyewitness principle' is introduced by E.H. Gombrich in his essay, 'Standards of truth' in *The language of images*, W.J.T. Mitchell (ed.), University of Chicago Press, Chicago 1980, pp. 181–218. As an example of the misunderstanding of artists' motives, an important recent paper on computer graphics by Cohen & Greenberg begins, '*The representation of a realistic image of both actual and imagined scenes has been the goal of artists and scholars for centuries*'. Cohen, M.F. & Greenberg, D.P., 'The hemi-cube: a radiosity solution for complex environments', *ACM SIGGRAPH Computer Graphics*, July 1985 (**19**) 3, pp. 31–40.

2. Lansdown, J., 'Design in computer graphics', *Proceedings BCS/ACM State of the art in computer graphics conference*, 1986.

3 Leler, W.J., 'Human vision, anti-aliasing, and the cheap 4000 line display', *ACM SIGGRAPH Computer Graphics*, July 1980 (**14**) 3, pp. 308–13.

4. For an outline of some of the methods of improving the computational efficiency of ray tracing see Kajiya, J.T., 'New techniques for ray tracing procedurally defined objects', *ACM Transactions on Graphics*, July 1983 (*2*) 3, pp. 161–81; Weghorst, H., Hooper, G. & Greenberg, D.P., 'Improved computational methods for ray tracing', *ACM Transactions on Graphics*, Jan. 1984 (*3*) 1, pp. 52–69; Glassner, A.S., 'Space subdivision for ray tracing', *IEEE Computer Graphics and Applications*, Oct. 1984 (*4*) 10, pp. 15–22; and Fujimoto, A., Tanaka, T. & Iwata, K., 'ARTS: accelerated ray tracing system', *IEEE Computer Graphics and Applications*, April 1985 (*5*) 5.

5. Sutherland, I.E., Sproull, R.F. & Schumacker, R.A., 'A characterisation of ten hidden-surface algorithms', *Computing Surveys*, Mar. 1974 (**6**) 1, pp. 1–55.

6. Requicha, a pioneer in the field, gives a good review of the theory, methods and systems of CSG in Requicha, A.A.G., 'Representations of rigid solids: theory, methods and systems', *Computing Surveys*, Dec. 1980 (*12*) 4, pp. 437–64.

7. A tutorial review of some of the features of computational geometry is given by Faux, I.D. & Pratt M.J., *Computational geometry for design and manufacture*, Ellis Horwood Chichester 1979; and Duncan, J.P. & Mair, S.G., *Sculptured surfaces for engineering and medicine*, Cambridge University Press, Cambridge 1983. Chiyokura, H. & Kimura, F. in 'Design of solids with free-form surfaces', *ACM SIGGRAPH Computer Graphics*, July 1983 (**17**) 3, pp. 289–98, propose a unified method of describing a range of shapes from the polyhedral to free-form. They point out too, that the best methods of describing a shape in its purely geometrical form may not be the best for making modifications to it as might happen in the process of designing.

8. Although fractals have a more widespread application than appears from many discussions in computer graphics literature, they are extemely valuable in making images of natural objects. Mandelbrot, B.B., *The fractal geometry of nature*, Freeman, New York 1982, discusses the theory and mathematics and shows striking examples of their use. Voss, who works closely with Mandelbrot, covers the fractal description of mountains and coastlines in Voss, R.F., 'Random fractal forgeries' in *Fundamental algorithms for computer graphics*, R.A. Earnshaw (ed.), Springer-Verlag, Berlin 1985, pp. 805–35. Aono, M. & Kunii, T.L. outline their way of generating the forms of trees and plants in 'Botanical tree image generation', *IEEE Computer Graphics and Applications*, May 1984 (**4**) 5, pp. 10–34. Gardner, G., 'Visual

simulation of clouds', *ACM SIGGRAPH Computer Graphics*, July 1985 (**19**) 3, pp. 297–303 shows how clouds can be modelled.

9. Some of the problems involved in modelling the human body are discussed in Badler, N.I. & Smoliar, S.W., 'Digital representations of human movement', *Computing Surveys*, Mar. 1979 (**11**) 1, pp. 19–38; and Lansdown, J., 'The computer in choreography', *Computer*, Aug. 1978 (**11**) 8, pp. 19–31.

10. Methods of dealing with lighting of images are given in R. Hall, 'Colour reproduction and illumination models', *Proceedings BCS/ACM State of the art in computer graphics conference*, Stirling 1986. Warn, D.R., 'Lighting controls for synthetic images', *ACM SIGGRAPH Computer Graphics*, July 1983 (**17**) 3, pp. 13–21, looks at ways of modelling different forms of lighting. Cook & Torrance discuss a widely-used reflectance model which now bears their name in Cook, R.L. & Torrance, K.E., 'A reflection model for computer graphics', *ACM Transactions on Graphics*, Jan. 1982 (**1**) 1, pp. 7–24. In their paper cited in Note 1 above, Cohen & Greenberg show the way in which reflected illumination from surfaces can be incorporated in a scene by using a technique somewhat different from ray tracing. Surface texture modelling is considered by Hayumara, S. & Barsky, B.A., 'Using stochastic modelling for texture generation', *IEEE Computer Graphics and Applications*, Mar. 1984 (**4**) 3, pp. 7–19; Peachey, D.R., 'Solid texturing of complex surfaces', *ACM SIGGRAPH Computer Graphics*, July 1985 (**19**) 3, pp. 279–86.

Notes to Chapter 16

1. Dürer, Albrecht. *Underweysung der Messung mit der Zirckel und Richtscheyt*, etc. . . . ., Nürnberg, 1525. Several of these drawing machines are illustrated in Dubery, F. & Willats, J., *Perspective and Other Drawing Systems*, London: The Herbert Press, 1983.

2. *Codex Atlanticus*, Ambrosiana, Milan.

3. Hooke, Robert. *Micrographia*, London: 1665.

4. Brook Taylor, *New Principles of Linear Perspective*, London: 1719.

5. Gibson, J.J. A theory of pictorial perception, *Audio-Visual Communications Review*, 1954.

6. Marr, D. *Vision: a Computational Investigation into the Human Representation and Processing of Visual Information*, San Francisco: W.H. Freeman, 1982.

7. Rivière, J. Sur les tendances actuelles de la peinture, *Revue d'Europe et d'Amérique*, 1912.

8. The idea that pictures are 'natural' is associated with J.J. Gibson, for example Gibson, J.J., Pictures, perspective and perception, *Daedalus*, **89**, 1960, especially p. 227. The idea that pictures are 'conventional' is associated with Nelson Goodman, for example, Goodman, N., *Languages of Art*, Indianapolis: Hackett, 1976. For a discussion and further references, see Wollheim, R., The philosophical contribution to psychology, in Butterworth, G. (ed.), *The Child's Representation of the World*, New York and London: Plenum Press, 1977.

9. Hockney, D. *David Hockney by David Hockney*, London: Thames and Hudson, 1976.

Notes to Chapter 17

1. Wittgenstein, L. (1953), *Philosophical Investigations*. Basil Blackwell, Oxford.

2. Kenny A. (1984), *The Legacy of Wittgenstein*. Basil Blackwell, Oxford.

3. Descartes, R. (1637). *La Dioptrique* (see *Philosophical Writings* transl. and ed. E. Anscombe & P.T. Geach (1954) London, Nelson).

4. Descartes, R. (1649), *Les Passions de l'Ame* (see *The Philosophical Works of Descartes I*, transl. & ed. E.S. Haldane & G.T.R. Ross (1911) Cambridge University Press, Cambridge).

5. The minutes of the June, 1986, meeting of the steering committee for the SDF Symposium on Computational Neuroscience were prepared and circulated by Professor Eric Schwartz of the New York University Medical Center in September 1986.

6. Young, J.Z. (1978), *Programs of the Brain*. Oxford University Press, Oxford.

7. Hacker, P. (1987). Languages, brains and minds. In *Mindwaves*, ed. C. Blakemore & S. Greenfield. Basil Blackwell, Oxford.

8. Woolsey, T.A. & Van der Loos, H. (1970). The structural organization of layer IV in the somatosensory region (SI) of mouse cerebral cortex. The description of a cortical field composed of discrete cytoarchitectonic units. *Brain Res.*, **17**, 205–42.

9. Kossut, M. & Hand, P. (1984). Early development of changes in representation of vibrissae following neonatal denervation of surrounding vibrissae receptors: a 2-deoxyglucose study in the rat. *Neuroscience Letters*, **46**, 7–12.

10. Barlow, H.B. (1981). Critical limiting factors in the design of the eye and visual cortex. The Ferrier lecture 1980. *Proc. Roy. Soc.* B **212**, 1–34.
    Barlow, H.B., (1986). Why have multiple cortical areas? *Vision Research*, **26**, 81–90.

11. Hubel, D.H. & Wiesel, T.N. (1977). Functional architecture of macaque monkey visual cortex. *Proc. Roy Soc.* B **198**, 1–59.

12. Albus, K. (1975). A quantitative study of the projection area of the central and the paracentral visual field in area 17 of the cat. II. The spatial organization of the orientation domain. *Experimental Brain Research*, **24**, 181–202.

13. Harris, L.R., Blakemore, C. & Donaghy, M.J. (1980). Integration of visual and auditory space in the mammalian superior colliculus. *Nature*, **288**, 56–9.
    King, A.J. & Hutchings, M.E. (1987). Spatial response properties of acoustically responsive neurons in the superior colliculus of the ferret: a map of auditory space. *J. Neurophysiol.*, **57**, 596–624.

14. King, A.J., Hutchings, M.E., Moore, D.R. & Blakemore, C. (1987). Developmental plasticity in the representations of visual and auditory space. *Nature*, **332**, 73–6.

15. Rose, D. & Blakemore, C. (1974). Effects of bicuculline on functions of inhibition in visual cortex. *Nature*, **249**, 375–7.
    Sillito, A.M. (1984). Functional considerations of the operation of GABAergic inhibitory processes in the visual cortex. In *The Cerebral Cortex*, vol. 2A, ed. A. Peters & E.G. Jones. Plenum Publishing Corporation, New York, pp. 91–117.

16. Calford, M.B., Graydon, M.L., Huerta, M.F., Kaas, J.F. & Pettigrew, J.D. (1985). A variant of the mammalian somatotopic map in a bat. *Nature*, **313**, 477–9.

17. Suga, N., Kuzirai, K. & O'Neill, W.E. (1981). How biosonar information is represented in the bat cerebral cortex. In *Neuronal Mechanisms of Hearing*, ed. J. Syka & L. Aitkin. Plenum Publishing Corporation, New York.

18. Zeki, S. (1983). Colour coding in the cerebral cortex: the reaction of cells in monkey visual cortex to wavelengths and colours. *Neuroscience*, **9**, 741–65.

19. Van Essen, D.C. (1985). Functional organization of primate visual cortex. In

Cerebral Cortex, vol. 3, ed. A. Peters & E.G. Jones. Plenum Publishing Corporation, New York.

Notes to Chapter 18

1. Roy, C.S. & Sherrington, C.S. *J. Physiol*, **11**, 850 (1890).
2. For a recent comprehensive review of this extensive literature including methods, the relationship of neuronal activity to blood flow and energy metabolism, and changes in blood flow and metabolism in the resting and activated normal human brain see: M.F. Raichle, *Handbook of Physiology, The Nervous System*, ed. V.B. Mountcastle & F. Plum (American Physiological Society, Bethesda, Maryland, 1987). Volume V, Part 2, pp. 643–74.
3. Fulton, J.F. *Brain*, **51**, 310 (1928).
4. Landau, W.M. *et al*, *Trans. Am. Neurol. Assn*, **80**, 125 (1955); and Kety, S.S. *Methods Med. Res.* **8**, 228 (1960).
5. Herscovitch, P., Markham, J. & Raichle, M.E. *J. Nucl. Med.*, **24**, 782 (1983); and Raichle, M.E. *et al.*, *ibid*. **24**, 790 (1983).
6. Fox, P.T., Perlmutter, J.S. & Raichle, M.E. *J. Comput. Assist. Tomogr.* **9**, 141 (1985).
7. Fox, P.T., Burton, H. & Raichle, M.E. *J. Neurosurg.*, in press.
8. For a review of this literature and a more detailed discussion of these experiments with PET see: Fox, P.T. *et al.*, *Nature*, **323**, 806 (1986); and Fox, P.T. *et al.*, *J. Neuroscience*, **7**, 913 (1987).
9. Petersen, S.E. *et al.*, *Nature*, **331**, 585 (1988).
10. Powers, W.J. & Raichle, M.E. *Stroke*, **16**, 361 (1985).
11. Engel, J., Kuhl, D.E., Phelps, M.E. & Mazziotta, J.C. *Ann. Neurol.* **12**, 510 (1982).
12. Foster, N.L. *et al.*, *Ann. Neurol.* **16**, 649 (1984); and Duara, R. *et al.*, *Ann. Neurol.* **16**, 702 (1984).
13. Sheehan, D.V. *New Engl. J. Med.*, **307**, 156 (1982).
14. Pitts F.N. & McClure, J.N. Jr., *New Engl. J. Med.*, **277**, 1329 (1967).
15. Reiman, E.M. *et al.*, *Nature*, **310**, 683 (1984); and Reiman, E.M. *et al.*, *Am. J. Psych.* **143**, 469 (1986).
16. Wagner, H.N. Jr *et al.*, *Science*, **221**, 1262 (1983); and Calne, D.B. *et al.*, *Nature*, **317**, 246 (1985).
17. This work was supported by NIH research grants NS 06833, HL 13851, NS 14834 and AG/NS 03991 and the McDonnell Center for Studies of Higher Brain Function.

Notes to Chapter 19

1. Levi, Primo (1984). *The Periodic Table*, Schocken, New York, p. 227.

Notes to Chapter 20

1. Gibson, J.J. (1950). *The Visual World*, Boston: Houghton Mifflin. 1(a), p. 14; 1(b), p. 20; 1(c), p. 142.
2. Gibson, J.J. (1986). *The Senses Considered as Perceptual Systems*. Boston: Houghton Mifflin.
3. Helmholtz, H. von. *Physiological Optics* (1867), and *Popular Scientific Lectures* (1903).
4. Berkeley, G. (1710). *A New Theory of Vision* and Berkeley, G. (1713). *Three*

Dialogues between Hylas and Philonous, (edt.) G.J. Warnock (1962), London: Fontana.

5. Gregory, R.L. (1980). 'Perceptions as hypotheses'. *Phil. Trans. R. Soc.* B **290**, pp. 181–97.

6. Gregory, R.L. (1981). *Mind in Science*. London: Weidenfeld.

7. Gregory, R.L. (1970). *The Intelligent Eye*. London: Weidenfeld. New York: McGraw Hill.

8. Locke, J. (1690). *Essay Concerning Human Understanding*. P.H. Nidditch, Oxford: OUP.

9. Marr, D. (1982). *Vision*, San Francisco: W.H. Freeman.

10. Ittelson, W.H. & Kilpatrick, F.P. (1952). 'Experiments in perception', *Scientific American*, **185**, 50.

11. Schumann, F. (1904). 'Einige Beobachtungen uber die Zusammenfassung von Gesichtseindruckern zu Einheiten', *Psychologische Studien*, I, 1–32. (Cited in: R.S. Woodworth (1938), *Experimental Psychology*, New York: Henry Holt, p. 636.)

12. Gregory, R.L. (1972). 'Cognitive contours', *Nature*, **238**, 51–2.

13. Dumais, T. & Bradley, D.R. (1976), 'The effects of illumination level and retinal size on the apparent strength of subjective contours', *Vision Research*, **19**, **4**, 339–45.

14. Coren, S. (1972). 'Subjective contours and apparent depth', *Psychological Review*, **79** (4), 359–67.

15. Which is why I called them 'Cognitive contours' in Gregory, R.L. (1972). 'Cognitive contours', *Nature*, **238**, 51–2.

16. Kennedy, J. (1979). 'Phantom contours', in: C.F. Nodine & D.F. Fisher (eds.) (1979) *Perception and Pictorial Representation*, (pp. 167–95). N.Y. Preager.

17. Lawson, R.B. & Gullick W.L. (1967). 'Stereopsis and anomalous contour', *Vision Research*, **7**, 271–97.

18. Pastore, N. (1972). *Selective History of Theories of Perception, 1650–1950*, Oxford: OUP.

19. This powerful technique for showing that a visual phenomenon is 'central', and not retinal in its origin or cause, goes back to Witasek, S.Z. (1899), *Psychol. Physiol. Sinn.*, **19**, 81. Pastore (18) in his use of it, was discussing Gestalt-type isomorphic brain field-type explanations, which place the origin centrally and not retinally.

20. Harris, J.P. & Gregory, R.L. (1973). 'Fusion and rivalry of illusory contours', *Perception*, **2**, 235–47.

21. Gregory, R.L. & Harris, J.P. (1974). 'Illusory contours and stereo depth', *Perception & Psychophysics*, **15**, 411–16.

22. It is interesting that such processing, which is equivalent to David Marr's (Marr, D. (1982) *Vision*) '2 $\frac{1}{2}$-D Sketch', can take place so early in the visual system. There is evidence (or rather negative evidence) from single-cell recording from the visual cortex that illusory contours are not produced retinally, or at the first stages of visual processing, for Baumgartner, G., von der Heydt, R. & Peterhans, E. (1984) ('Anomalous contours: a tool for studying the neurophysiology of vision' *Exp. Brain Research*, Suppl. 9, 413–19) found that neurons in area 17 did not respond to stimuli that in man produce illusory contours; though activity was found in area 18 of rhesus monkeys (*Maccaca mulatta*). We (see Note 25) found no activity in area 17 of the cat. Unfortunately this study was not completed to find whether there is related activity further up the cat's visual system.

23. Gregory, R.L. (1964). 'Stereoscopic shadow images', *Nature*, **203**, 1407.

24. Bradley, D.R. & Dumais, S.T. (1975). 'Ambiguous cognitive contours', *Nature*, **258**, 582–4.
25. Sillito, A., Gregory, R.L. & Heard, P. (1982), 'Can Cognitive Contours Con Cat Cortex?' Talk presented to Exp. Psychol. meeting, 1982, at St Andrews.

Notes to Chapter 21

1. Lakatos, I. 'History of science and its rational reconstruction' in R.C. Buck & R.S. Cohen, eds., *Boston Studies in the Philosophy of Science*, **8** (1971), p. 91.
2. Dietz, R.S. & French, B.M. 'Two probable astroblemes in Brazil', *Nature*, **244** (1973), 561.
3. Conklin, H.C. & Pinther, M. 'Pseudoscopic illusion', Letter to *Science*, **194** (1976), 374.
4. Tolansky, S. *Optical Illusions* (Oxford: Pergamon Press, 1964), figs. 79–80.
5. Dragesco, J. 'La vision dans les instruments astronomiques et l'observation physique des surfaces planétaires', *l'Astronomie* (1969), 355, 399 and 439. See too the classic works by Stoney, G.J., 'Telescopic vision', *Philosophical Magazine*, **16** (1908), 318; and by Vorhies, F.W., 'Telescopic vision of an illuminated surface', *Astrophysical Journal*, **40** (1914), 311.
6. Wilkins, H.P. *Our Moon* (London: Frederick Muller, 1954), p. 139.
7. Wilkins, H.P. & Moore, P. *The Moon* (London: Faber and Faber, 1955), p. 202.
8. Ashbrook, J. 'Is there a bridge on the Moon?', *Sky and Telescope*, **13** (1954), 205.
9. Quoted in Copeland, L.S. 'Illusions that trap lunar observers', *Sky and Telescope*, **15** (1956), 248.
10. Moore, P. *Survey of the Moon* (London: Eyre & Spottiswoode, 1963), p. 149.
11. Oberguggenberger, V. 'Statistische Untersuchungen zum Problem der Sternketten, I', *Zeitschrift für Astrophysik*, **16** (1938), 323.
12. Quoted in Struve, O. 'Star chains', *Sky and Telescope*, **13** (1954), 181.
13. Edgeworth, K.E. 'Some aspects of stellar evolution', *Monthly Notices of the Royal Astronomical Society*, **106** (1946), 470, 476 and 484.
14. Hahn, G. & Haupt, H.F. 'Physical investigations of star chains', *Astronomy and Astrophysics*, **41** (1975), 447.
15. Lindemann, E. & Burki, G. 'Rings and chains in simulated stellar fields', *Astronomy and Astrophysics*, **41** (1975), 355.
16. Isserstedt, J. 'Stellar rings', *Vistas in Astronomy*, **19** (1975), 123.
17. Uranova, T.A. 'Statistical study of stellar rings', *Soviet Astronomy*, **18** (1975), 746.
18. Shane, C.D. & Wirtanen, C.A. 'The distribution of galaxies', *Publications of the Lick Observatory*, **22** (1967), pt. 1.
19. Seldner, M., Siebers, B., Groth, E.J. & Peebles, P.J.E. 'New reduction of the Lick catalog of galaxies', *Astronomical Journal*, **82** (1977), 249.
20. de Lapparent, V., Kurtz, M.J. & Geller, M.J. 'The Shane-Wirtanen counts: Systematics and the two-point correlation function', *Astrophysical Journal*, **304** (1986), 585; also their earlier paper Geller *et al.*, 'The Shane-Wirtanen counts', *Astrophysical Journal*, **287** (1984), L55.
21. The subject is too vast to dwell on here; but see, for example, Arp, H., 'Evidence for non-velocity redshifts – new evidence and review' in J.R. Shakeshaft, ed., *The Formation and Dynamics of Galaxies* (Dordrecht: D. Reidel, 1974), p. 199; Burbidge,

G., 'Evidence for non-cosmological redshifts – QSOs near bright galaxies and other phenomena' in G.O. Abell & P.J.E. Peebles, eds., *Objects of High Redshift* (Dordrecht: D. Reidel, 1980), p. 99.

22. de Lapparent, V., Geller, M.J. & Huchra, J.P. 'A slice of the Universe', *Astrophysical Journal*, **302** (1986), L1.

23. Maddox, J. 'Galactic voids may be statistical', *Nature*, **319** (1986), 445.

24. Burns, J.O. 'Very large structures in the Universe', *Scientific American*, **255**, no. 1 (1986), 30.

25. Land, M.F. 'Vision in other animals', this volume, p. 202.

26. Cairns, I., McCusker, C.B.A., Peak, L.S. & Woolcott, R.L.S. 'Lightly ionizing particles in air-shower cores', *Physical Review*, **186** (1969), 1394; also McCusker & Cairns, 'Evidence of quarks in air-shower cores', *Physical Review Letters*, **23** (1969), 658.

27. Adair, R.K. & Kasha, H. 'Analysis of some results of quark searches', *Physical Review Letters*, **23** (1969), 1355.

28. Rahm, D.C. & Louttit, R.I. 'Comments on "Evidence of quarks in air-shower cores"', *Physical Review Letters*, **24** (1970), 279.

29. Imhoff, C.L. & Grady, C.A. 'Science fiction with IUE, I', *IUE NASA Newsletter* no. 26 (1985), 66.

30. Quoted in Ordway, F.I. 'The legacy of Schiaparelli and Lowell', *Journal of the British Interplanetary Society*, **39** (1986), 19.

31. E.g., Lowell, P. *Mars* (Boston: Houghton, Mifflin & Co., 1895), *Mars and its Canals* (New York: Macmillan, 1906), *Mars as the Abode of Life* (New York: Macmillan, 1908).

32. Sagan, C. & Pollack, J.B. 'On the nature of the canals of Mars', *Nature*, **212** (1966), 117.

33. Sagan, C. & Fox, P. 'The canals on Mars: an assessment after Mariner 9', *Icarus*, **25** (1975), 602.

34. Maunder, E.W. & Maunder, A.S.D. 'Some experiments on the limits of vision for lines and spots as applicable to the question of the actuality of the canals of Mars', *Journal of the British Astronomical Association*, **13** (1903), 344; see too Evans, J.E. & Maunder, E.W. 'Experiments as to the actuality of the "canals" observed on Mars', *Monthly Notices of the Royal Astronomical Society*, **63** (1903), 488.

35. Millman, P.M. 'The traditional features of Mars compared with the geologic map of the planet', *Journal of the Royal Astronomical Society of Canada*, **67** (1973), 115.

36. Quoted in Burnett, J. 'British studies of Mars, 1877–1914', *Journal of the British Astronomical Association*, **89** (1979), 136.

37. Antoniadi, E.M. (transl. P. Moore) *The Planet Mercury* (Shaldon, Devon: Keith Reid, 1974).

38. DeLamater, E.D. 'A new cytological basis for bacterial genetics', *Cold Spring Harbour Symposium on Quantitative Biology*, **16** (1951), 381.

39. Dawkins, R. *The Blind Watchmaker* (Harlow, Essex: Longman, 1986), ch. 3.

40. Bisset, K.A. 'Do bacteria have mitotic spindles, fusion tubes and mitochondria?', *Journal of Genetic Microbiology*, **8** (1953), 50; also his 'The cytology of *Micrococcus cryophilus*', *Journal of Bacteriology*, **67** (1954), 41.

41. DeLamater, E.D. 'Withdrawal of the concept of the occurrence of classical mitosis in bacteria', *Nature*, **195** (1962), 309.

42. See Hillman, H. & Sartory, P. 'The unit membrane, the endoplasmic reticulum, and

the nuclear pores are artefacts', *Perception*, **6** (1977), 667; their paper 'A re-examination of the fine structure of the living cell and its implications for biological education', *School Science Review*, **62** (1981), 241; and Hillman's *Cellular Structure of the Mammalian Nervous System* (Lancaster: MTP Press, 1986).

43. Darius, J. *Beyond Vision* (Oxford: Oxford University Press, 1984), p. 140.

44. Carr, M.H. *The Surface of Mars* (New Haven: Yale University Press, 1981), ch. 10.

45. Special thanks are due to Kenneth Bisset, Don Davis and Bernard Dixon for helpful discussions.

Notes to Chapter 22

1. *The Mind's New Science* (Basic Books, Inc. New York. 1985), p. 6. Two chapters of this book are especially relevant to our present discussion: Chapter 1, on the distinguishing features of cognitive psychology, and Chapter 11 on the question whether mental images are themselves mere 'figments of the imagination'.

2. On verbal images see further Nelson Goodman's *Of Mind and Other Matters* (Harvard University Press, Cambridge, MA, 1984), pp. 21–8. The present paper is a sequel to that discussion, titled 'On Thoughts without Words'.

3. The ensuing discussion applies an idea explained and developed in my papers 'On Likeness of Meaning' (1949) and 'On Some Differences about Meaning' (1953). Both are reprinted in Chapter V of my *Problems and Projects* (Hackett Publishing Co., Indianapolis, 1972), pp. 221–38.

4. After writing this paper, I found that a central thesis – the assimilation of image-talk to fiction – and some other points had been included in two of Daniel Dennett's writings: *Brainstorms* (Bradford/MIT Press, 1978), Chapter 10, 'Two Approaches to Mental Images', pp. 174–80; and 'How to Study Human Consciousness Empirically, or Nothing Comes to Mind', *Synthese*, **53** (1982), pp. 159–80. My own development of these ideas grew out of my earlier work on likeness of meaning, fictive representation, and 'thoughts without words', and is integrally related to my whole treatment of the ways fictional, and other, symbols function.

5. And later writers such as John Updike!

6. For further discussion of the general nature of rightness see Nelson Goodman, *Ways of Worldmaking* (Hackett, 1978), Chapter VII, 'On Rightness of Rendering', pp. 109–40.

7. Those who feel handicapped by being denied a license to talk as if there are images, may still say there are images, provided that is understood as saying that at least someone has an image, and this is interpreted in the way outlined above.

8. 'On Thoughts without Words', cited in note 2 above. A reading of that discussion should aid understanding of the present paper.

9. I am indebted to Catherine Elgin for her cooperation in the work on this paper; and I have profited from Robert Schwartz's brilliant 'Imagery – There's More to it than Meets the Eye' in *PSA 1980*, 2, ed. P.D. Asquith and R.N. Giere (Philosophy of Science Association, East Lansing, 1981) pp. 285–301.

Notes to Postscript

1. Place, U.T. (1956), 'Is consciousness a brain process?' *British Journal of Psychology*, **47**, 44–50.

   Shepard, R.N. (1978), 'The mental image.' *The American Psychologist*, **33**, 125–37.

   Smart, J.J.C. (1959). 'Sensations and brain processes.' *Philosophical Review*, **68**, 141–56.
2. Podgorny, P. & Shepard, R.N. (1978). 'Functional representations common to visual perception and imagination.' *Journal of Experimental Psychology: Human Perception and Performance*, **9**, 380–93.

   Shepard, R.N. & Podgorny, P. (1986). 'Spatial factors in visual attention: A reply to Crassini.' *Journal of Experimental Psychology: Human Perception and Performance*, **12**, 383–7.
3. Shepard, R.N. & Metzler, J. (1971). Mental rotation of three-dimensional objects.' *Science*, **171**, 701–3.
4. For an overview see: Cooper, L.A. & Shepard, R.N. (1984). 'Turning something over in the mind.' *Scientific American*, **251**, 106–14; and Shepard, R.N. & Cooper, L.A. (1982). *Mental Images and Their Transformations*. Cambridge, Massachusetts: MIT Press/Bradford Books.
5. Kubovy, M. (1983), 'Mental imagery majestically transforming cognitive psychology.' (Review of Mental images and their transformations), *Contemporary Psychology*, **28**, 661–3.
6. Preparation of this Postscript was supported by the National Science Foundation (Grant Number BNS 85–11685).

Index